LIVING IN THE SHADOW OF DEATH

LIVING
IN THE SHADOW
OF DEATH

Tuberculosis and the Social Experience

of Illness in American History

_____

SHEILA M. ROTHMAN

BasicBooks
A Division of HarperCollinsPublishers

Designed by Ellen Levine

Library of Congress Cataloging-in-Publication Data
Rothman, Sheila M.
    Living in the shadow of death : tuberculosis and the social experience of illness in American history / Sheila M. Rothman.
              p.   cm.
    Includes bibliographical references and index.
    ISBN 0–465–03002–5
    1. Tuberculosis—United States—History.   I. Title.
RC310.R68 1994
616.9'95'00973—dc20   91–59017
                                                             CIP

94 95 96 97 ❖/RRD 9 8 7 6 5 4 3 2

For Micol

As she begins a career dedicated to caring and healing

CONTENTS

PART IV
BECOMING A PATIENT, 1882–1940

ACKNOWLEDGMENTS

IN THE COURSE OF RESEARCHING AND WRITING, I RECEIVED ASSISTANCE from a number of foundations and individuals and I am delighted to acknowledge their contributions. A multi-year research grant from the National Endowment of the Humanities (RO 21349-06) freed me from other responsibilities and I particularly appreciated the counsel of my program officer, Daniel Jones. Matching funds were provided by the Samuel and May Rudin Foundation; Jack Rudin was a constant source of encouragement and friendship.

I relied heavily on archivists to locate manuscripts and it is a pleasure to acknowledge their assistance. Barbara Neilon, Virginia Keifer, and Deborah Saito at the Special Collections of the Tutt Library in Colorado Springs facilitated my long periods of research in that library. At Columbia, Walter Barnard and Michael Stoller cheerfully gave me access to the manuscript database whenever I needed it, often assisting me in the process. So too Kenneth Lohf and his staff in the Rare Book Room were equally generous. I spent several weeks at the American Antiquarian Society, where Barbara Trippel Simmons and Keith Arbour tolerated my constant searching for one more collection from a family decimated by consumption. (After I finished, the staff added tuberculosis to its catalogue and listed the collections I used.) Sheila O'Neill at the Brancroft Library of the University of California at Berkeley located several collections in advance of my visit. Virginia Rust and her staff at the Huntington Library in San Marino, California, and Judith Ann Schiff and her staff at the Yale University Archives patiently assisted my efforts to locate in their vast collections records of those who had consumption and tuberculosis. Both repositories have many important collections and I value the efforts of their staffs on my behalf. So too do I appreciate the assistance of Adelaide Elm and her staff at the Arizona Historical Society. Sandy Schmidt at the Connecticut Historical Society, Faye Phillips and her staff at the Louisiana and Lower Missisippi Valley Collections of the Louisana State University Library, and Elaine Trehub and Patricia Albright at the Mount Holyoke Archives not only scoured their collections during my visits but continued to search for material on persons with the disease even after I returned to New York. I made several visists to the Trudeau Institute at Saranac Lake where I always received a warm gracious welcome from the staff and was given complete access to their material. My work in Denver was facilitated by Jeanne Abrams, who opened the archives of the Jewish Consumptive Relief Society, and by Michael Schonbrun and his staff at the National Jewish Hospital. Their own knowledge of the influence health seekers exerted on the growth of Denver was also valuable. Finally, Richard Wolfe of the Harvard Medical Library, informed me of one or another yet-to-be-catalogued document which, in several instances, proved particularly helpful. During my work in several archives I met other researchers and staff who offered transcripts of private letters, diaries, and memoirs of a family member who had the disease, certain that they too would want their story told.

My colleagues at the Center for the Study of Society and Medicine formally and informally gave valuable suggestions about the work in progress and I would like to thank Sherry Brandt-Rauf, Rita Charon, Nancy Lundebjerg, Stephen Hilgartner, and Robert Zussman. Eric Foner was important in the conception of this study and assisted me in linking the history of medicine to social history in the pre–Civil War era. Richard Bushman and Jim Shenton read an early draft of the first chapters and gave me many helpful comments. My colleagues at the Columbia College of Physicians and Surgeons and other medical schools assisted me in evaluating the treatment regimens of nineteenth-century physicians. Paul Brandt-Rauf, Edgar Leifer, Robert Michels, Constance Park, Harold Neu, and John Stoeckle were always ready to answer yet one more question about the disease. The manuscript benefited greatly from the careful readings provided by Paul Edelson, Daniel Fox, Sandor Gilman, Margaret Heagarty, Bert Hansen, Emily Marks, Regina Markell Morantz-Sanchez, and Nancy Tomes. My editor, Susan Rabiner, provided particularly helpful suggestions and made significant editorial changes. Martin Rivlin patiently checked my citations and managed to locate even the most obscure documents.

I enjoyed the opportunities to present various sections of the study to colleagues in the fields of history and medicine at Brown University (Edward Beiser), the University of California at San Francisco (Guenter Risse), Cornell University (Sandor Gilman), Johns Hopkins University (Gert Breiger), Payne Whitney Clinic of Cornell University Medical School (Leonard Groopman), New York State Psychiatric Institute (Peter Schapiro), and the Woods Medical Institute (Charles Rosenberg). I also presented papers at the annual meeting of the American Association for the History of Medicine in 1991 and 1993, the Smith-Kline Beecham meeting on Controversies in Infectious Disease 1992 (courtesy of Harold Neu), and the meeting on tuberculosis of the Society for Law and Medicine 1992 (courtesy of Nancy Dubler and Larry Gostin). I also had the privilege of writing a section of this book at the Villa Serbelloni in Bellagio, Italy. I wish to thank the Rockefeller Foundation and the staff at the villa for their generous hospitality.

Once again, family conversations and work in progress blurred. My husband, David Rothman, my frequent collaborator, cheerfully became a research assistant and was always ready to read or listen to a section. I benefited greatly from his insights, keen sense of history, and editing skill. My son, Matthew, took part in many of the lively dinner conversations about the book. Although his own career will be in economics, he had more to say about tuberculosis and medicine than he expected. My daughter, Micol, is now about to enter medical school and so it is with particular delight that I dedicate a book about both mothers and daughters and doctors and patients to her.

INTRODUCTION

WHEN I BEGAN THIS BOOK, THERE WERE MANY HISTORIES THAT CELE-brated the achievements of innovative physicians and prize-winning inves-tigators, but few histories looked at the world of medicine from the per-spective of the patient. There was no shortage of accounts of eminent hospitals or of remarkable diagnostic and therapeutic advances, but the lit-erature paid scant attention to the experience of those who entered the facilities or took the cure. I was determined to fill the gap, confident that the story would be fascinating. But I underestimated, at least at the start, just how challenging the assignment would be.

To move patients to the center of a history requires breaking out of the language and constructs of medicine. By definition, to be a patient is to be under a doctor's care. Not surprisingly, then, it is the doctor's voice that has been heard most often and most clearly. Case histories composed by physi-cians abound in medicine, psychiatry, and neurology. What is missing are the life histories that capture the patient's voice. A simple exercise demon-strates the point. Consult a library card catalog and you find a plethora of entries under "physicians." Look under "patients," and you are likely to find nothing.

I quickly came to understand that to grasp the patients' experience, I had to leave medical archives—their story was not to be found in hospital charts or physician records—and explore general archives, collections of family papers, diaries, and memoirs. I was not disappointed. These sources, which I will refer to as "narratives of illness," turn out to be as textured as the lives that they portray.

The narrative of illness is very different from the case record. Although both report the origins, symptoms, and progress of the disease, each has a particular structure, perspective, tone, and plot. Arthur Kleinman, trained in psychiatry and anthropology, characterized the "illness narrative" as a written or oral response of the sick person and his or her family to illness and disability. The illness narrative, he observes, is intimate, emotive, and deeply personal. By contrast, the case record, as Kathryn Hunter, a literary critic, has maintained, is "objective, detached, impersonal, unemotional," far more intent on understanding the disease than the patient's experience of it.[1]

The distinction is critical to this book. A medical chart might well describe Deborah Fiske (1806–44) as a thirty-five-year-old poorly nourished white female, married with two children; chief complaints—chronic cough, persistent aches, shortness of breath, and severe weight loss; examination was remarkable for diffuse crackles in both lung fields. In Deborah Fiske's narrative of illness—the letters she wrote to friends that were, by her instructions, carefully preserved—she is a mother who is desperately trying to prepare her two daughters for their future as orphans and who finds solace in a circle of female friends, many of whom shared her disease and her religious faith. As her narrative makes clear, illness set the parameters of her life but was not its sum. Deborah's letters were precisely the type of source I was seeking, and with some detective work, good luck, and the assistance of archivists, I located over one hundred relevant collections.

I soon made a second decision: I would focus not on several illnesses but on one, tuberculosis. The choice was an easy one, for tuberculosis was the leading cause of death in the United States throughout the nineteenth century and well into the twentieth. From 1800 to 1870 tuberculosis was responsible for one out of every five deaths. Paying little attention to geography, social class, or age, it struck rich and poor, young and old, and urban and rural residents. After 1870 mortality rates in the general population declined, but the disease became endemic among immigrants living in ghettos. Well into the 1930s it continued to be the disease that set the pattern for both personal habits and public policy, influencing everything from the length of women's skirts to the design of tenement houses.

Given my interest in the social history of patients, tuberculosis had the added advantage of being a chronic disease. Individuals lived with it for years, sometimes even for decades; families were haunted by its specter for two or three generations. Those who struggled with the disease were likely to leave a rich record, and they did.

Although I did not know it at the outset, tuberculosis turned out to be not one disease but several—even as we now encounter it in still another guise. It is not merely that the name of the disease changes over time, from consumption in the nineteenth century to tuberculosis in the twentieth. More important, the perception and treatment of the disease changes from era to era. As I read the life histories—and, more generally, as historians of

medicine from Charles Rosenberg in his examination of American materials to Megan Vaughan in her analysis of African ones, began to analyze and
debate the degree to which disease categories are socially constructed—it
became clear that tuberculosis could not be examined outside of its societal
frame. Each generation has its own way of defining the etiology, transmission, and appropriate therapy for a disease, and these definitions reflect not
only medical technologies and concepts but also, as we shall see, broader
influences, including religious beliefs, gender obligations, and community
responsibilities.[2] None of this is to say that a disease like tuberculosis does
not have a material base; the bacillus is real enough. I stop short of accepting the notion that historians should treat all medical diagnoses as con-
structions, as though they had no intrinsic reality. But to ignore the frame
in which a disease is defined and treated is to ignore the powerful interplay
between medicine and society.

From this vantage point, it became apparent that the narratives of illness
varied from generation to generation and were highly sensitive to considerations of space, gender, and time. The particular climatic attributes of
Massachusetts, New York, Colorado, and California affected the tone and
the plot of the narrative. It mattered whether the diary was written in the
gloom of winter in Saranac Lake or in the spring sunshine of Colorado
Springs. So too, as the narratives of illness make clear, men experienced and
recorded consumption in very different terms than women did, particularly
in the nineteenth century. Even medical prescriptions, as we shall see, were
gender-specific. Finally, early-nineteenth-century invalids held a very different conception of their illness and their obligation to improve than did
their counterparts who several decades later went West in search of health
or who in the twentieth century became patients in the new sanatoriums.
And social class mattered as well. In the nineteenth century consumption
affected everyone, but those with greater resources were able to pursue the
optimal cures. Even in the twentieth century, when access to the preferred
treatment was greater and facilities intended primarily for the poor were
established, individual and family wealth still counted. Those with the most
money lived in the shadow of the facilities, those with less became patients
in not-for-profit sanatoriums, and the very poor entered large public institutions. Thus, to analyze the experiences of patients requires a detailed
understanding of who contracted the disease, when and where they contracted it, their sex, and the resources they had to seek a cure.

The book opens with the invalid encounter with consumption. For most of
the nineteenth century, physicians considered the disease hereditary and
noncontagious, presuming a familial predisposition (as in the case of insan-
ity) and finding no evidence of transmission from person to person (unlike

the case of smallpox). They defined the symptoms of consumption in terms of readily observable physical changes—the body was literally consumed by the disease. Descriptions in the medical texts of the era are vivid and evocative, not distant and neutral. The cough in its early stages was "frequent and harassing" and later developed into "hollow rattles" and "graveyard coughs." An initial "ruddiness" of the face gave way to a "deathlike paleness," which, at the very last stages of the disease, was masked by a "glowing hectic flush." The mucous discharge changed color and texture from "green" to "blood streaked"; hemorrhages, measured by teaspoons and cupfuls, occurred more frequently.[3]

Diagnosis was more easily accomplished than therapy. Physicians believed that the disease originated in "irritations," the sources of which were to be found in the interaction of an inherited constitution with a particular life-style and environment. Among the most "irritating" occupations were such sedentary and bookish ones as law, ministry, and teaching, and among the most "irritating" climates were those with cold, wet, and windy weather. The only way to reverse the course of the disease was to counter the irritants—changing diet (it should be "mild" and "unstimulating"), routine (follow a regimen of "gentle exercise"), and residence (go to a "mild and uniform" climate).

Those who contracted consumption were considered "invalids." The term was as much a social as a medical category, defining the responsibilities of the sick even as it freed them from fault. Invalids were obliged to seek cures and in turn were permitted, even expected, to modify social obligations in order to fulfill this special task. In the language of the day, invalids had a lifelong obligation to improve—with all the nuances of the phrase intended.

Although consumption was found in every region, it was considered particularly endemic to New England (which seemingly had the worst social and environmental irritants), and the first life histories we shall explore are of young, educated New Englanders—both men and women. Through their highly introspective and exceptionally intimate narratives, we learn what it meant for men to contract consumption as students in college, to leave home and friends and seek a cure on a whaling voyage or to forgo a career in the ministry to become a farmer. And because the experience of illness in this period was so gender-specific, we will also learn what it meant to New England women to try to pursue a cure even as they remained at the hearth, to fulfill the duties of parenting, and to satisfy Christian precepts as they confronted their own mortality. Through the letters and diaries of parents and siblings, we will also explore how family and community coped with the death of children, parents, and spouses, and how they fulfilled deathbed wishes.

The next part of the book, covering the period 1840–90, takes us from

New England to the western frontier. Some earlier precepts continued to hold during this period—hereditary influences and constitutional and environmental irritants were still viewed as the primary causes of consumption. However, new patterns of migration transformed the experience of the sick. Invalids turned into health seekers, searching for their cures in the American southwestern plateau, in the mountains and deserts of Colorado, New Mexico, Arizona, and California. Indeed, it was men, and to a lesser extent women, with the symptoms of consumption who were among the first settlers to populate these regions. Pioneers, explorers, and health seekers were practically interchangeable.

Popular fantasies joined with medical precepts to attribute to the West therapeutic powers. The region exerted its hold on the imagination not only in dreams of personal wealth (finding gold) but also in desires for physical renewal (finding health). The climate itself, its pure air and wholesome atmosphere, was restorative, as testified to both by travelers' accounts and by physicians who organized a climatological association. But even more health giving was the western way of life. Taking its inspiration from the trapper and the Indian, the cure became hunting, camping, fishing, and hiking.

The western narratives of illness, like so much else of western literature, was often brash, boastful, and optimistic. In the 1840s and 1850s explorers who had gone West to map the territory and find a cure experienced an extraordinary restoration of health, which they attributed to a natural lifestyle as exemplified by horseback riding and eating buffalo meat. Their hyperbole was soon matched by those who went West in wagon trains, and later by those who traveled on the intercontinental railroad. As settlements became more dense and the availability of amenities increased, successive waves of newcomers had to stretch to achieve a "natural" life. But the hallmarks of the cure remained vigorous outdoor exercise in this Eden-like region.

The endorsements that came from successful migrants were echoed and reenforced by the autobiographical accounts of physicians. They presented themselves as the "living proof" of the adage "Come West and Live," in the process wedding medical theory to popular perception. In towns like Colorado Springs doctors donned the garb of the trapper and served, quite literally, as wilderness guides to health seekers. And all the while, the railroad and the town developers added their paeans of praise, as they aimed their message at invalids back East. Come West—by train—and live—in our particular town.

Thus, the tone of the narratives, whether published or unpublished, in letters or in books, is almost always confident and hopeful, telling of bodies restored and fortunes made. To be sure, there are occasional references to separation and loss, to the pain of men dying far from home, puzzled at their bad luck. But it is the success stories that dominate the literature, as though each settler struck his vein of gold and each health seeker found his mine of health.

The final section of the book (1882–1940) opens with Robert Koch's discovery of the tubercle bacillus and his proof that the disease was communicable. Consumption now gave way to tuberculosis. No longer the symptoms of illness, as revealed on the body of the sick, but the presence of the bacillus in the sputum, as revealed on the laboratory slide, was the marker of the disease. The prestige of medicine expanded with these scientific breakthroughs. It appeared that transmission of the disease could be controlled and a cure fashioned. However, tuberculosis brought with it a nearly total reordering of the relationship between the sick, their doctors, and their communities. When health seekers became patients, exuberance gave way to frustration, and the open space of the West narrowed to the confines of a facility.

The threat of contagion fostered a significant expansion of public health mandates. Departments of health gained new authority to order diagnostic tests and chest X rays, to inspect and fumigate the lodgings of those with tuberculosis, and even to ban spitting in public places. Officials could also commit those with tuberculosis, even against their will, to sanatoriums. Their powers were all the more extensive because tuberculosis was found most often among the poor, in particular among immigrants living in tenements and working in sweatshops.[4]

What medicine defined as a crusade for supervision and cure, the sick frequently experienced as stigmatization and confinement. The twentieth-century narratives of patients with tuberculosis are often self-deprecatory and angry. They refer to themselves and are referred to by others as "lungers," or "tbs," as the disease subsumes their identity. Patients' descriptions of life in the sanatoriums are suffused with bitterness. They complain of boredom, the meanness of their fellow patients, and the condescension and conceit of the nurses and doctors. Indeed, for the first time the narratives of illness are coterminous with disease itself; little margin is left for a life outside it.

Nevertheless, the narratives also testify to the ingenuity with which the patients manipulated the system. They knew which sanatoriums gave better treatment and how to persuade a charitable society to send them to the preferred facility. They learned how to cope with the staff and manage stigma while preserving some degree of autonomy and integrity. But most of all, and despite the unwillingness of the staff to confront it, patients in the facilities recognized that they were living on the frontier of death. Their narratives of illness recount how a patient subculture articulated what the staff would not. The coping mechanisms included black humor and initiation rites for newcomers (like taking the route to the sanatorium that went past the cemetery). It also included "cousining," their term for sexual liaisons, which were officially prohibited but nevertheless flourished. No matter that the affair might be brief or doomed—at least for a moment one escaped the grimness of an institution permeated by death.

Several themes cut across all these encounters with illness and are of especial importance to understanding the patient experience. First was the challenge that uncertainty posed for the sick, their families, and their doctors. With consumption as with tuberculosis, there was no way of knowing whether a remission might last for months, years, or decades. Lives were lived in the shadow of the disease, as decisions had to be reached about careers, about marriage, and about childbearing. Thus, in the 1840s the community expected those with consumption to marry and bear children; relatives, with no irony intended, readily concluded that the groom would make a fine husband—that is, if he lived. In the 1930s, by contrast, physicians strongly discouraged marriage for the tubercular and insisted that women patients not bear children. To make exquisite calculations about risk has a modern ring to it, but in fact, each generation has had to make its own hard choices.

Second, across all periods, gender attributes altered and were altered by medical prescriptions.[5] New England women invalids, for example, opted to take their cures at home; although the medically preferred choice was to travel for health, women placed their domestic duties above medical prescriptions and physicians deferred to them. Among the western health seekers, women, particularly single women, were more common, but this cure, too, was primarily the province of men. It took bacteriology to override gender—the sanatorium was prescribed for both sexes.

Third, the balance of authority between patients and doctors changed over time.[6] In the early period medical textbooks were written in a style that made them readily accessible to an educated public. By the 1930s the texts used a technical language that was obscure to lay people. By the same token, in the 1830s patients were not uniformly passive, or physicians, unassailably authoritarian. In the lives of most New England invalids, the physician as compared with ministers, family, and friends, was a peripheral figure. Invalids were told to travel for health, but it was up to them to select the destination and devise the regimen most suitable for their particular constitutions. In the lives of health seekers, physicians appeared more as companions than authorities and dispensed counsel informally. Doctors suggested a daily routine (often modeled on their own) and might even serve as guides, but health seekers had ample room to improvise.

Medical authority was far more intrusive in the lives of persons with tuberculosis than it had been in that of consumptives. The physician pronounced the diagnosis (only he knew whether the bacillus was present), defined the precise character of the cure (the number of hours to be spent resting on the sanatorium porches), and decided on the time for discharge. But even here, some room for maneuver existed, notwithstanding the insistence by such sociologists as Talcott Parsons that the sick did, and should, adopt a passive role.[7]

Fourth, the psychological and social support that the sick received from each other and from their communities varied over time and by place. New England families did everything to prevent a loved one from dying alone. A father who received a letter that his son was nearing his end in a southern town immediately booked passage to be with him, sometimes, but not always, beating the angel of death. At home, the dying chose which neighbors were to "watch" with them; and those who were asked considered it a privilege. Later, when a more heterogeneous society confronted a contagious disease, the sick experienced illness as stigma and treatment as banishment.

In exploring all these themes, I have tried to correct the powerful stereotypes that have obscured the lives of the sick, to liberate them not only from the confines of the case record but also from literary constructs that have distorted their experience. Susan Sontag's path-breaking study, *Illness as Metaphor*, has made us aware of how the language used to describe illness can distort reality—illness is not a war, the sick are not guilty. I hope that my analysis of the narratives of illness will in turn, demonstrate the gap between the actual experiences of the sick and literary depictions of illness. Thus, for example, although death from consumption was frequently a powerful spiritual experience, it was not, as literary conventions describe it, beautiful or painless. The incessant coughs made talking and eating almost impossible and breathing, painful; the swelling of the joints and the loss of weight precluded walking; and the dying often subsisted on opium and whiskey. By the time death was at hand, emaciation was so complete that it appeared as if a cadaver had already replaced the human form. By the same token, the sanatorium was not a "magic mountain." Life inside was cruel and dismal, not bewitching or seductive. In reality, if not in fiction, the facilities dispensed less magic than mischief.[8]

A few qualifications are in order. This book is not an institutional history. Its vantage point is that of the patient, not the hospital or sanatorium superintendent. Nor is it an evaluation of outcomes or an examination of the usefulness of any one therapeutic intervention, whether leeching, a climatic cure, or a sanatorium stay. So, too, it does not pretend to tell the story of all Americans who contracted tuberculosis. I have not included the narratives of illness of miners, of African Americans or Native Americans, even though large numbers of them suffered from the disease. Miners were believed to have a special variety of consumption, called miners' phthisis, which often confused silicosis with tuberculosis; their experience has been the subject of a separate and fascinating historical investigation.[9] So, too, although many African Americans and Native Americans contracted the disease, the medical understanding of their condition and the resources devoted to their treatment were so different as to require their own special analysis.[10] My hope, of course, is that the approach I have taken here will encourage other historical investigations into the experiences of these groups.

Taken together, the narratives of illness that I examine are poignant as biographies and illuminating as social history. They demonstrate how cultural ideas on gender duties, religious obligations, the magic of the sea, the west as Eden, and the dangers posed by new immigrants all gave a particular cast to medical prescriptions. And in turn, medical ideas on healthful occupations, climate, exercise, rest, and cleanliness profoundly altered social habits. Finally, this is a history that reminds us that ours is not the first generation to have to cope with the death of the young, or with a stigmatized disease, or with the limits of medical authority. But just as persons with chronic illness today demand that their voices be heard, so, too, their historical predecessors are entitled to the dignity of explaining in their own words how they lived life in the shadow of death.

PART I

THE INVALID EXPERIENCE: NEW ENGLAND MEN, 1810–60

1

The Dreaded Disease

DURING THE FIRST HALF OF THE NINETEENTH CENTURY CONSUMPTION was America's deadliest disease, responsible for one out of every five deaths. It crossed all boundaries of geography and social class, affecting residents in rural as well as urban areas, the prosperous as well as the poor. It struck the young even more notably than the old, females more often than males.[1] In 1844 the town clerk of Amherst, Massachusetts, recorded 51 deaths in a population of 2,550; 14 died from consumption, most of them married women over the age of thirty. In 1852, when Franklin Pierce was elected president, his new vice president was in Cuba unsuccessfully trying to cure his consumption, the secretary of state was in mourning for his son, who had just died from the disease, and there were rumors that Jane Pierce, the president's reclusive and sickly wife, was also suffering from it.[2] "*Consumption*, that great destroyer of human health and human life, takes the first rank as an agent of death," declared Lemuel Shattuck, one of the country's earliest and most prominent epidemiologists, in 1849. "Any facts regarding a disease that destroys *one-seventh* to *one-fourth* of all that die, cannot but be interesting."[3]

Although consumption has often been labeled "the great white plague," in reality it bore little resemblance to the epidemics that had earlier ravaged Europe. Consumption did not suddenly appear, devastate a population, and then abruptly recede.[4] Its course was at once less precipitous and more tenacious, taking a grim toll year after year. Its sufferers did not usually succumb within a matter of days. Acute attacks alternated with remissions; the process of wasting and dying could take a few years or span several decades. In effect, consumption was a chronic disease, not a plague.

Consumption, or "phthisis" as the Greeks termed it, is one of the oldest and most persistent diseases known to civilization. Skeletons found in Neolithic burial grounds and mummified bodies preserved in ancient Egyptian tombs reveal evidence of it. We know little about the impact of the disease from the medieval to the early modern period. There is conjecture that it was more widespread in urban than rural settings, but its prevalence is not well documented. By the seventeenth century, however, consumption had become so common that John Bunyan in 1680 labeled it "the Captain of all these men of death."[5]

Whatever its antecedents, it was not until the beginning of the nineteenth century that consumption became pervasive and feared in the United States. It was present in the colonial period, and there is evidence that some men and women from prominent families died from it, including Lawrence Washington (the brother of George Washington), one of the daughters of Cotton Mather, and the famous missionary David Brainerd. But not until the beginning of the nineteenth century is there reference to an increase in the number of those contracting the disease and a concomitant sense of panic. In 1816 Dr. Joseph Gallup reported that since 1810 he had "three times as many cases" of consumption among his patients as he had "had for sixteen years before."[6]

By the 1830s, most Americans, and certainly all New Englanders, had a firsthand familiarity with its symptoms. It was an era when the ill were nursed at home not in hospitals, indeed, when most people died at home. Everyone understood that a hollow cough, an emaciated body, night sweats, and daily intermittent fevers were marks of consumption. This recognition did not make the illness any less baffling, however. There was no predicting who would be struck. The popular and medical conception was that consumption was hereditary: those whose parents or siblings had contracted it were predisposed to the disease; and it haunted some families for generations, like a deadly curse. But then it attacked some members of a household while sparing others and also struck some with no family history of it at all. No one was considered safe from its ravages. To be robust and strong was no guarantee that a fever and cough would not linger and turn into consumption.

The unpredictable and deadly character of the disease terrified many Americans. As Orra Hitchcock, the wife of Edward Hitchcock, professor and then president at Amherst College, watched several neighbors die of consumption, she became convinced she would be next. Even as she tried to console a friend dying of consumption, she could not hide her own fears. "I think I feel better than usually prepared to sympathize with you," she wrote. "For many thoughts which may be passing through your mind have so lately occupied by own, viz consumption which may be marching forth [through] this land to seize me with that firm grasp which will surely (though it may be slowly) lead me to the grave."[7]

Americans in the antebellum era were surprised by the spread of the disease. They recognized that consumption had been decimating English families for the preceding century and a half, but they found little evidence of it in their own colonial past. How accurate their impressions are is difficult to gauge. It may well be that the colonists, not recognizing its symptoms, attributed death from consumption to a "fever" or to malaria. But it is true that English physicians in the eighteenth century were far more concerned and alarmed about it than their American counterparts. Thomas Beddoes was one of many noted London physicians who observed that the number of Englishmen dying of consumption was so great that "the members of the two houses of Parliament, who have lost neither father, mother, brother, sister, or child, by consumption, could I suppose be ascertained without much difficulty."[8] Americans did not have such a legacy. Perhaps life in scattered agricultural settlements with relatively high levels of nutrition minimized the disease. But whatever the explanation, the nineteenth-century mortality statistics seemed by contrast all the more frightening.[9]

Theodore Parker, a prominent Unitarian minister in Boston, was one of those New Englanders convinced that death from consumption had increased dramatically. After carefully examining the genealogical tree of the "P's" (a thin disguise for his own family), he concluded that the first six generations of his colonial forebears had been healthy and long-lived, free of the illness—until an abrupt change occurred. About 1800 one of his grandmothers contracted consumption and died from it, and in short order eight of her eleven children succumbed to it before the age of forty. The disease struck the next generation even harder. All six children born to one of Parker's relatives died of consumption, and in Parker's own family line, eight brothers and sisters died before he himself contracted it. He was short on explanations for the change, but of its extraordinary implications for the health of the citizenry he had no doubt.[10]

It was not only the increased number of cases in the population but also the very course of the disease in the individual that made consumption so thoroughly mysterious. Some died quickly, within months, but many suffered a severe attack that was followed by a respite which could last ten years, even twenty or thirty. How then was one to plan a career or think about marriage and children? Thus, almost every aspect of consumption was marked by an uncertainty that bred apprehension and bewilderment.

Medical practitioners tried valiantly to make sense of the odd epidemiology and morphology of consumption and to provide advice on prevention and treatment. A disease that would eventually be identified by the presence of the tubercle bacillus was defined throughout these years in terms of a constellation of symptoms that doctors, and for that matter lay people, could observe. Consumption was a term that drew on an image of a body wasting, quite literally being consumed, before one's eyes, and the language of the medical texts (at one, as we shall see, with the accounts of those suffering from the disease) was explicitly and graphically descriptive of what they called "harassing," "mournful" and "frightening" changes. (The marker for tuberculosis, by contrast, was an organism visible only when properly stained and viewed under a microscope; the language turned objective and neutral, charted the course of a microbe through tissues, and no longer spoke of a body in decay.)

Despite the disturbing visibility of the symptoms, the diagnosis of consumption, particularly in its early stages, and predictions about its course, at least in any single case, were exceptionally difficult to make. Physicians divided consumption into three separate stages, but the earliest signs of the disease might easily portend another, much less serious ailment, and the fact that each stage merged imperceptibly into the next undermined efforts at prognosis. In textbook presentations the first stage was marked by a dry persistent cough, an irritation in the throat, pains in the chest and shoulders, a slightly accelerated pulse, and some difficulty in breathing, particularly during exercise. But the very commoness of these symptoms made it almost impossible to say with certainty that the person had consumption.[11]

The second stage brought more intense and debilitating symptoms. The cough became increasingly "severe, frequent, and harassing," as Dr. William Sweetser, a noted American physician, observed; it produced mucous materials and pus, which as the disease advanced became "thicker, more opaque, greenish . . . [with] fine streaks of a yellow color."[12] A "hectic fever" periodically broke out, spiking twice daily and marked by a rapidly accelerating pulse (to a rate of 120 a minute). The fever often lent a ruddiness to the complexion of consumptives, giving them a deceptive appearance of good health. "This red tint," as Sweetser described it, "often appears as though it had been laid on with a brush. . . . A deathlike paleness is often seen alternating with a glowing hectic flush. . . . Such complexions are generally esteemed handsome, but to the experienced eye, it is a beauty fraught with the mournful associations of its transitory nature."[13] During this second stage ulcers appeared in the throat, causing a continual hoarseness and making it painful to eat or speak above a whisper. Even with all these markers present, however, doctors were reluctant to pronounce a firm diagnosis of consumption: the cough and fever might still be indications of bronchitis, and the pains, signs of neuralgia or rheumatism.

Diagnosis became more certain in the third and terminal stage. "The emaciation is frightful," noted Sweetser, "and the most mournful change is witnessed in the whole aspect. . . . The cheeks are hollow. . . . The fat of the face being most absorbed . . . rendering the expression harsh and painful. The eyes are commonly sunken in their sockets . . . and often look morbidly bright and *staring*. . . . All the comeliness and pleasing symmetry of the human form are destroyed." The body "is wasted away." The lungs now sounded hollow (either to the ear or through the stethoscope), and the cough, known as the "graveyard cough" or "death rattle," was distinctive and unmistakable, enabling physicians to say that the disease had spread to the lungs.[14] The pain in the joints was constant, the pulse accelerated and then became weaker, diarrhea broke out and became uncontrollable, and the legs swelled. All these changes gave a ghostly and cadaverous appearance, indicating that the person had "gone into a consumption."

The death was anything but beautiful, as physicians described it in their texts. "Different phenomena and degrees of suffering mark the termination of consumption," wrote Sweetser in almost excruciating detail. In some cases, "life, wasted to the most feeble spark, goes out almost insensibly." But in others the symptoms were "painful and exhausting," including "excessive sweats and diarrhoea . . . with colic pains." The victim might also suffer from a choking and suffocating sensation, lacking the power "to free the lungs of the matters accumulated in them." At still other times, "a profuse hemorrhage comes on at once, pouring from the mouth and nostrils, and causing an almost instant suffocation." Without euphemism or the cover of medical jargon, Sweetser closed his account by noting that "in the majority of instances, the mind maintains its integrity to the last."[15]

For all their immediacy and particulars, the descriptive categories did not enable physicians to give a time frame to the progress of the disease. They could not tell someone whose cough had turned mucosal how many months he or she had left. Indeed, even the debilitating process in the final stage of the illness might be suspended for a period lasting as long as a year. In effect, one had to live *with* the disease and make life plans without knowing whether they would ever come to fruition.

Physicians, by their own lights, had more to offer in terms of prevention and therapeutics. They based their therapeutics on a venerable and ancient tradition of humoral medicine; the balancing of elements within the body framed their interventions accordingly.[16] The disease, they believed, had its origins in "irritations," the causes of which were both internal and external to the individual and linked to constitutional makeup and interaction with the environment. As the historian John Warner so aptly notes, nineteenth-century medical advice was expected to be "sensitively gauged not to a disease entity but to such distinctive features of the patient as age, gender, ethnicity, socioeconomic position, and moral status, and to attributes of place like climate, topography and population density."[17] Thus, nineteenth-century American physicians, following the tradition of their European counterparts, presumed that repeated and increasingly severe respiratory ailments, particularly those that could not be countered by purgatives and emetics, pointed to a tenacious inflammation or irritation in the body that, if not eliminated by countering the irritants, might well develop into consumption.

To identify the causative factors of the irritation, the physician first conducted an extensive inquiry into the details of the person's life history and social circumstances, looking particularly to occupation, daily habits, and place of residence. The irritating elements identified, he would then propose a regimen—or "constitutional treatment" as it was known—to reduce or eliminate them. Almost inevitably, the prescriptions had the most far-reaching consequences for everything from attending college to earning a living.

But the focus of the medical inquiry, its point of departure, was the male, not female, consumptive, indeed the male with sufficient financial resources and the ability to leave family and friends for indefinite periods of time. The disease did strike women as well as men, laborers as well as those in the professions. The texts, however, address treatment almost exclusively from the perspective of the middle- and upper-class male, not that of the female or the lower classes.

Since English physicians had been concerned with consumption for a longer period than their American colleagues, their medical texts set the pattern for therapeutics. Dr. Charles J. B. Williams, a prominent British authority on pulmonary disease and the author of the widely read *Lectures on the Physiology and Diseases of the Chest*, advocated an interventionist approach. "Even in the cases in which the phthisical [tubercle] lesions are most limited," he explained, "we are never to forget that it is not these lesions alone that we hope to remove. Their very presence in the system, or the operation of the cause that produces them, may lead to the formation of more." The physician's task, therefore, was to prescribe specific anti-inflammatory agents to heal the presenting lesions (for example, bleeding or leeching the individual); then, more broadly, he was to outline the particulars of a "constitutional treatment." He was to identify "all those circumstances and agents that may best promote and set forth the due action and balance of all the functions," those that would "remove those low degrees of vascular irritation, or that unhealthy condition . . . which, singly or combined, occasion the deposition of tuberculous indurations." Three considerations in particular were to guide his efforts: climate, exercise, and diet. The physician was to prescribe "the purest air and the most suitable climate for regular and ample exercise in it—the most nutritious food that the digestive organs can easily assimilate, and that the vascular system can bear without excitement. . . . [These] are the means which are rationally indicated to fulfill the object of improvement of the general health."[18]

Of the three considerations, physicians gave most prominence to climate, although its benefits were almost inseparable from exercise and, curiously enough, from the very act of travel itself. Consumption was considered especially likely to originate in the cold, bracing climate of the North, particularly England and New England—hence, the belief that individuals could halt its progress and prolong their lives if they traveled to warmer, in medical terms, less irritating, settings.[19] "If the individual dwells in a cold and variable climate, and is consequently restrained within doors, and abridged of his needed exercise," Sweetser advised, "the vital energies will more quickly decline, and the disease proceed more rapidly than under the softer and more equable skies, where he can daily exercise his limbs abroad, and inhale the fresh air of heaven." Or as Dr. John Eberle, a professor at the Ohio Medical College, put it: "The most efficient of all measures for counteracting the tendency to phthisis, or arresting its development or progress, is a removal to, and residence in, a mild, genial, uniform, and salubrious climate."[20]

Physicians endorsed a variety of destinations, but the most popular prescription was for a sea voyage to a temperate climate. The purity of the sea air along with gentle motion of the ship would soothe an irritated constitution. "Nothing appears more salubrious to the lungs than the pure air of the sea," counseled Dr. Samuel Morton. "I should say that in a great majority of cases, life is much prolonged, and in many instances the very seeds of disease are to appearance eradicated by sea-voyaging and foreign travel." Sir James Clark was also convinced that the advantages of a sea voyage far outweighed any possible discomforts. "An objection to sea voyages is the length of time that the patient is necessarily confined to the close and relaxing air of the sleeping places," he acknowledged. "But this is far more than compensated for by the facilities which he enjoys of being constantly on deck during the day, and there breathing the purest and most salubrious air." Physicians even believed in the therapeutic value of seasickness. "Short voyages on sea have been much recommended to consumptive persons, under the idea that sailing is of all modes of conveyance the smoothest," explained Dr. Robert Thomas. But, he continued, the positive effects depend "chiefly on the purity of the air, assisted somewhat probably by the occasional vomiting, which persons unaccustomed to be on board of a ship usually experience."[21]

The sea voyage had the potential not only to cure consumption but also to prevent it. Physicians frequently advised those with a hereditary predisposition to the disease to consider a maritime occupation. "A sea-life," contended Dr. Thomas Trotter, appropriately enough the physician of the fleet of the British Navy, "has often been considered a preservative against pulmonary consumption, and a voyage in a ship frequently recommended as a cure for the complaint." Even physicians with a less immediate interest in the sea shared his enthusiasm. "Sea voyaging in warm latitudes," wrote Sweetser, "I conceive to be one of the most effective means in eradicating, or at least, keeping dormant the tuberculous disposition. Phthisis is not commonly developed, even in the predisposed, during long voyages, and it is not frequent among sailors during their seafaring life."[22]

Many physicians were almost as enthusiastic about prolonged overland voyages, provided the journey did not take place in a closed conveyance such as a stagecoach or in damp weather. Given the lineage of the therapeutic regimen, it is not surprising to learn that a treatment devised in the seventeenth century would be reinterpreted to fit the needs and circumstances of nineteenth-century Americans. So it was with overland voyages. The idea seems to have originated with Dr. Thomas Sydenham, the seventeenth-century English physician. He advised consumptives, particularly those who had been unsuccessful in finding a cure, to take long horseback journeys. John Locke testified that Sydenham's prescription had cured his consumptive nephew. The young man, "soe weak . . . he could hardly walk," left on a horseback journey of one hundred and fifty miles. When he returned to London several weeks later, he was, Locke reported, "perfectly cured."[23]

The enthusiasm for such journeys persisted and become part of the accepted therapeutic armamentarium of American physicians. Dr. Henry Bowditch of Boston reported to his colleagues that his father, Nathaniel Bowditch, a renowned navigator, cured his consumption on a 748-mile journey through New England in an open chaise.[24] His colleague, Dr. Sweetser, agreed: "Long journeys pursued on horseback, through pleasant countries, and during the warm season, are often of peculiar advantage to those strongly predisposed to consumption, and may likewise be useful in its incipient stage."[25]

Although these prescriptions for constitutional treatment were at the core of the system of therapeutics, physicians were not precise about either the optimal length of the trip or the ideal destination. "With respect to the length of time requisite for a consumptive invalid to pass in a mild climate," James Clark noted, "no general rule can be given." In some cases, one winter was sufficient but in others, he contended, "several years may be requisite, and . . . it may be necessary to reside permanently in a mild climate." For his part, Dr. Robert Thomas counseled patients living in regions like New England to go "to a warm climate before the winter comes," for they "might escape an attack . . . and by continuing there for a few years, may be perfectly recovered." But since any change of air or of residence might be therapeutic, still other physicians prescribed a short trip along the seacoast or a stay of several months in the country, breathing its "pure air."[26]

Once in the new location, the individuals were to subsist on a bland and "unstimulating" diet and follow a regimen of outdoor exercise. Clark advised that even in a warm climate the person with consumption "must adhere strictly to such a mode of living as his case requires; he must avail

himself of all the advantages which the climate possesses." Thus, "neither
traveling nor climate, nor their combined influence will produce much permanent benefit, unless directed with due regard to the nature of the cases,
and aided by proper regimen." In sum, halting the tendency to consumption and countering the irritating process was a demanding and lengthy
procedure.[27]

Given the life-and-death character of the decision, physicians were anxious about their ability to identify the most healthful place for each individual. No sooner did Dr. Charles Williams finish writing about the power of
constitutional treatment to effect cures than he lamented: "How vague is
this statement! How little can it guide us in particular cases! And so it must
be: the means must be varied and adapted to the diversified forms of particular subjects, and it is in the study of individual cases, and in the power of
discovering their conditions and of adapting means to them, that the ability
of the practitioner is displayed."[28] Sidestepping this dilemma, many practitioners made the choice of location a rote exercise and recommended the
same destination to all their patients. "The common practice of sending all
cases of the disease to some one favorite place," Dr. D. T. J. Francis
charged, "furnishes one reason why faith has been shaken in the sanative
properties of foreign mild climates in consumption. Madeira is a good climate, and Nice is a good climate, but each of these is good in different
cases; and a patient who would derive benefit from the one would, in all
probability, lose ground in the other."[29]

To overcome these limitations, some physicians pursued the study of climatology, in hopes of making a science of environmental cures. They carefully measured basic meteorological elements (rainfall, changes in temperature, wind velocity) and then compared the irritating elements in the
climate (fierce winds) with the ones that would counter these irritants (mild
sunny days). They also mixed in crude epidemiological data about the
ostensible rate of consumption among the local inhabitants; after all, if the
climate was so efficacious, then those who experienced it from birth ought
to be immune to the disease. But having gathered all this information,
physicians nontheless continued to hold contradictory notions about the
curative value of one location over another. Clark, for example, was convinced that Madeira offered "the best" climate for consumptives but saw
little to commend the West Indies. (He also cited data that "twice as many
cases of consumption originate among our troops in the West Indies as at
home.") But other New England physicians downplayed the climatic value
of Madeira. Sweetser remarked that "consumption is quite common among
the natives of this island, and that there is, indeed, some vice about its climate, rendering it actually prejudicial to the phthisical." Still other New
England physicians championed the West Indies, along with Cuba, but
again there were dissenters. "Dr. Jackson of Boston, U.S., whose experience

has been somewhat large," noted Clark, "thinks favorably of the West Indian climate in consumption . . . but he does not define the periods of the disease in which he finds it most useful." Clark would not send his British patients there, convinced that "the cases of pulmonary consumption . . . in which the climate of the West Indies promises advantage are very few, and their character scarcely ascertained; while those in which it produces mischief are numerous, and generally well marked."[30]

These conflicts over the curative elements of any one location persisted despite the concerted efforts of physicians and a rapidly growing library of climatological treatises. Apparently, one or another physician would have a patient return from a locale feeling much better, or they themselves might benefit from a trip South. Excited about this preliminary finding (just as their counterparts today would be about initial reports of the efficacy of a new drug), they would gather meteorological information about the location, ask about others who had been cured there, and then publish a pamphlet announcing their "discovery." A flurry of rival claims conveyed two seemingly contradictory messages: no one climate was right for everyone, yet almost any climate might prove efficacious for someone.[31] The net impact was to send consumptives scurrying first to one island and then to another in search of a cure.[32]

For most of the nineteenth century men and women with chronic and debilitating respiratory ailments, carrying the harbingers of consumption or already afflicted with the disease, defined themselves and were defined by others as invalids. The term originated in the seventeenth century to identify soldiers and sailors unfit for active duty. Because of their wounds, or the loss of a limb, or persistent illness, invalids were excused from military service and might, depending on time and place, be eligible for a pension. By the nineteenth century the term came to encompass *all* persons, military or civilian, who were weakened by disease and lacked the strength to participate fully in daily activities. Robert Louis Stevenson, himself an invalid, brought the older and newer definitions together when he labeled the group "the wounded soldiery of mankind."[33]

Invalidism was as much a social as a medical category. The symptoms that a doctor might emphasize—like a deep, mucosal cough—were certainly distinguishing characteristics, but so were more amorphous if no less evident characteristics—a general physical frailty or debility that signaled an incapacity to carry out daily tasks. To be classified an invalid was by definition to be excused from fully complying with social expectations. Invalids were allowed to modify, or in the extreme case, to avoid the obligation to earn an income or to fulfill the duties of wife and mother. But at the same time, invalids had a very special duty to meet: they had to do everything possible to reverse the course of the illness, to rid themselves of the malady.

Invalidism, no matter how enfeebling, might well be susceptible to a cure. Alice James, herself an invalid, spoke on behalf of several generations when she declared that invalids had the "life long occupation of improving."[34]

Hence, as one begins to explore the experience of invalids, particularly consumptive or pulmonary invalids, one enters the home, school, work-place, and church—but not, of course, the hospital or the almshouse, except in the case of the unworthy poor. To understand how invalids went about fulfilling their obligation to improve, how they attempted to comply with medical prescriptions and satisfy community expectations, requires understanding not only the underpinnings of the system of therapeutics but also the religious, social, and economic imperatives of the larger society.

The power of cultural assumptions is evident in almost every aspect of the lives of nineteenth-century New Englanders who contracted consumption. They ordered their routines with an eye not merely to this world but the next as well. They shared a belief that the sea was health giving as well as animating and exhilarating. Perhaps the most important stamp of the culture on their behavior was in the matter of proper gender behavior. Male invalids with consumption followed different routines than did their female counterparts—almost as if they had different diseases.

Physicians in their practices were sensitive to the separate spheres of activity of each sex and the privileges and obligations of each. They recommended markedly different regimens for men and for women. Women, insofar as possible, were expected to restore health within the family and in ways consistent with their domestic responsibilities. Physicians assisted them in devising daily schedules that allowed them to pursue a cure even as they remained within the household and community. At the very same time, however, physicians encouraged male invalids with similar symptoms and levels of debilitation to leave the home and community and travel in search of health. "Sex, moreover, ought to influence the decision," Sweetser proclaimed.

> Females, from their nature, as well as the customs of society, are far more dependent beings than ourselves. Man may roam the seas and the earth at his pleasure, hardship and change are his enjoyment, and the world his home. But woman is more the creature of domestic life, and her happi-ness is more intimately blended with its quiet comforts and tender associ-ations, and the sacrifice of these—especially when her body is sensitive and infirm—often casts a deep shadow over all her feelings. Hence to her, travel is ofttimes a painful task—a series of inconveniences. All circum-stances of the disease then being alike, it might be proper for a male to go abroad, when it would not be proper for a female.[35]

To be an invalid, male or female, was to confront a series of wrenching choices. While living with an extraordinary degree of uncertainty, they had to decide just what level of sacrifice their illness required of them. Since they could not know with assurance when a dry, hacking cough would turn moist and blood streaked, or when an intermittent fever was actually consumptive, they had to make decisions with qualms and misgivings, never confident they had made the right choice. Indeed, the oscillation of acute attacks and periods of remission in which there was semblance of well-being made these life choices that much more difficult. For the moment, their health seemed to have been "confirmed," their strength "recruited," and they immersed themselves again in domestic duties or educational or vocational enterprises. But then chest pains, deeper and more hacking coughs, intermittent fever, and even hemorrhages would recur and force another withdrawal from school or career. Thus, invalids continually wrestled with the "silent destroyer." Locked in combat they groped for an occupation or a life-style that would satisfy their ambitions or duties but not endanger their health. The opponent was tenacious and capricious, at times appearing subdued and defeated, but then reappearing unexpectedly with unassailable furor to shatter the most carefully constructed plans.

The dilemma was frustrating and ongoing: how to reconcile an invalid's moral and medical obligations with personal ambitions and goals. Was it necessary for those who yearned to become ministers or teachers to take up farming? More poignantly, should invalids with unmistakable evidence of consumption avoid engagement and marriage? Religion and social mores provided some answers, particularly as they distinguished between duties (that is, marriage and childbearing) and privileges (higher education and a professional calling). Because marriage was a duty, the answer to the question of whether to avoid it was a resounding no. Thus, when the aunt of Jane Pierce, the president's wife, was engaged to be married to a consumptive widower with three grown children, a friend wrote that if the groom's "health should be restored, he will be an excellent husband," but such a fate seemed "extremely doubtful."[36] (In fact, he died soon after the wedding.) By the same token, no one made adverse judgments when Ralph Waldo Emerson married Ellen Tucker when she was in the final stage of consumption. Indeed, it was a commonplace of popular literature for a bride to die of consumption on or immediately after the wedding day, the bridal dress turned into a shroud or winding-sheet.[37]

The dictates of invalidism manifested themselves with particular clarity in the life choices of educated men and women of New England. To judge by the surviving medical and biographical materials, its residents were the most apprehensive about contracting it, the most preoccupied with preventing and curing it, and the most articulate in writing about life with it. They left poignant and very detailed diaries and letters—life histories really—in which they chronicled their encounters with consumption. These narratives do not isolate the sick in their illness but reveal, often painfully, how the disease affected the decisions of everyday life, from educational and career choices to marriage and child rearing. They are the invalids' reports to their friends, and to God, of their efforts to improve. They also recount how the burdens of invalidism affected not only the sick but also their families, friends, and neighbors. Fathers were deeply involved in their invalid sons' every educational and occupational choice, and they readily spent their savings to provide sons with every opportunity to regain their health. Because invalids frequently died in the prime of life and had not hesitated to marry, they left behind widows, widowers, and orphans. Deathbed wishes were clearly articulated and dutifully followed. It was not unusual for brothers to raise their orphaned nieces and nephews, or even to marry the widows.[38]

The narratives of illness in this period, even more consistently than the medical texts, describe the course of disease in highly evocative language—the report of the first hemorrhage spares no detail about how copiously the blood flowed or how distraught the individual was. In the narratives the sick are the subjects and not the objects of discourse, engaged in a vigorous and energetic battle to conquer disease, fulfill domestic and economic responsibilities, and tame the terror of death.

2

Manhood and
Invalidism

THE NARRATIVES OF ILLNESS COMPOSED BY EDUCATED NEW ENGLAND
men often began in adolescence, precisely when the privileges of their class
and gender exemplified by a college education were shaping their future.
Just as their brothers and friends were trying to unite their talents with
their aspirations, to select a college and career, male invalids were becoming acutely aware of the fetters of disease. Just when contemporaries were
asserting their independence, they were forced to cope with the constraints
of an intermittent illness. In the diaries kept by young male invalids during
these years, they confided their anguish at the "wretchedness" of their
predicament even as they tried to shape an uncertain future. Instead of
developing an adult identity consonant with their social class and intellectual abilities, they undertook long and agonizing consultations with physicians and family about their ongoing "fitness" for college and the suitability
of their aspirations in light of their poor health.[1]

Invalids recognized that every aspect of college life, social and intellectual, posed very particular risks to their health and that this level of intense
intellectual activity was suitable only for the physically fit. In New England
colleges, for example, the dormitory rooms were frigid and damp, and the
campus diet was spartan. Classmates presented yet another danger, what
one invalid called "the rough handling of college society." And there were
also the long hours of study, "sedentary labor" in poorly ventilated rooms.
Thus, for invalids, the decision to enter college took on the character of a
great gamble.[2]

The pages of the diary of Nathaniel Cheever II, written in 1829 when
he was fourteen years old, poignantly set out the tribulations of one of
these frail and ambitious young men. Nathaniel, whose father had died
from consumption, very much wanted a college education, but recurring

and severe colds and coughs prevented him from attending an academy in his hometown of Hallowell, Maine, and even ruled out retaining a tutor. Instead of spending his days studying alongside his brothers and sister, he had to engage in "mechanical pursuits." By the time he began his diary, Nathaniel already knew that his poor health was likely to thwart his ambitions. In its pages, he recorded his repeated frustrations. While his siblings were "rapidly advancing in their studies. . . . I am making no progress,nor have I advanced in any degree to compare with them. If I had been in health . . . how much might I have learned and how many books read in the time that I have been unwell." Nathaniel sometimes fantasized that his ailments would suddenly disappear, that his delicate frame would miraculously become muscular, and he would be able to study and become "fit" for a ministerial career. But then he would quickly return to the reality of his predicament. "Unless my health is restored very soon," he sadly noted, his hopes to study for the ministry "would never be realized. . . . There is a possibility yet, but rather a faint one, that a thing I so desire may be." Periodically, he felt better and believed it possible to reach his goals; but with the next attack, he would note in his diary: "The bright hopes that I cherished a week since have been sadly disappointed even beyond what I had any idea of, for I have been almost as unwell as ever." Nathaniel had no choice but to adapt to the life of an invalid; instead of entering Bowdoin as his brothers had done, he undertook the occupation of "improving."[3]

Joseph Kimball, who was to become a prominent antislavery agitator and author of a widely read tract on slavery in the West Indies, was especially bitter that his poor health precluded a collegiate education, and he too recorded his despondency. In 1833, when he was fifteen years old, his tutor, aware of the keen ambitions of this precocious and diligent student, urged him to apply to Dartmouth or Harvard. But his family, fearful that he had the symptoms of incipient consumption, begged him to find a vocation more suited to his health. Kimball reluctantly obeyed, noting in his diary that he had "yielded to the importunities of my friends and advice of my physicians and concluded to forgo that privilege."

Three years later, on a visit to Dartmouth, he still could not suppress his envy of "the health and vigor of my friends." "Had my health been spared," he wrote,

> I should have with them enjoyed the privileges and pleasures which are now denied. . . . I looked forward to the happiness of spending four years of study amid the halls of Harvard or Dartmouth. . . . But they are sealed now to me forever! Poverty I could have struggled with, the buffeting of business opposition, I could have withstood, but who can contend with disease, who can strive for the high attainments of intellect with the strong and swift around him when he feels his countenance sinking day

after day in weakness and weariness? Who would not shrink when his friends and his physicians and sometimes his own heart tell him of brief days?

Walking around the campus and listening to students' discussions, Kimball wondered if he had been too cautious. "And yet I wish sometimes that I had persevered that I had gambled with death amid the glorious exertions of mind, in the study with the treasures of learning around me and lain down, if so it must have been, in the field of intellectual strife." But these thoughts were potentially so devastating that Kimball repressed them: "When I meet old friends, as I have met them today rebellious feelings are stirred in my bosom. But they must be hushed and subdued."[4]

The diaries of male invalids repeatedly expressed the idea that only the most physically fit and intellectually talented were suited to be ministers. Indeed, "bookish" occupations that we assume are chosen by those with less physical stamina were considered by New England educated men as prizes for the most robust. This standard underlay the life choices of John Gould, the son of Judge John Gould, one of the founders of the law school in Litchfield, Connecticut. His older brother, Edward, later recorded the frustrations that dogged John as he tried to reconcile his ambitions with his health. Like other invalids, John's health was so poor that he had to be educated at home. When he was thirteen he seemed so frail, his chest so "narrow" and his coughs and colds so persistent, that his family had him "undertake the labors, privations and hardships of a farmer's boy." Following a regimen of outdoor labor, John gained weight and appeared stronger. He tried to persuade his parents to let him enter a seminary to study for the ministry, but they insisted that he attend the Oneida Institution, where "manual labor formed a part of the scholar's regular duty." At Oneida, however, John's symptoms returned, and violent attacks of coughs and lingering colds forced him to withdraw. In 1833, when he was seventeen years old, John acknowledged he was an invalid and that all formal education was beyond his strength.[5]

Even those who seemed healthy when they entered college might soon evince the symptoms of consumption. Parents, recognizing that the disease struck apparently "strong and swift" as well as frail and sickly undergraduates, admonished their college-bound sons to balance hours at the desk with outdoor activity. Samuel A. Eliot counseled his son Charles (who later became president of Harvard) to guard his health as he improved his mind. "Remember the object, health, to enable you to study with advantage, and you will not neglect it. It is impossible for you to have health long without exercise, constant and active. . . . You are forming your habits for strength or for weakness in both, not only for college, but for all your after life."

Eliot was acutely sensitive as to how precarious and transitory the state of good health was. "I dare say," he told Charles, "you will find . . . students who do not appreciate the importance of attending to the vigor of the body and who consider all time lost which is not spent over their books. . . . In a few years they are apt to become warnings; and either lose their health, or perhaps their lives."[6]

Looking back, we know that some undergraduates probably suffered a relapse of the consumption that had been latent since childhood. The stress of college life, including the poor diet and crude living arrangements, reactivated the disease. Others, living and studying in poorly ventilated rooms with students who had active cases of the disease, may well have acquired a new infection. In either event, an encounter with consumption at college or immediately after graduation had devastating consequences. To the dismay of those who contracted the disease, the business of "improvement" now became their career.

Howard Olmsted was apparently in good health when he entered Yale in 1837. During his freshman year, however, after a series of protracted fevers and violent coughs, he experienced the most dreaded symptom of consumption—a hemorrhage. Howard's father, Denison Olmsted, a professor of astronomy at the college, became alarmed. Believing his son had a hereditary predisposition to the disease (consumption had claimed his mother a decade earlier), he urged Howard to give up his "sedentary pursuits for a more active life . . . best adapted to his health." At first Howard resisted, maintaining that the hemorrhage was an isolated incident. After all, he had not been a delicate child, and for years he had wanted to become a mathematician.[7]

Soon, however, in the course of a visit home, he was "overtaken by an attack of bleeding at the lungs." Howard said nothing to his family and tried to ignore it, but one evening as he prepared for bed,

> the hemorrhage returned in all its violence. . . . I was seized with difficulty of breathing, with coughing and spitting blood. . . . Frank [his older brother] ran downstairs and called Papa, while Fisher [his younger brother] ran for Dr. Tully. The doctor came and gave me a powerful astringent that stopped the bleeding, but my lungs were so that I could not lie down, but had to remain all night seated in my chair. The bleeding returned at intervals for several days, but gradually grew less and less until it ended. However for several weeks I could not lie down at night, unless my pillow was raised, without experiencing a difficulty of breathing, owing to phlegm collecting on my lungs.

With this attack, Howard knew that he would have to withdraw from Yale. In his diary he recorded his despair at having been forced by his physical frailty to forgo the privilege of higher education and a profession suitable to someone of his background: "My whole prospects for life have suddenly been changed. My future path will be those of the man . . . who has to . . . earn his living by the sweat of his brow."[8]

Even after he withdrew from college, Howard still chafed at his invalid status and its obligations. "It is now Sabbath," he wrote in September 1840. "All is comparative stillness about me. But I can hardly keep myself composed in union with the occasion. . . . I am now out of health. I have for some time past experienced considerable weakness at my chest, brought on by close confinement to the desk writing, which warns me to do something for my health immediately." But it was the very uncertainty of his future that troubled him most. "My thoughts wander off to what I have been about, and to what I am likely to do in the future. I know not what profession I may be directed to in the Providence of God; all is mysterious and unknown to me."[9]

John Todd, who came from a poor farming family in northwestern Connecticut, had never been frail prior to entering Yale in 1818. But two years later, after months of severe chest pains and coughs, he was forced to withdraw from college. The decision, he wrote in his diary, like a "gloomy cloud, which at first was hardly noticed in my sky, has been continually blackening." Cyrus Bradley from Canterbury, New Hampshire, was similarly infuriated when lingering and debilitating respiratory complaints compelled him to leave Dartmouth. Like Howard Olmsted, Cyrus also had a family history of consumption. One sister had already died from it and another had its unmistakable symptoms. But these facts did not lessen his resentment or despondency. "Shackled and oppressed by the most tedious and vexatious complaint that ever cursed human nature, I have been obliged to . . . relinquish my studies and overthrow and destroy some of my fondest and darling expectations."[10]

Even the most bitter and acerbic of complaints were tempered by intermittent articulations of hope. As the diaries make clear, although the men knew that the odds were against them, they also knew that remissions occurred and symptoms dissipated. Any one of them might be among the fortunate few who improved and realized their ambitions. "On Tuesday and Wednesday," Nathaniel Cheever II wrote in his diary on April 13, 1843, "my sputum was quite tinged with blood. . . . I felt this to be a solemn warning to be ready for my summons to the eternal world for it may at any moment come." He feared that consumption might have "already commenced its fatal ravages and may very soon hurry me to an early grave." However ominous the symptoms, he nonetheless tried not to give in to his despair. "To be sure, it is not necessarily fatal by any means; many persons . . . have it to quadruple the extent that I ever suffered and yet live twenty to thirty years afterwards and enjoy good health."[11]

* * *

The very desperation of their situation led these young men to an urgent search for a cure. For Cheever, as for the others, no intervention was too drastic or too burdensome. If it appeared to have any efficacy they were willing to give it a try. In this spirit, invalids consulted physicians, friends, and kin, indeed, almost anyone who had had firsthand experience with the disease, to learn about regimens that had proved successful. The advice they most often received from physicians and lay people was to change climate and life-style, and the prescription of choice for those of sufficient means was to go on a "voyage for health." These prescribed voyages were anything but frivolous ventures or an excuse to wander about Europe or sail the seas. A physician's prescription to travel for health indicated the gravity of the condition and the need for immediate compliance. Indeed, the voyage for health disrupted lives and shattered dreams even as it held out the promise of recovery.[12]

The narratives of illness record the diligence with which invalids complied with the prescription. The hallmark of these accounts is the way they interweave the events of a sea voyage such as might be recorded by any traveler with an almost obsessive attention to the way every aspect of the trip affected their health. "A consultation of Doctors was called on Tuesday," Henry Russell Cleveland informed his brother, Horace, from Cambridge on October 20, 1842.

> They examined me with great care for more than an hour. . . . There are strong indications that my lungs are attacked though not yet in such a way as to be at all alarming. But I am in just such a condition that if I were to remain here I should be in great danger of falling into a consumption, whereas by going away, I am almost sure of getting entirely well. I am therefore earnestly advised to go to the West Indies immediately and not come back till next summer. I shall therefore be off by the first of November if possible.[13]

The speed with which the male invalids complied with medical advice does not mean that physicians exerted absolute control over them. They quickly learned that there was no one correct destination; finding the right climate and regimen was inevitably a matter of trial and error. The medical advice was vague, variations on the theme of "go southward." It was up to the men to fill this broad prescription in a specific and individual way. Nor was there any single type of conveyance that guaranteed a cure. The invalids heard stories of men who restored their strength on horseback or stagecoach trips on overland routes. Physicians and invalids generally agreed that the optimal course was a sea voyage. It was not only easier to arrange and less fatiguing than overland travel, but as the narratives of illness indicate, it had a very exceptional psychological and physical appeal.[14] The sea voyage transformed a medical prescription into an almost mythical quest. These ventures very tangibly allowed the physically frail to pursue a curative regimen that incorporated the attributes of courage and daring and gave a man the chance to throw off the shackles of invalidism and identify with the strongest and most ambitious members of his sex, from courageous sea captains to fearless missionaries.[15]

New England maritime routes were so extensive as to give invalids wide leeway in choosing an itinerary. When Cuba opened its ports to foreigners in 1818, Boston merchants immediately began to trade New England furs and timber for its sugar and molasses. As the Spanish Empire crumbled, the merchants shrewdly expanded their Caribbean routes to include all the ports of South America. With similar ingenuity, they augmented the already flourishing trade with Great Britain by creating American markets for British exports. Ships sailed regularly from New England ports not only to Charleston, Savannah, and New Orleans but also to Cuba, the West Indies, and St. Croix. On very short notice, an invalid could book passage and head South. Indeed, by the 1830s it was as simple to arrange to sail from Boston to Havana as from Boston to Portland. Nor was it difficult to find accommodations on ships heading to the West Indies, the Sandwich Islands, Rio de Janeiro, or, for that matter, China.[16]

All New England ports had a resplendent display of brightly colored barks, brigantines, and schooners providing invalids with a great variety of accommodations. There were fleets of regular oceangoing packet boats, which ranged from small single-sail sloops to majestic schooners. The 1850s saw the appearance of the prized clipper ship. This vessel so effectively joined utility with beauty that the ship and its designer, Donald McKay, came to symbolize the extraordinary inventiveness of American engineers even as it marked the apogee of American domination of maritime commerce. It was a portrait of McKay, not Ralph Waldo Emerson or Walt Whitman, that F. O. Matthiessen chose for the frontispiece of his classic study of the antebellum literary renaissance. Indeed, the link between ship design and cultural creativity was a powerful example of the hold the sea had on both the American economy and the American culture.[17]

The precise itinerary an invalid organized for his voyage for health balanced his own social, economic, religious, and political considerations. Those with links to the shipping industry or with substantial financial resources almost always chose a sea voyage; those of lesser means selected an overland route or a shorter coastal trip. Given the fragile health of the voyagers, even the well-to-do tried to arrange an itinerary that maximized the opportunity to meet friends and relatives. It was less lonely and frightening to travel with companions or go to a region where one had acquaintances. If an invalid knew others going to Charleston, particularly on a voyage for health, he, too, might choose that city, even though he had heard many tales about the salubrious climate of Savannah.

In 1836 Joseph Tuckerman, a prominent Boston Unitarian minister, consulted his physician, Dr. John Warren, about his worsening cough. "Dr. Warren thinks me *now* in the best possible state for recovery," Tuckerman wrote his sister, Elisabeth Salisbury, "if the winter and spring shall be passed under a tropical sun." The doctor had recommended St. Croix, but other invalids told Tuckerman of their successful recuperation in Cuba. Before reaching a final decision about where to go, he consulted his colleague and friend William Ellery Channing, who had spent a winter on each of the two islands. The choice, Channing explained, was difficult.

> The difference between St. Croix and Cuba, I suppose to be considerable. The former has the more uniform warmer temperature and far drier atmosphere. . . . It hardly ever rained while we were there. The dry heat was withering to me . . . but my wife luxuriated in it and is the better for it to this day. . . . Cuba has a lower temperature, more variable, moister, such as would suit me better . . . but would suit my wife much less. You see how much depends on the patient's constitution.

In the end, Tuckerman opted for the drier climate of St. Croix.[18]

Jeremiah Day, who eventually became president of Yale, decided to go to Bermuda in 1801 on his voyage for health, a decision based on ease of travel to the island and his own social connections. Two fellow students from Yale were from Bermuda, and by coincidence, their father, a wealthy merchant, was visiting New Haven and invited Jeremiah to accompany him back on his boat.[19] For his part, John Todd settled on Charleston because Jeremiah Evarts, a distant relative and Todd's trusted adviser, had gone to Charleston on his first voyage for health. Evarts not only encouraged Todd to go there but also helped him plan the trip and arranged for him to lodge in the same boardinghouse that he had used. And in much the same fashion, Henry Cleveland chose Cuba over the West Indies: his father had been vice-consul in Cuba and so the family still had many friends on the island and there were familiar places to revisit. Indeed, one old friend, a local physician, invited Cleveland to live on his sugar plantation.

Invalids who could not afford a sea voyage grasped at any other opportunity to travel in search of health. When James Colt, the brother of Samuel Colt, the inventor of the revolver, began to suffer hemorrhages, he returned to his family in Hartford. "We felt very anxious about him," his mother wrote to Samuel, "knowing the predisposition of our family to consumptive complaints." Feeling better, James took a position as a clerk in New York City, but his modest three-hundred-dollar annual salary left him with few options should his health decline. Then, unexpectedly, as his mother related, "a gentleman merchant in Savannah came into his store, wanted a clerk to go with him to Savannah, made James an offer of six hundred dollars a year. . . . He concluded to go, to sail that day, two o'clock and he was off." The rapid decision, and the delight with which the family greeted it, demonstrates the extent to which New Englanders esteemed a trip southward.[20]

The readiness of invalids to go to sea also reflected a deeper psychological attraction to the power of the sea itself and to the thrill of a seafaring life. Even as passengers, they mingled with courageous men and experienced, albeit vicariously, the romance inherent in the enterprise. To men frail in body and disheartened in spirit, the appeal was almost irresistible.[21]

The narratives of illness that recount these voyages incorporate as well the invalids' fantasies about the sea. These fantasies were fed by the nautical tales of the era that were avidly read by many New England men. Sea stories combined romantic adventure with realistic detail. The reader learned the technicalities of the craft of sailing and the courage and camaraderie of the crew. The sea yarns glorified the skilled captain, able to navigate through the strongest gales and maintain order during the long and often tedious voyage; ordinary crew members became daring mariners who exemplified the rugged spirit of the nation. James Fenimore Cooper's sea stories, like his frontier stories, were populated with men who thrived on adventure and were willing to endure hardship to obtain it. "I love suspense," said a mariner in Cooper's *Red Rover*. "It keeps the faculties from dying, and throws a man upon the better principles of his nature. . . . Calms may have their charms for your quiet spirits; but in them there is nothing to be overcome."[22]

Like other men of their generation, invalids viewed the sea as both medicinal and magical. But as we shall see in the narratives, all the powers of the sea—the potent air, the rocking waves, the salt water—inspired an invigorated sense of self and took on novel meanings. Male invalids were convinced that this environment was the elixir that would strengthen their frail bodies. The choice of destination almost paled in comparison to the exhilaration of the journey itself. Indeed, the fantasies were so compelling that they led the men to discount the dangers and the inconveniences inherent in the trip.

Even before the voyage began, invalids learned that the expansion of routes and the competition among the various shipping lines did not necessarily mean punctual departures or arrivals. The words "weather and wind permitting" in the advertisements of oceangoing ships meant that the vessel could leave two or three days after a scheduled departure or that an eight-day voyage might take ten or twelve. Moreover, the first few days at sea could be terrifying. Invalids were advised to head South in the late fall or early winter to avoid the storms so common on the Atlantic. Even so, they often encountered turbulent weather, including gales that lasted for days. The boats never seemed as sturdy as their registered weight suggested, and the best crafted among them were overturned by waves, or wrecked by icebergs, shoals, and submerged reefs.

The case of Jonathan Smith, Jr., a New Hampshire lawyer who traveled for health in a brig from New York to St. Croix in November 1836 is not atypical. His ship was first delayed for several days due to bad weather. Once it set sail, gales caused the boat to heave on enormous waves for almost a week. Smith and most of the other passengers were confined to their berths, and almost all of them became seasick. Torrents of water occasionally swept through the cabin, keeping the floor wet and the passengers scared and shivering. Smith was convinced that on a voyage designed to improve his health, he would "perish with cold." "The above four days may as well be lumped together," Smith wrote in his diary when he was strong enough to hold a pen. "My movements are such as could be made in a box 6 ft by 3 ft by 2 ft in height." On the fifth day the weather abruptly changed, the sun shone brightly, and Smith observed: "We suffered infinitely more from the heat than we could have suffered from the cold." Indeed, the voyage led him to empathize with the plight of others, as he concluded, with no sense of irony: "I never before fully realized the sufferings of the poor inmates of the Black Hole of Calcutta."[23]

Nathaniel Cheever, the father of Nathaniel Cheever II, undertook a sea voyage for health in 1818, and he, too, found the eight-day trip from Boston to Charleston more of an ordeal than he had anticipated. The first four days were cold and stormy, and the tossing of the boat left most of the passengers seasick. As the winds pitched and rolled the vessel around on the waves, the frightened travelers huddled together below deck. During a temporary lull Cheever and some of his fellow passengers ventured on deck; a strong wind unexpectedly came up and knocked a mate off the rig. The passengers watched with horror as the crew vainly attempted to save him from "a watery grave." When Cheever finally arrived in Charleston, he reported being "more enfeebled and debilitated than when I left Boston."[24]

Once the ships were south of Bermuda, the winds dropped and the sea calmed. The gentle rolling movements of the vessel soothed the spirits of the invalids, and the sea air, laden with salt and moisture, suffused and intoxicated their senses. Invigorated and enchanted, they groped for words to convey the potency of the experience. Their vocabulary emphasized strength, autonomy, and self-reliance and was replete with images that invoked the beauty and force of nature.

A week out of New York, Jonathan Smith found himself entranced by the motion of the boat gliding through the "wilderness of waters." "I fairly confess," he wrote in his diary,

> that I never had my sensitivity to the beauties of nature so strongly excited before. . . . At first the motion of the vessel was fearful through the waves. Every sail was set and she moved swiftly through the water. As she channeled into the trough of the sea, she seemed to be going to the bottom, for the waves broke over the stern and came more than half way to the stem—but she rose again majestically to the summit. Our course was south east—against the rising sun—and the appearance of the sea as the vessel rose was splendid beyond anything I ever witnessed.[25]

Smith, long intrigued by sailing, was an inveterate reader of sea fiction. Having already read James Fenimore Cooper and Washington Irving, he took along the sea novels of Sir Walter Scott. Standing on the deck, Smith recalled Cooper's imagery, but metaphors that had seemed compelling from the vantage of his armchair at home were now inadequate. "Our Mr. Cooper," he noted, "has given the most elaborate descriptions of sea scenery—but they all fail and come short of the reality." Where Cooper had compared the sea to "molten silver," Smith saw its colors as far more varied and subtle. "As the ship rose from the trough our course being toward the sun, the deep blue gradually changed—one shade following another, till, when she reached the summit of the wave, the whole surface of the ocean glowed and sparkled with a splendor that language cannot describe."[26] The salt air and mild wind seemed to strengthen his body, and he relished the night air that had frightened him at home. "Stayed upon deck a part of the evening—had no fear of taking cold, though there was a strong breeze. There was delicious softness and sweetness to the air." In such a setting cure seemed altogether feasible. [27]

Other invalids also drew strength from the sea voyage. "I sincerely believe it is the very best thing I can do for my health," Henry Cleveland wrote to a friend from Cuba. "The sea, you know, is like a mother to me, so gentle and kind are its influences upon me. My heart really leaps for joy at the thought of being again on the bounding waves. I feel as if I were going home."[28]

Sailing on the high sea also invigorated Nathan Fiske, a professor of classical languages at Amherst. Sitting on deck and staring out into the broad expanse of waters, he conjured up gods and spirits whose power to control the force of the sea might also regenerate him. "I no longer wondered," he wrote in his diary, that the Greeks imagined the goddess of beauty and pleasure to be begotten of the sea-foam. Repeatedly, I seemed almost to see her, rising up on a distant wave, and standing in her scallop, wringing out her silver tresses, and half-revealing her charms . . . but in a moment she sank out of sight dissolving in the very instant of birth, into the elements that gave her being. . . . The wind was balmy and soothing. . . . The sun was giving out his mildest beams; the ship moved easily and proudly through the gently swelling waves, while around me was spread out a scene of novel beauty, on the surface of the vast sea.

In so fantastic a scene Fiske "soon forgot that I had any such organs as lungs, or any such work as breathing to do." Surely he had found his cure.[29]

If a voyage to a particular destination could be so health giving, some invalids were tempted to increase the dosage, that is, to spend a few years, rather than a few weeks, at sea. Those who made this choice were generally men who had been delicate and sickly children, had a strong hereditary predisposition to the disease (more than one member of their immediate family had already died from it), and were already experiencing its unmistakable symptoms. They opted for the most drastic and risky intervention because they were certain it was their only chance.

A seafaring life posed very different challenges from those of a sea voyage, for it was not only physically but also morally dangerous to live in an isolated, self-contained, and at times disorderly and violent all-male society. In the preface to his first sea novel, *The Pilot*, James Fenimore Cooper told would-be women readers that the book "had little interest for them"; he intended "to illustrate vessels and the ocean, rather than draw any pictures of sentiment or love." If women appeared in these novels at all, they came in disguise, cross-dressing, or in the role of an Amazon. Not only in fiction, however, but also in real life women were normally denied access to life at sea. Occasionally, a captain's wife accompanied her husband on a voyage, but she remained a shadowy figure, confined to the officers' quarters. Absent women as crew, it was men who carried out domestic chores. In the "wooden world," as a seafaring life was sometimes called, men did the sewing, knitting, cleaning, and cooking. They mended the sails and washed the decks.[30]

The sea yarns made clear that the wooden world had its own code of behavior, language, rituals, and rites of passage. This code was often at odds with the rules that governed life on land, and it violated Christian precepts. Sea tales exposed the brutality and disorder of ship life—unruly and drunken sailors, tyrannical captains who repeatedly flogged crew members, violent encounters with pirates, bloody mutinies, and even a degeneration into cannibalism after a shipwreck.[31] So, too, the reports of benevolent organizations (like the American Seamen's Friend Society) and newspaper accounts gave full details of mutinies along with the depravity and cruelty of both officers and crew.[32]

The invalids' imagination, however, was captured not by these grim reports but by the testimonials of the healing and regenerative power of the sea. Invalids from the most respectable families were ready to brave the physical hardships and moral perils for the recuperative benefits of a seafaring life. They signed up as sailors on commercial voyages, and some even became crew on whaling vessels. The invalids who took up these options were, to be sure, a very small percentage of the sick, but their impact on other invalids, and in some cases the broader society, was considerable. For one, they took the medical dictum about travel for health to its farthest limits, wrote extensively about their experiences, and helped to pattern the curative regimens of invalids. For another, their testimonials had a significant impact on social attitudes toward sailors, captains, and shipowners.[33]

An invalid willing to sign on as crew had a greater choice of destinations than ordinary passengers. Ships regularly left Boston for the ports of South America (looking, for example, to purchase hides for the leather and shoe industry), and the long voyage across the equator to Buenos Aires, Rio de Janeiro, and Santiago allowed the invalid to test the effects of a number of climates. Invalids who wanted to travel for still longer periods of time could join the crew of a whaling ship. Although all commercial maritime ventures were perilous, whaling was considered the most hazardous of all. Expecting to capture their cargo and fill their holds with whale oil, the ships set sail with only a crew and provisions. The voyages were for an indefinite period—the men signed on for two or three years— and the date of return depended not on weather but on the success of the hunt. As tirelessly and tenaciously as the crew hunted whales, the invalids pursued health.

The speculation and risk inherent in whaling and the owners' and captains' reputation for brutality meant that these ventures attracted the toughest and most unruly seamen. The crews consisted of unemployed immigrants, millworkers, and recently released prisoners. On these long voyages the discipline required to sail the ship was always tenuously established. Order competed with chaos, spilling over into brutality. The elements of the seamen's subculture that bound the men together and gave them a pride in their work could, with repeated provocation from officers, turn them into a mutinous mob. Life on board these ships was so violent that a large number of sailors deserted these "floating hells" at foreign ports, preferring to forfeit wages rather than make the return trip. To fill their places, the captains recruited Polynesian or Sandwich Island natives, who had no idea of shipboard conditions.[34]

Male invalids and their families, knowing the hazards that were posed when a delicate young man became a "sailor before the mast," tried their best to gain a protected situation on board. The ideal solution was to occupy a position midway between passenger and crew that afforded the invalid a berth on the upper deck. Families also sought out "Christian" captains, and packed letters of introduction to American consuls in distant ports into the invalid's sea chest. They also made personal visits to the captain before the vessel sailed and promised extra money for the safe return and special care of their kin.

These strategies were shrewd, albeit not always successful. Some invalids were able to secure a degree of protection from the captain or find a position that avoided the rigorous and difficult physical labor demanded of an ordinary seaman. But others were not so lucky, and the results were disastrous, particularly for those who were physically weak. Not only did they lack the stamina for the work, but they were also often whipped and abused.

Francis Allyn Olmsted, the older brother of Howard Olmsted, was an invalid who decided to stake everything on a voyage for health. Two generations of his family had already been decimated by the disease, so his own delicacy and recurring ailments convinced him that he, too, was "destined to be a victim of consumption." These circumstances led him to roll high, in his words, "to experiment" with a whaling voyage.

Both Frank and his father, Denison Olmsted, were fully cognizant of the risks involved. Denison Olmsted conceded that a whaling voyage, at least "at first view," might seem less suitable for "a young man of education who wished to see the world than a trip to Europe or the Mediterranean." And the dangers confronting those who did become crew were so great that father and son agonized over the decision. "From an erroneous prejudice against whalers," Frank later wrote, "it was with great reluctance that I determined upon embarking on this voyage, and many of my friends made sage predictions of the wretched life to which I was consigning myself." Nevertheless, the excitement and potential benefits of such a trip induced him to go: "A love of the adventurous inclined me to a voyage in preference to any other plan for the recovery of my health."[35]

Denison Olmsted did everything possible to minimize the risks. He arranged for Frank to sail on a ship of which his uncle was part owner, and this uncle vouched for the Christian qualities of the captain. The uncle also had Frank appointed the ship's physician, receiving no pay but a free passage. (Frank was not a doctor but planned to enter the profession if his health was restored.) By the time the ship set sail, father and son were convinced that the decision was right. Frank would test various climates and learn some medical skills. Most important, he would improve his health.

Shortly after he returned home in 1841, Olmsted published *Incidents on a Whaling Voyage*, describing life on a whaling vessel and evaluating its benefits for other invalids. Olmsted presented himself as the "living proof" that such a voyage could restore health without corrupting the invalid. Throughout the book Olmsted emphasized the journey's therapeutic character. A whaling ship, he insisted,

> offers many inducements over any other mode of conveyance. The excitement of whaling operations; the preparation of the boats and their armaments . . . the breathless anxiety stimulated by hope. . . . The lowering of the boats—the dash of the oars and the fearless attack, all combine in a variety of highly interesting scenes, such as cannot but be favorable to the health of the invalid.

Even the excitement of closing in on the whale was therapeutic: "I still recollect with pleasure the first time we took whales, and the very favorable effect it had upon my health; my bodily ills were forgotten in the engrossing interest of the novel scenes then presented."[36]

Olmsted acknowledged that deprivations existed, but he insisted that they were trivial. "I came to sea to recover my health and not in pursuit of luxuries; and while participating in our frugal meal with the captain and his officers, whose openhearted kindness has made me almost forget my wide separation from home, I do not envy the luxurious epicure whose companions may indeed be more polished, but possibly less noble and disinterested." Olmsted repeatedly expressed his respect for the sailors, to the point of insisting that the very aspects of sea life that many educated men found offensive were physically invigorating and uplifting. "Living upon an element, every aspect of which is an object of solicitude to him, the sailor becomes a close observer of what takes place around him; and accustomed to face danger in some of its most terrific forms, he acquires a hardihood of character, an independence of mind, which the circumstances in which he is placed are so well fitted to produce."[37]

Olmsted included detailed accounts of the pagan beliefs and odd rituals of seamen, but he presented them as entertaining diversions in a community in which moral order ruled supreme. He acknowledged that the sailors tenaciously held superstitions that often ran counter to Christian precepts, but at least as he presented them, they become a colorful and exotic part of a life at sea, not a subversion of Christian values. Sailors, he casually informed his readers, believed it was bad luck to begin a voyage on Friday, but they were happy to set sail on Sunday; moreover, Christmas was barely acknowledged on board his whaler. Perhaps most intriguingly, he provided an unusually graphic account of the classic "sailor's baptism" that many other travel accounts preferred to omit.

The appearance of "Neptune's light" as the boat crossed the equator was the occasion for an elaborate and exotic saturnalia to initiate the greenhorn into maritime culture. The central figure in the ceremony was the sailor who was crossing the equator for the first time, and the main protagonists were the king and queen of the sea. At the start of the ceremony, the novice was dunked and held down in salty water; then, "he is blindfolded to await the awful presence of the king and *queen* of the ocean." Neptune appeared bedecked "with long streamers of seaweed entwined in his hair and bearing on high his mystic trident" and the queen, a cross-dressed sailor, came wearing "finery appropriate for the Queen of the Mermaids." They were "hailed with enthusiastic devotion by all the genuine salts who have passed through the ordeal of initiation." With assistance from "mischievous attendants," the king and queen subjected the candidate to a variety of humiliations, from shearing his hair to forcing him to eat garbage. At the culmination of the ceremony the sailor was "*keel-hauled*"—that is, a rope was tied around his body and he "is thrown overboard to be drawn under the ship and hauled up on the other side!" If he swore "to observe all the requisitions of the sea god," he was released from his ordeal and given the title of "sea-man." The account may indicate why families worried about a seafaring life (the ritual obviously mocked Christian baptism), but Olmsted reported the ceremony as a prank, an event that amused the invalid.[38]

Incidents of a Whaling Voyage was finally a report on sea life as viewed from the upper deck. Olmsted was protected by the captain and allowed privileges denied to ordinary crew. When the heat became oppressive, Olmsted slept on the deck, and he was the only one on board allowed to remain idle, amusing himself by assisting others or studying the functions of "mechanical contrivances." He acknowledged all these advantages, but was hopeful that his book would "secure to the whaling business, that share of respectability which has been withheld from it through ignorance or prejudice," even as it encouraged invalids to take to the sea to regain their health.[39]

Those who took Olmsted's advice without enjoying his privileged position typically underwent a very different experience. Invalids who occupied berths in the forecastle soon realized that they had entered an alien world which had none of the sensibilities and religious mores that guided society on land. To survive they had to become one with their mates, speaking the language of the sailors and satisfying the expectations of the officers. Unlike Olmsted, these invalid-seamen experienced the penalties for disobeying or ignoring arbitrary authority.

When these invalids wrote fictional and autobiographical accounts about life on board ship, they looked to accomplish two seemingly different ends: to promote the therapeutic value of the voyage and to champion the cause of the sailors. Their narratives and short stories are an accepted part of the sea literature of the period, but it is not always appreciated that their writing is part of the genre of invalid narratives (endorsing the curative quality of the journey), as well as a contribution to the genre of reformist tracts by giving a firsthand account of the plight of the seamen. By virtue of both their illness and their position, invalids tended to empathize with the underdog. Those among them who joined the crew of a commercial ship or a whaler understood, and later depicted, their fellow sailors not as rowdy pagans but as men who were subjected to cruelty and abuse. Even as their testimonials celebrated the health-giving power of the sea, they urged greater protection for the well-being of the sailor.

The best-known work is Richard Henry Dana's *Two Years before the Mast*. Dana, an invalid albeit not a consumptive, went to sea in search of health. "I made my appearance on board at twelve o'clock, in full sea-rig, and with my chest, containing an outfit for a two or three years' voyage, which I had undertaken from a determination to cure, if possible, by an entire change of life, and by a long absence from books and study, a weakness of the eyes, which had obliged me to give up my pursuits, and which no medical aid seemed likely to cure."[40] Dana, who had an uncanny knack for survival, very quickly became adept at satisfying the expectations of both captain and crew. Still, his voyage was traumatic, as he was forced to witness the brutality inherent in the life of a "sailor before the mast." Although he had not gone to sea in order to write an exposé, his book became a powerful indictment of ships' officers as despotic and a vindication of seamen as victims. Reviewers believed that it would "serve to dissipate all the illusions about the sea, which most young men are wont to cherish; they will learn from it, that the forecastle of a ship is the most undesirable of asylums, to anyone who has had even a moderate share of comforts at home." But for all the hardships, Dana returned healthier than when he had left, so that despite the book's shocking revelations, invalids had one more example of the potency of the sea voyage.[41]

Narratives of other invalid-seamen of the era also reported on the darker aspects of a seafaring life as well as its regenerative powers. In 1833, when he was nineteen years old, John W. Gould realized that unless he undertook this drastic constitutional treatment, his health would never improve. He decided, as his older brother Edward reported, "to attempt the trials and perils of a sea-voyage as a sailor boy before the mast—that humble capacity being considered as, on the whole, best fitted to furnish a decisive remedy for his disease." The desperate character of his choice, and his determination "to be *nothing but a sailor*," prompted his family to find a "suitable vessel, a proper voyage, and a competent and *kind* captain." Believing they had located all three, they allowed John to sign up for a voyage to Canton on the ship *Commerce*. John's parents took comfort in "the captain's personal and reiterated assurances" that John "should be used and dealt with as his situation required" and "the fact that several of the passengers knew John's social position at home and understood his motives in going to sea." Nevertheless, despite their efforts, or perhaps because of them, John suffered "such personal indignity and cruelty, that but for the encouragement and kindness of the carpenter of the ship . . . he might never have returned alive."[42]

John's reports of his adventures appeared in a series of short stories, really sea yarns, in the *New York Mirror* and the *Knickerbocker Magazine*. In one tale, "My First and Last Flogging," which was replete with sailors' vernacular to document its authenticity, he recounted the beating of a young crew member who, after being "properly stripped," was "seized up to the Jacob's ladder" and "hoved" with the "cat" by a sadistic officer. Fearing for his life and in great pain, the young man, together with another sailor, managed to escape the boat and through the interventions of benevolent strangers to survive a hazardous trip back home. The story's hero then has a fortuitous meeting with the despotic captain and gains his revenge. As the protagonist relates, he struck the captain in the face crying, "Take that, and *that, and THAT!* He struggled violently, but it was in vain—for, nerved with passion, I had the strength of twenty men,—and continuing my merciless battery . . . I showered my blows upon his visage until it was bruised out of the form of humanity, and he, entirely senseless, was only upheld by my arm."[43]

The inspiration for the story, of course, was John's own experience. On board the *Commerce*, John had been the object of a particular officer's sadism. Repeatedly harassed and occasionally whipped, he did, with the aid of a boatswain on a naval vessel, gain a "discharge" and returned home as a "landsman" under protection on a naval ship. He and his family were outraged by Captain Christianson's breach of trust and brought legal proceedings against him. But unlike his fictional counterpart, his revenge was far less sweet. Although Christianson pleaded for leniency and offered a "*very ample apology*," the family insisted upon a trial and his public humiliation. "I wish sea captains to learn," John declared, "from the example of Christianson, that they cannot with impunity treat their people like dogs: and because I wish the poor, desolate sailor boy, abroad and friendless on the ocean to know from *my* example that the majesty of THE LAW will protect even his poor rights, and punish the scoundrel who tramples on them." But the case meandered through the courts and John died from consumption before justice was done.[44]

But however treacherous long sea voyages might be, invalids continued to pursue them. No undertaking was too risky and no venture too demanding if it held out the promise of cure. These New England men readily made it the "business of life to live," not debilitated by the shadow that chronic illness cast over their lives.[45] It was not passivity or resignation but tenacity and resolve that marked their response to consumption.

3

The Pursuit of Health

To BE A MALE INVALID REQUIRED A REORDERING OF LIFE'S PRIORITIES: the pursuit of health had to compete with other personal values and aspirations. Men whose talents led them to consider entering the fields of science, law, medicine, and the ministry were warned by family as well as by physicians that these professions were too dangerous for them. To improve, they were to work out-of-doors, using their "muscle to earn bread." Educated New England men chafed at this decree and often resisted it, loath to abandon grander aspirations and goals.[1] But even as they considered the prudence of such a trade-off, they had to make their decisions in the face of extraordinary uncertainties. Although some invalids never regained even a semblance of health—no matter what cures or occupations they followed—still others, and there was no way to calculate their numbers, lived with their disease for decades. Were they, therefore, to presume longevity or an abbreviated life? Should they enjoy what time they had or make plans as though they were to be the fortunate ones?

It is hardly surprising that college-educated men who enjoyed intellectual discourse and the companionship of equals did not easily reconcile themselves to becoming farmers or entering other manual occupations. Conceding the wisdom of being physically active in the open air, they still balked at a routine of monotonous chores, isolation from people, and distance from the bustle and stimulation of city life. Most troubling of all to them was the fear that their talents would not be fully utilized in such pursuits, that they would never make their mark.[2]

Joseph Emerson was a graduate of Harvard and an ordained minister, but in 1810 after the deaths of his first two wives from consumption and the appearance of signs that he, too, might have the disease, he gave up his

pulpit and set about the business of improving. He rejected his family's urg-
ings to become a farmer and instead set off to travel for health. After several voyages and a third marriage Emerson returned to New England.
Once again his family urged him to take up farming but Joseph became an
educator and established the Saugus Academy, one of the first Protestant
seminaries for women in the country.[3]

Although he disregarded his family's wishes, Emerson self-consciously
devised a routine of diet, dress, and exercise that would ostensibly bring
him the benefits of a farmer's life without its drudgery. Each day he allotted
time for prayers and manual labor, as diligent in the one activity as in the
other. "Though pressed with business," he wrote, "I have endeavored to
practice, what I have so often repeated to brother invalids, 'Do thyself no
harm.' I have about two cords of wood, almost wholly sawed, split and piled
with my own hands. . . . I do indulge the hope that my health is substan-
tially improved. But as long as I continue in this tabernacle, I shall doubtless have occasion to take up the lamentation, 'Lord what a feeble piece.'"[4]

In 1834 Joseph succumbed to consumption, leaving his family convinced
that his health would have improved and his life been prolonged had he
only followed their advice. "Had he labored longer on the farm," his
brother insisted, "and become more familiar with the complicated routine
of its manly, invigorating, and improving occupations, it might have given
him more vigor of constitution, while it could not have failed to benefit his
practical judgment in all human affairs."[5] But Joseph's friends, many of
whom were themselves invalids, were unable to accept so harsh a judgment.
As Zilpah Grant, who joined him in his seminary work, pointedly reminded
the family: "It was with him an established principle, that it was his duty to
prolong his usefulness in this world, as many years as possible." His regimen, she believed, had added to his years. "Had he taken no more care of
himself than even conscientious invalids generally do, he would have been
lost to the world . . . at least ten years sooner. . . . How much, then, do
mankind owe to his peculiar watchfulness and singular fidelity in relation to
every thing that could affect his physical system."[6] The minister who could
not become a farmer should not be blamed for his early death.

When Howard Olmsted, who had been forced to leave Yale after
repeated hemorrhages, returned from his voyage for health still debilitated,
his father pressed him to become a farmer. "I had some conversation with
him respecting his going to Missouri and turning farmer," Denison Olmsted wrote in his diary in 1840, "believing that this profession may be more
favorable to the enjoyment of sound health. . . . I told him he should have
his choice among our Missouri lots, if he chooses to settle there, but should
especially commend to him a 240 acre tract in Shelby County." Howard
himself conceded that "the prospect of going to the west and establishing
my health and fortune on a secure basis seemed inviting." And he recog-

nized the pointlessness of denying his invalid state. "How fatal could be the discouragement to all exertion," he admitted, "if one who should enter upon such a course were to be met, at the outset, by the appearance that he was aiming at a goal which he would certainly never attain. How palsying to all mental action the thought as he pored over his books, or bent in profound thought over his mathematical calculations, that he was causing his already shortened sand to flow more rapidly by the process." Nonetheless, he could not muster any enthusiasm for the plan.[7] His ambition was to return to Yale "to pursue my studies and live for the remainder of my life not altogether in vain." To abandon his goals was more unbearable then the prospect of a foreshortened life.

Given the apparent symptoms of consumption and his infirmities, Howard could not totally disregard his father's advice. He countered with another proposal, really a plea. He would return to Yale but in the interest of health pursue a different course of study. Instead of mathematics, he would learn surveying and upon graduation join a team and live outdoors. Howard did return to Yale but never became a surveyor. Shortly after graduation he died from consumption.[8]

Invalids discovered yet another disadvantage in farming. Those whose health left them little choice but to abandon their chosen careers learned that the steady routine of agricultural life did not fit well with the uncertain course of their illness. How could they carry out the duties of farming when remissions so often gave way to fresh attacks? Repeated hemorrhages or weeks of racking coughs accompanied by severe pains made it impossible to carry out farm chores and set them off on yet another voyage for health. Invalids were often in motion—even the most responsible of them were forced to lead, as Frederick Law Olmsted phrased it, "a decently restrained vagabond life." Their lives became a series of disruptions, hastily planned and executed voyages interspersed with semesters at college and short and unsatisfying stints at farming. They were, in effect, hostage to the mysterious course of the disease.

However dispiriting the invalids' plight, many among them joined personal aspiration to the restoration of health. Those who succeeded became examples to other invalids that a vagabond life could be satisfying. One of the models that kept hope alive was Jeffries Wyman, who combined a curative regimen with a creative career. Wyman accepted the invalid's need to improve but fulfilled his duties without sacrificing his own intellectual preferences.[9]

Wyman first exhibited the symptoms of consumption in 1833 while a student at Harvard.[10] He managed to graduate and then immediately embarked on a voyage for health. He felt well enough upon his return to enter Harvard Medical School, complete the course of study, and graduate in 1837. His interests lay in research more than in clinical practice, particularly in the study of human and comparative anatomy. But for all his accomplishments, his health was frail and he did evince the symptoms of incipient consumption. Rather than remaining at Harvard and suffering the New England climate, Wyman accepted a professorship at a medical school in Richmond, Virginia; the milder winters might retard the progress of his continuing colds and lingering coughs.

A few years in Virginia did seem to improve his well-being, and when invited to become a professor of anatomy at Harvard Medical School, he accepted the position. But how would he cope with the Boston winters? Wyman arranged through lectureships and the generosity of friends, most notably George Peabody, the founder of the museum of ethnology and archeology at Harvard, to undertake regular scientific expeditions to warmer climates. Almost every winter Wyman left his family to travel, conduct his research, and regain his strength. His was a life of perpetual movement, but always with a purpose. He set a route for his journeys that fit both with his professional goals and with the precepts of invalidism.[11]

Wyman's regular destination was the St. John's River in the Florida Everglades. This choice had both medicinal and scientific value. The climate was reputed to be restorative. Sidney Lanier, the poet who was also consumptive, was one of many who observed: "Consumptives are said to flourish in this climate and there are many stories told of cadaverous persons coming here and turning out successful huntsmen and fishermen of ruddy face and portentous appetite after a few weeks."[12] As for science, Wyman's laboratory, the St. John's River, was a naturalist's paradise. Freshwater fish and alligators lived in its waters, and deer roamed its shores. The dense forests of oak and moss-draped magnolia that lined the banks afforded Wyman endless opportunities for observation of the wildlife. Thus, he collected, classified, and labeled botanical and zoological specimens and carried out a daily regimen of exercise designed to improve his health.

Since Wyman lacked the strength to row for hours, set up camp, and gather food, he brought along a companion-aide. In his later years, it was George Peabody who not only shared his adventures but covered all expenses. During the winters they spent together, Wyman searched for shell heaps and mounds, and Peabody assisted him with the digging and maintaining the camp. In 1871 the two spent several months camping on the riverbank, and as Jeffries proudly informed his brother: "I have not been sick a day since leaving Hibernia, have slept with and without the tent, have gained strength, have taken long rows in the boat once of nine and twice of ten miles each without fatigue. My cough has not gone but is greatly diminished and my appetite is always good." His research needs fit perfectly with his health needs. "Besides the rowing I ought to mention the digging in the mounds, which though it cannot well be measured, amounts to a good deal of muscular labor, more than that of all the rows long and short together."[13]

The combination of the scientific explorations and the opportunity to "rough it" and "knock around" invigorated Wyman. To be sure, his health occasionally waned. "On the last day of the voyage," he wrote his brother in the course of a trip southward in the winter of 1854, "I had another chill but much less severe than the one before I left. Having determined to push on to Florida at once, I, of course, saw but little of Savannah. . . . I thought it best to save my strength as much as possible." And he did complain that his health sometimes interfered with his ability to carry out his research. "Thus far I have done nothing in the way of natural history; but my strength is now so far restored, that I feel able to accomplish much more in the way of labor and hope to collect something of value before I leave Florida."[14]

Winters in Florida, or occasionally in even more exotic places like South America or Java, followed by summers in Cambridge, punctuated by camping and hiking trips to the White Mountains, constituted Wyman's regimen. Though pleased with the health he gained from these trips, he knew that sooner or later the disease would take its toll. In 1872 he reported to his brother that he had had several hemorrhages. Visitors might remark on his "improved appearance," but "the trouble is there where it has been and I see no reason why I should ever be free from it again."[15]

Wyman did not alter his routine, even though he did not experience its same invigorating effects. "My health holds its own," he wrote to his brother, "and I recognize a strong contrast between my present condition and the state of things before leaving home." He conceded that "I have done less work than last year, my longest row being five miles, but this and shorter distances both rowing and walking I get through without fatigue."[16] He knew that time was running out, and within two years he died. But Wyman had managed, with more than a measure of good luck, to find a solution to the invalid conundrum. He had been able to integrate a satisfying career with the precepts of invalidism. As an invalid-scientist, his vagabond life made eminent sense.

Other invalids, including those who had access to similar resources, were not so fortunate. John Hull Olmsted, the cousin of Howard Olmsted and the younger brother of Frederick Law Olmsted, was as resolute as Wyman, but however many plans he devised or however decisive his efforts, he was not able to reconcile his ambition to be a physician with the constraints of invalidism. His life was a series of forays and disappointments. In the course of twelve years, from the time he first evinced the symptoms of consumption until his death at the age of thirty-two in 1857, John took six lengthy voyages for health and interspersed them with stints at farming. Every time some semblance of strength returned, he resumed his medical studies, only to be forced to suspend them once again. In John's letters to his brother Frederick and to his other friends, we have another intimate narrative of illness in which determination is not compromised by defeat.[17]

Both John and Frederick had been sickly children, carrying what they believed to be an inherited predisposition to consumption. Fred was spared, but John showed the first symptoms of the disease as an undergraduate at Yale. In 1845, he took a leave of absence, booking passage on a winter voyage to the West Indies, and then returned to spend the summer hunting and camping with Fred. This regimen improved his spirits but not his health and, uncertain whether he would ever be fit enough to graduate from Yale, he considered abandoning his medical school plans to become a farmer. Deeply ambivalent about making such a choice, he turned, as he frequently did, to his brother for advice. Frederick enthusiastically, perhaps too enthusiastically, endorsed the advantages of farming. If pursued properly, it was, he believed, the most suitable profession for an invalid with intellectual ambitions. "Rural pursuits," he insisted, "tend to elevate and enlarge the ideas, for all the proudest aims of Science are involved in them. They require a constant application of the principles and objects of the Chemist, Naturalist, Geologist, Mechanic, etc.. More than all of *them*, it cultivates, or should, the taste and sentiment." The steady routine of farm life would spare a man of "the annoyances . . . [inherent in] most other active occupations." At the same time, the "manual exertions" required would be "healthful." Farmers, he concluded, were "the most contented men in the world."[18]

It was a convincing defense, and John joined Frederick on the farm purchased for them by their extremely generous and devoted father, John Olmsted senior. Indeed, the decision was all the easier because their father was both a shrewd businessman and an insightful parent. He knew that whatever his sons' rhetorical commitment to farming, their temperaments and aspirations would not leave either of them content with it as a full-time commitment. Accordingly, he hired an Irish immigrant to carry out the daily chores and left his sons with only a general responsibility for managing the property. In this way they seemingly enjoyed the health benefits of "rural pursuits" without its most tedious burdens.[19]

But the plan did not work. Even the life of the gentleman farmer proved too physically demanding and confining for John, and too dreary for Frederick. Frederick pursued any opportunity to travel or write that presented itself, leaving his father or brother to supervise the help. John, for his part, found that a farmer's life did not fit with either his well-being or his ambitions. "Farming does not suit my health at all," he declared, "at least to judge from experience. I have been twice or more down with sick headaches the regular old style and am just recovering from the effects of an attack of dysentery—looking as pale and thin as you please." In fact, John's routine on the farm approximated that of a scholar on a vacation. "I generally study past the forenoon," he continued, "then work in the garden and go sailing, fishing, etc. same in the afternoon, the evenings are nothing as we go to bed at nine (or pretend to) and get up at five, breakfast at six." Even with so light a schedule and so limited a number of chores, he could hardly wait to regain enough strength to return to college.[20]

John's health did soon take a turn for the better. He was able to go back to Yale and graduate in 1847. In fact, he felt well enough to begin the study of medicine in New York under the supervision of one of its most celebrated doctors, Willard Parker. But then in 1849 his symptoms returned and he was forced to leave medicine and go to live with Frederick on yet another family farm, Southside, located on Staten Island. It was an unusually beautiful and well-situated property; one hundred acres were already under cultivation with fruit trees, and it also had "two excellent gardens, with profusely bearing grape vines." The land bordered on Raritan Bay near the mouth of Great Kills, "with a wide front on the water, in which there is a great abundance of fish and clams." The property also contained a "mansion house" and two new barns on what was, according to its former owners, an "uncommonly healthy" site.[21]

However luxurious the environment, life at Southside did not improve John's health or spirits. "I am so wretched usually that I excuse myself from all hard labor physical or mental," he wrote to his friend Fred Kingsbury in July 1849. "The fact is I am beginning to lose all spunk. I had calculated to do a great deal this summer both in the way of strengthening my body and increasing my stock of useful information. But except for a day or two ever since I have been on the Island, I have been *sick* not unto death but quite weak."[22]

In an effort to revive body and soul, John undertook a sea voyage with Fred, leaving their father to manage the farm. Returning home in a much improved condition, he resumed study for his medical examinations and was able, in the summer of 1851, to take a post as a physician at the Seamen's Retreat, a hospital for sick and disabled sailors on Staten Island. But then he began to hemorrhage. He consulted Dr. Parker, who informed him straight out that he had "consumption in its earliest stages."[23] And John himself, because of his training and experience at the Seamen's Retreat, knew just how grave and ominous a hemorrhage was. "Lots of them I've seen die here this summer," he wrote to Kingsbury. "They have died strangled with blood in a fortnight. I held one in my arms the day before I bled myself, while he died, and his lungs were little more diseased than I suppose mine to be." After a hemorrhage, the chances for long-term survival even "with the very best treatment are frightful."[24]

Shaken by these events, John decided to put health before career. I am going "to see how long I can live," he wrote Kingsbury. "I have good ground to start upon. Good appetite strength and cheer." Perhaps I will "sell all my medical books and retire on my muscles for bread." This new course may, in fact, have been prompted by John's rather sudden decision to marry Mary Perkins, a young woman whom he had been courting for some time. John had vacillated about the decision. "There is a continual dropping of yeas and a loud occasional thundering no." But for him as for other invalids, consumption's course was so erratic that it did not preclude marriage. In October 1851 John and Mary took a wedding trip to Europe, really a voyage for health for the bridegroom. When they returned home, John had to wrestle again with his predicament.[25]

Although John still clung tenaciously to his dreams of a medical career, he was now convinced that he did not have the strength to practice full time, at least not in New England. But instead of changing his profession, he thought of changing residence. With Mary at his side, leaving home and family did not seem quite so grim. "I've a mind to go into *Tennessee* and half-farm and half-medicate," he told Kingsbury. And Mary's grandfather had some land in Florida. "I think it is not under cultivation. . . . I've a good mind to go and look at it this winter. . . . I don't know about Montreal. It's so cold there. . . . Yet I would prefer it to a regular hot debilitating climate like New Orleans or Havana I think. I was all ready to go to the Sandwich Islands, [but the] prices are very high there."[26]

Uncertain of where to go and whether he had the capacity for so drastic an uprooting, in November 1853 John joined Frederick on an overland trip to Texas to scout out its possibilities. John carried the "hope of invigorating weakened lungs by the elastic power of a winter's saddle and tent-life." Maybe Texas was the elixir he sought, a place where he could prolong his life and where he and Mary could raise their children. The brothers spent the winter traveling across the state on horseback and camping out. To cover their costs, Frederick had accepted a contract for a book about slavery in Texas, but he soon lost interest in the project and gave his notes over to John to edit. The book that resulted, *A Journey through Texas; or, a Saddle-Trip on the Southwestern Frontier,* was really John's more than Frederick's. It was in part a pro-free-soil tract and in part a guide for invalids about the benefits of overland travel through the southwest.[27]

A Journey Through Texas, like the narratives of invalid-seamen, described and evaluated the health-giving aspects of a particular environment —in this case, Texas. It contained detailed information on the amount of sun and rainfall as well as the velocity of the wind, and with their beneficial ratios established, went on to recount the availability of food, horses, and guides. John touted the curative value of the trip, even as he conceded that it had not improved his own health.

For ourselves, we had derived less physical advantage, from our two thousand miles of active exposure, than we had buoyantly anticipated. The abominable diet, and the fatigue, sometimes relatively too severe, had served to null the fresh benefits of pure air and stimulating travel. Lungs, oppressed at home, played, perhaps a little more freely; but the frame had not absorbed the sanguine sturdiness that should enable it to resist subtle tendencies and get itself rudely superior to circumstances.

Indeed, at one point, "the hot, soggy breath of the approaching summer was extremely depressing; so much so, as to cause me once a fall from the saddle in faint exhaustion. . . . I lay half an hour alone, face to the ground, hardly breathing and unable to speak."[28]

Nevertheless, John insisted, perhaps at the urging of the publishers, that his experience had been atypical and that other invalids would benefit greatly from the journey. "To a pulmonary invalid, who can throw off cares, and who has any recuperative elasticity in him," he declared, "I can recommend nothing more heartily than a winter's ride or sporting trip upon the Texan prairies." It would be of most help to those whose symptoms were "incipient" and who had the means to supply themselves with all necessities. "With money and sufficient pains-taking, it is possible to command a wholesome diet; with clothing and patience, the northers [winds] are easily endured."[29] *A Journey through Texas* concluded on a very positive note: "Six months of leisurely prairie-life . . . would, for many a man, now hacking away at his young tubercles in hot rooms, and a weary routine of business, double not only the length but the enjoyable value of life, at no greater outlay than the sum of his medical bills."[30]

In any case, the trip convinced John that migration was not the answer to his predicament. He returned to his family and once again lent a hand in the management of Southside. But the stint was brief. In 1855 he, Mary, and their two small children set off on what would be his last voyage for health. In 1857 in Nice, France, at the age of thirty-two, John Hull Olmsted died from consumption.

Other invalids also acted on the hope that migration, particularly to a warm Caribbean climate, might enable them to practice their profession without sacrificing their health. Prepared to exchange life in a tightly knit community of kin and acquaintances for a chance to realize career ambitions, New England men still found the experience excruciating. To uproot themselves from family and friends and settle in a foreign land among people who spoke a different language, had different customs, and practiced a different religion turned out to be far more difficult than they had imagined.

The experiences of Nathaniel Cheever II exemplify the difficulties encountered by these invalids. Although he had not been fit enough to attend college, Nathaniel did manage to muster enough strength as a young adult to apprentice to a local physician in Hallowell, Maine, and then attend the Columbia College of Physicians and Surgeons. But as graduation approached, Nathaniel's health became more precarious; he obtained his medical degree but never had the stamina to practice his career in New York or New England. "I must seek a milder climate before another winter, for I have barely survived this," Nathaniel wrote to his sister, Elizabeth, shortly before graduation. To do otherwise, "with my present health . . . would be folly and madness." Cheever was not altogether unhappy with this decision, for before entering college he had taken several long voyages for health to Malaga and Gibraltar that had rendered him fluent in Spanish and familiarized him with Spanish customs and Catholic practices. Based on these experiences, he settled on Cuba. Though he had never visited the island, it was Spanish, not that far from home, and the destination of a goodly number of men in search of health. Once there, he planned to obtain a medical license and open a practice that would cater to Cubans and to those invalids who came for the winter. In November 1843, with all his worldly possessions in tow and his medical chest filled with surgical instruments, patent remedies, and opiates, Nathaniel set sail for Cuba to cure his disease and to practice his profession.[31]

He took up residence in Trinidad de Cuba, a small town two days' journey (by boat and mule) from Havana. Getting there was no small feat. "My baggage of which I unfortunately have an enormous quantity," the intrepid invalid recounted in his diary, "was mounted in different parcels on the backs of four horses; I mounted a fifth and my two guides each another, making in all seven horses and three horsemen—quite a caravan. I trembled for the safety of the contents of my medicine chest, when I saw it mounted and jolting upon horseback but there was no remedy. Jolt it must as well as everything else."[32]

Nathaniel quickly settled into a boardinghouse and embarked on his own curative regimen. He bought a horse and rode for several hours each day. As he had anticipated, his skills in Spanish enabled him to integrate more fully into the life of the island than most other invalids could. He used all his letters of introduction to meet prominent and influential Cubans, visited their estates, and learned about the economics of growing sugar. He was never comfortable in Cuba—he remained contemptuous of Catholicism and of the monarchy—but his sentiments did not interfere with his sense of purpose. He had come to Cuba to prolong his life and practice medicine, and nothing would deter him.

Shortly after arriving, Nathaniel arranged to take his medical examination to obtain a license. But just as he was making his plans, he began to hemorrhage more frequently, which he viewed with some sense of irony. "I have not been at all well today having had some bloody sputa and considerable uneasiness in my chest," he wrote in his diary. "My cough continues very bad and expectoration is enormous." Was it wise to pursue his career? "It will cost me about 300 dollars to take out my license and perhaps I may not live to earn even that sum." Nevertheless, he might enjoy yet another remission. "But what can I do?" he wondered. "I cannot practice at Trinidad without a license and if my life should be spared I may get into business and soon more than earn that amount." And so he, like his fellow consumptives, formulated an invalid's creed: "We must act as though we expect to live, although we may be taken from this world at any moment."[33]

A constant cough, hoarse voice, frequent sweating, and bloody sputa did not deter Nathaniel from submitting to a three-day oral examination by several prominent physicians. The event was an ordeal, and the coughing invalid received little sympathy from his examiners. He passed the examination and soon submitted an article to the *Boston Medical and Surgical Journal* encouraging other invalid-physicians who wanted to practice medicine to come to Cuba.[34]

For all his enthusiasm, Nathaniel enjoyed little professional success. Unlike Northern Europeans, the Spanish held that consumption was contagious in its final stages; not only did they burn the belongings of consumptives after death but shunned them while they were alive. In North America and Northern Europe the disease was presumed to be hereditary and consumptives were not discriminated against; nor was their movement restricted. In Cuba avoidance was the norm, as Nathaniel discovered not long after he received his license. He accompanied two Spanish physicians to confirm a diagnosis of yellow fever on board a newly arrived vessel. The doctors made it clear that they considered Nathaniel's consumption more of a threat to them than the yellow fever. "The Spanish physicians and all others here are contagionists," Nathaniel reported. "The people have much more dread of taking consumption than they do yellow fever. When a person dies with consumption, his clothes and all the furniture of the room, bedding and all are immediately burned."[35]

Nathaniel ran up against these same sentiments at his boardinghouse. The residents did not want a coughing and hemorrhaging consumptive in their midst. "The other customers seeing that I suffer with a complaint of the chest are afraid I shall give them the consumption!" In fact, their fears were so strong that they asked him to move out. "The circumstance hurt my feelings excessively and I have today passed some very, very sad moments. It is true that my cough and expectoration are dreadful and a nuisance to myself and everybody else who chooses to esteem it so." To avoid being evicted from his next boardinghouse, he intended to have his food sent to his room, "and eat alone where I shall annoy no one but myself."[36]

Not surprisingly, Nathaniel did not build up much of a practice. Cubans would not come to him, and not many Americans did either. Over the course of the next few months, he had only two patients: the consul general of the United States consulted him once, and the consul's servant required thirty-five visits for the treatment of a wound. In an effort to expand his practice, Nathaniel published an article in a New York newspaper promoting the salubrious effects of wintering in Trinidad de Cuba—if pulmonary invalids came to Cuba, perhaps they would seek out his services. But as summer drew near, Nathaniel himself became the main consumer of the medicines in the chest he had so carefully transported. Despite the daily rides and nutritious diet, he became more and more frail. To relieve an almost constant pain and hoarseness, he began to take the laudanum he had brought for his future patients. Soon the syrups and opiates became the staple of his diet, and before the winter migration of invalids occurred, Dr. Nathaniel Cheever was dead.

4

Body and Soul

THE FIRST DECADES OF THE NINETEENTH CENTURY WERE A PERIOD OF intense religious fervor. Revivals swept the country, affecting the well-established settlements of New England as well as the frontier. The evangelical spirit reinforced many traditional religious obligations. Newly professed Christians, like their Calvinist forebears, attended church regularly, prayed daily, and engaged in ongoing self-examination. But evangelicalism also brought new doctrines and attitudes, softening the harsher elements of Puritan theology. An image of a loving and tender God replaced the more forbidding Calvinist deity, and revivalist sermons devoted more attention to salvation with its promise of a heavenly reunion with family and friends than to damnation and the specter of a fiery pit of hell.

Evangelicalism had a particular appeal for invalids, and its influence in their life histories is marked. Weighed down by the burdens of disease and deeply apprehensive that their present afflictions were punishment for past sins, many of them participated actively in the revivals. The experience not only provided personal comfort but enabled some of them to turn a vagabond life and voyage for health into a spiritual odyssey.[1]

The routines prescribed for invalids on a voyage for health might have posed conflicts for religious men. To sail for weeks on the open sea, or to spend days exercising on horseback might be equated with idleness and frivolity. Thus, to obey both their ministers and their doctors, to serve body as well as soul, invalids made themselves into penitent pilgrims in search of redemption.[2] Since the voyage for health was uncharted, newly professed Christians anticipated spiritual challenges in addition to the physical ones. The trip was bound to be filled with unexpected obstacles and temptations to test the faith of the most resolute Christian. Invalids who were condemned to

leave family, church, and community were certain to encounter morally corrupt travelers and witness spectacles that would offend both moral and religious sensibilities. Most important, they realized that the journey might not
be successful, that the end might come hundreds of miles away from family,
friends, and ministers, leaving them to travel alone through the Valley of the
Shadow of Death. Their journey required a faith that brooked no spiritual
infirmity and would not falter in the face of adversity.

The intensity with which professed Christians confronted these challenges is apparent in their daily journals and diaries. Some of them, following the habits of Puritan ancestors, actually kept two journals: One recorded
the temporal journey and was to be read by family and friends to learn how
they carried out their daily duties; the other, which charted the spiritual pilgrimage, was a private document filled with laments about their sins and
doubts about their ability to submit to God's will.[3]

Invalid men also brought along other books to provide them with spiritual guidance. For many, the favorite text, kept alongside their Bible, was
John Bunyan's *Pilgrim's Progress*. This account of one man's search for
redemption, whom Bunyan called Christian, had a particular appeal to
invalids. The allegorical significance of Christian's perilous travel
through a seemingly never-ending wilderness with his burden of sin
weighing heavily on his back and the vivid personifications of human
nature (Mr. Malice, Mr. Love-Lust, and so forth) set the frame for their
own journey. The similarities between the text and the hardships of their
errand led some among them to blur the distinction between allegory and
experience and to use the text as a guidebook. Joseph Emerson kept a
copy of the book with him and maintained that he "believed every word
to be literally true."[4]

By fusing Christian's quest for the Celestial City with their own search for
renewed health and spiritual redemption, the invalids translated medical prescriptions to travel into a religious quest. Christian's anguish at having to
leave his family and his determination to persevere despite trials and despair
was a model by which invalids judged the strength of their faith. They, too,
had to leave family and friends on a voyage of unknown duration to an
unknown destination, and along the way they, like Christian, might be
seduced by temptation. They might become mired in a "Slough of
Despond," or relax their vigilance and succumb to the false hopes incurred by
following a shortcut through a seemingly bucolic "By Pass Meadow." When
most weary and doubtful of the meaning of the journey, invalids might see
looming before them the narrow and treacherous path through the Valley of
the Shadow of Death. They had to avoid the traps that ensnared thousands of
travelers before them in order reach the Celestial City.

*   *   *

Nathaniel Cheever's lone voyage for health in an alien land exemplifies how invalid men joined medical and religious prescriptions and retained a resolute faith even as death neared. Nathaniel Cheever, the father of Dr. Nathaniel Cheever, was a bookseller and publisher in Hallowell, Maine. A devoted admirer of *Pilgrim's Progress*, he not only read and reread it but also published a new edition of it in 1817. The very next year Christian's ordeal became all too relevant to Cheever. In 1818, when he was thirty-nine years old, he could no longer sleep at night because of his chronic cough, and his voice became so hoarse that he was unable to speak audibly. As his discomfort became more acute, Cheever consulted a local physician, who warned him that he was in imminent danger of contracting consumption and advised him to leave for a warmer climate. The advice made sense to Cheever. His brother-in-law, George Barrell, had experienced similar symptoms and improved his health in this way. Cheever wrote to Barrell, who heartily endorsed the prescription. "Let me advise you my dear friend and don't slight my advice," Barrell responded.

> The climate is the most wretched in creation where you now are, and altogether unfit for human beings much less for invalids. . . . Leave it for a season, take your passage at once for a warmer and a better air—take a trip to sea—go to Madeira, to Bermuda, Savannah. . . . Take passage for it will add thirty years to your life and give happiness to your wife and children. . . . A change of air is necessary for you and you must not neglect this imperious duty.[5]

At first Cheever resisted so drastic an uprooting, reluctant to leave behind his wife, his five children, and his church. He was particularly hesitant to go southward even for a season to live in a region "dependent on the evils of slavery." To Cheever, the South seemed to bear an uncanny resemblance to "Vanity Fair" that Bunyan so graphically described. In the southern states, Cheever declared, "a man of fortune would find a hotter climate and better servants, but his ear would be often assailed by the gloomy groans of the African slave, and his eye would be cheered by less beautiful prospects and improvements than appear in this northern section; and in that part of the country the ornaments of education, religion and morality are less valued or cultivated than in New England." His antipathy to the South ruled out taking his family along. They would be deprived not only of New England schools but also of "religious exercise, and . . . good examples." More, "if disease deprives a man of health or life, his children have no longer the blessing of his parental care to look to, in a land of strangers, where every thing is new, and every thing beset with difficulties, uncertainty and dangers; and in case of his loss, none are left to advise or help them."[6]

All his doubts notwithstanding, the duty to "improve" compelled him to act quickly. Within a month after consulting his Hallowell physician, Cheever was traveling alone on a brig heading to Charleston. But each step in the journey posed conflicts, and it was religion and family that gave him guidance and strength.[7] Cheever knew he would miss his family, but the intensity of his feeling after the separation surprised him. "The very first glance at your last kind letter," he wrote to his wife, Charlotte, "had the effect of exciting all the tender sensibilities of my heart, and I am not ashamed to own to you, my dearest friend, that my eyes immediately over-flowed in tears, to repress them I had no desire, for I found pleasure therein. With some this would be called weakness; yet *I* would not wish to exchange one moment of such tender melancholy for hours of heroic insensibility."[8]

Cheever conceded that Charleston was more heterogeneous than he had expected, and the planter class, more diverse. "Much dissipation prevails among the higher classes, and yet there are many, very many I believe truly pious people."[9] But the institution of slavery was as corrupt and depraved as he had anticipated. "This subject of slavery," he wrote, "so disgusting to my mind, would soon fill my sheet if indulged in; I will therefore desist." Indeed, the longer he remained the more repulsed he became. "No tempta-tion could induce me to take up a permanent residence in this country. The customs and practices that prevail here are peculiarly disagreeable to my mind."[10]

Determined to avoid any temptations that might deflect him from his mission, Cheever spent a lonely winter in Charleston. He purposely chose a lodging house that was "not crowded with boarders," and the few visits he made were to other New Englanders who had come "on the same errand as myself, the recovery of health."[11] Each day he took his exercise by riding along the wide and dusty streets and fording the marshy swamps and shal-low creeks that crisscrossed the city. But his mind was not on the sights. He was most concerned with comporting himself in a way that would allow God to smile on his efforts. "I still feel, as if an all wise God will bless the means that I have resorted to for recovery and again return me to my beloved wife and children with renovated health and strength," he assured Charlotte.[12]

Cheever was prepared nonetheless for the possibility that his mission might not have the conclusion he so wanted. "I desire to be patient and rec-onciled under a trial and affliction, and above all things I do believe I am sincere when I wish that my mind may be prepared through the abundant grace of God, to meet my last, my solemn charge, come when it will. . . . My constant prayer is that this event may be prolonged; but I hope to be able to meet it with fortitude and resignation, in the firm hope that the exchange may be happy and glorious."[13] When his spirits flagged, as they often did during the nights alone in his boardinghouse, Cheever reminded himself of the gravity of his situation and the importance of his mission. "In some solitary moments," he confessed to Charlotte, "I wish myself home again; but having come here under a sense of impious duty, I check those feelings as they rise and determine within myself to make the days of my sojourning as pleasant as possible."[14]

As the weeks passed and his health did not improve, Cheever grew impatient. The climate of Charleston did not seem suited to his constitution—the dust of the streets irritated his throat during the day, and the dense humidity that hung in the air made him perspire and kept him from sleeping at night. He decided to take an overland journey to Augusta, Georgia, having heard that its climate was less humid and the cost of living lower. More, his stepbrother, Samuel Weston, was a merchant in Augusta and was ready to rent him a room in the boardinghouse in which he lived. Cheever also hoped that Weston's presence would alleviate his abiding loneliness.[15]

The ten-day journey to Augusta was worse than he had anticipated. He began the trip in the warm and sunny climate of Charleston, but as he headed inland it became "cold and very windy." One day took him through "a most violent *snow storm*," and only the chance hospitality of a widow provided him with shelter. But the fact that his health did not deteriorate further encouraged him to believe that his strength might well be returning. Once arrived in Augusta, he wrote Charlotte: "It certainly can be considered no indication of declining health when you learn that I have borne this long and lonesome and tedious journey without fatigue; and have rather increased in strength. But the ugly cough continues, more especially in the night . . . together with that disagreeable hoarseness."[16]

In Augusta, Cheever took long walks daily, continued to ride his horse even in inclement weather, and ate a bland vegetarian diet; and he did enjoy the companionship of his stepbrother. But the regimen and climate did not restore his health. On January 30, 1819, after almost a month's residence in the city, he wrote to Charlotte, "Toward night, I feel very tired." And he complained of the "continued hoarseness of my voice—I can only converse in a whisper." As the days wore on and he knew that the disease was steadily consuming his body, he began to question his own judgment in undertaking the trip. "In looking back on my journey, I am forced to reflect that, in my situation, it was imprudent, undertaken and prosecuted alone as it was, through a perfectly strange land, destitute of decent accommodations for travellers, invalids especially."[17]

Over the next month, despite his fervent efforts to counter the wasting process, the disease progressed. On March 4, 1819, James Bates and Samuel Weston informed Charlotte Cheever that "before this trembles in your hand, every symptom warrants that probability, that the man you have held so dear will be with us no more." Weston assured her that in his determination to prolong life, Nathaniel Cheever had not fought God's will. "Death with him had no terrors for he firmly believed he would be admitted to the mansions of the blessed." Like other pious pilgrims, Cheever had not allowed his afflictions or the obstacles of a pilgrimage to interfere with his desire for eternal salvation. He had undergone his ordeal with unquestioned faith and perhaps gained admission to the Celestial City.[18]

Evangelical Protestantism inspired invalids in still another way: since sin and depravity were omnipresent, a voyage for health could become the occasion to spread the reach of the Empire of Religion. Evangelicalism enthusiastically espoused the linkage between public missions to do good and the achievement of personal salvation. "The American people, if not blind to their own permanent interests," maintained Jeremiah Evarts, corresponding secretary of the American Board of Commissioners of Foreign Missions and editor of its newspaper, the Panoplist,

> can perform wonders in the accomplishment of the grandest designs . . . of no less magnitude than the establishment of schools, churches, and the regular ministration of divine ordinances, in all the destitute places of our country; the distribution of the Bible, and the support of missionaries to preach its doctrines in every part of the globe; the alleviation of human suffering of every kind wherever men are found—in a word, the entire subjugation of the world to Christ, and of course the eternal salvation of unnumbered millions in all future generations.

Evarts insisted that "the welfare of immortal souls ought to be the ultimate object of every Christian's labors. This obligation does not lie upon a minister . . . but it is binding upon . . . every Christian." God was calling Christians to become "co-workers with him in doing good."[19]

The spirit of millennialism turned voyages for health into missions and invalids into missionaries who took up the call to purify the world. It allowed them to link their "errand" directly to the goals of the evangelical crusades and gave the vagabond life a religious imperative. Invalids responded with particular energy, the very precariousness of their earthly probation making their participation the more urgent. Whatever the invalids' destination or talents, they could help promote the establishment of a "righteous" Protestant Empire. Accordingly, they set out to proselytize and gather souls for Christ. They collected Bibles, tracts, and sermons from a temperance society to distribute to seamen, and they continued their conversion efforts among the heathens on shore as well. In each instance, the medical and religious missions merged, elevating the significance of both.[20]

A number of tracts, often in the form of Christian biographies, guided the invalids in their efforts. Evangelical-minded texts recounted the tales of praiseworthy individuals who had endeavored that "earth should be made more like heaven, in its joys and its occupations." (One author of this genre declared, "Biography is prized in heaven.")[21] Older biographies like John Bunyan's *Pilgrim's Progress* had its hero seek personal salvation. The evangelically oriented versions joined personal redemption to the creation of a benevolent Protestant Empire.

The prototype of such biographies was *An Account of the Life of the Late Reverend Mr. David Brainerd* by Jonathan Edwards. Although written in 1749, it did not become a "spiritual classic" until almost a century later. Between 1833 and 1892, the American Tract Society distributed seventy thousand copies, which elevated Brainerd to "an exalted place in evangelical hagiography."[22] Edwards's account of this missionary who suffered from consumption became a source of spiritual inspiration for other invalids because Brainerd's life, in a number of ways, exemplified their own dilemmas. Despite his poor health, Brainerd was determined to serve God. He entered Yale in 1739 to study for the ministry but within a year was forced to leave to regain his strength. "I grew so weakly and disordered by too close application to my studies," he wrote in his diary in August 1740, "that I was advised by my Tutor to come home and throw off that oppressing care as much as I could, for I was grown so weak that I had spit blood more than once." In November 1740 Brainerd returned to Yale, obtained his degree, and in 1742 became a missionary of the Society in Scotland for Propagating Christian Knowledge. Between 1743 and 1747 he traveled on horseback across New York, New Jersey, and Pennsylvania, saving souls and seeking converts. Brainerd's diary revealed both the course of his inner journey—from doubts and perplexities to sincere piety—and the course of his illness—from bouts of pain and occasional bloody coughs to hemorrhages. As Brainerd's body became more frail, his faith became more resolute. In 1747 he died, secure in the belief that he had gained admission to the Celestial City.[23]

Jeremiah Evarts was a nineteenth-century version of David Brainerd. A studious young man, Evarts intended to become a minister. He also graduated from Yale, but incipient pulmonary disease convinced him that he was not physically fit for the calling. "Almost every minister whom I have known," he wrote to a friend in 1803, "who has engaged in that arduous work with a feeble constitution, has been obliged to leave it. . . . I conscientiously believe I could not recommend any society to settle a man of so frail a constitution as I possess, even should I be able to preach at first." He served as a principal in a grammar school but did not find it spiritually rewarding. ("The health of my soul, which is of vastly greater importance than that of my body, is also languishing.")[24] After months of indecision, he made the odd and ill-suited choice to read for the bar and become a lawyer. Evarts opened an office in New Haven but even in a community with a strong church, he had, according to a colleague, "too much unbending integrity to be a popular lawyer." He was both a "zealous partisan" and a "conscientious one," never able, regardless of his client's circumstances, to "be diverted, by any consider-ations, from the support of what he believed to be the real moral inter-ests of the country."[25]

Unsatisfied professionally and without clients, Evarts next became the editor of a missionary journal, *the Panoplist,* and moved with his wife and small children to Boston. From 1810 until 1817 Evarts edited the journal and promoted evangelical crusades. He sponsored the distribution of Bibles among prisoners and led the fight against intemperance. "Every-thing which has a direct tendency to promote the salvation of immortal souls is great beyond the power of language to express, or imagination to conceive," he declared. "Who shall adequately declare the magnitude of an attempt to evangelize whole nations and ultimately to renovate a world?"[26]

Evarts's health along with his zeal turned him from editor to missionary. His respiratory symptoms returned with renewed intensity in 1817, and Dr. John Collins Warren, one of Boston's most prominent physicians, recom-mended a trip South for the winter. Evarts combined the journey with an assignment from the Board of Foreign Missions "so as to make his absence, while securing the great object of health, as subservient as possible to its interests." Evarts intended to "avoid the evils of a northern climate, and to gain strength by a tour on horseback." At the same time, he planned to visit the homes of pious southern Christians, inform them of the work of the Board, and solicit donations. He also intended to take an overland journey to Chickamaugah, Georgia, to visit the Moravian mission to the Cherokee Indians.[27]

This last stop altered Evarts's life. "I could not but reflect on the digni-fied character and noble employment of the consistent and devout mis-sionary," Evarts recounted. "Happy are they who sustain this character and spend their lives in this employment." Evarts was so impressed that he considered joining the mission himself, but the thought of living in a slave state dissuaded him. "This county is very new; the climate is healthy and I should think very well of it as the place of my future residence, in case I leave Boston, were it not for the existence of slavery, which is a much greater evil than I ever conceived it to be before my visit to the south."[28]

Evarts returned to Boston with renewed energy and clear goals. He set about expanding the efforts of the Board among the Cherokees, and with his training in law, he become an advocate for their rights. But his periodic visits to the mission were what most excited him. Evarts lived at the mission (which was renamed Brainerd) and delighted in meeting the converted Indian children, who sported such names as David Brainerd and Lyman Beecher. These trips convinced him that Indians could become educated Christians and then counter the spread of slavery. Thus, Evarts and his missionary allies vigorously opposed southern efforts to move the Indians west of the Mississippi.[29]

Although this work fortified Evarts's spirit, his health became more frail. "As I am so weak and have so little flesh, it is to be expected that my progress will at first be slow," he wrote to his wife in 1831, on what would be his last voyage for health.

> I have a thousand things to be thankful for; and it is my daily prayer, that if my health should be fully restored, I may be more entirely consecrated to the service of God than at any previous period in my life. . . . I seek restoration for the sake of laboring in the missionary cause. . . . I now consecrate myself to God for this cause. If he needs or designs to accept my services, he will retain them; if not, it will be for reasons infinitely good and wise.

Evarts died that very year. His search for health had been a failure, but like Brainerd before him, his faith was secure.[30]

The abolitionists' passion to purify the nation by freeing slaves was at one with the missionaries' determination to purify the world by saving souls. Just as some invalids had combined a voyage for health with missionary zeal, so others linked their travel to promoting the antislavery movement. The commitment of the invalid-abolitionists, like others in the movement, had an extraordinary intensity. They pursued their cause with a reckless devotion. So single-minded was their resolve to abolish slavery that for some it overrode considerations of both health and family. Invalidism and a sense of impending death made them altogether impatient with compromise. Armed with a steadfast belief in the righteousness of their cause and a sense that they had little to lose, they confronted angry crowds and risked their lives to aid escaping slaves. Better death from the stones of a mob or in a vermin-ridden jail than a death in bed.[31]

Amos Augustus Phelps exemplified the fervor that invalids brought to the movement. Despite a familial history of consumption, he graduated from Yale and became an ordained Congregational minister. But when his health became too poor for him to continue in his post, he decided to use his remaining time to serve God and country by promoting immediate emancipation. Phelps became so committed to the antislavery cause that it overwhelmed all other responsibilities.

In 1835, when his wife, Charlotte, was dying at home (also from consumption), he undertook a dangerous assignment for the Massachusetts Tract Society. Leaving his wife and son with his widowed mother, he went to upstate New York to distribute tracts and urge immediate emancipation. Phelps recognized that his health might not withstand the demands of his work and that he was ignoring his obligations to his family, but he preferred to die fighting to free the slave. As his wife neared death, she asked him to return home to care for her and their son. It is clear from her pleadings that she feared he would refuse her request:

> My daily prayer is that I may be fitted for life or for death and I do hope that some arrangement can be made so that you can equally promote the cause of abolition and still be with your family. . . . I do not say, *leave the work*, by no means, for I know you are needed at this important crisis, but [I] only ask whether you cannot as well do some other part while I live and while our dear boy needs your attention which you could give him when at home. I know that the interest of a small family is small indeed compared with 2,000,000 perishing souls. I would not lose sight of the great cause but does not the peculiar circumstances in which your family are placed make it a duty to give them a share of your time and attention?[32]

Phelps, however, ignored the plea. He reminded her that he, too, faced imminent death from angry proslavery mobs. "In regard to our cause, you see the enemy is raging on all sides and foaming out his wrath and shame. . . . This cause will never terminate without the shedding of martyr blood. . . . Never were men called on to die in a holier cause and better die in the faithful discharge of duty as the negro's plighted friend."[33] But Phelps died not in the call of duty but in a sickbed wasted from consumption. Just before his death, he asked God to forgive him for ignoring his wife's last wish. "My *heart was on fire for the slave*," he confessed in his diary, "and *my dear wife* sacrificing feeling and with a *cheerful* and ready heart said 'go' and with the impression that the cause of the slave demanded it, I went, but in so doing did not do justice to myself, my son and my dear wife. . . . God forgive me and also the dear saint who would *never allow her infirmities* to keep me from what she or I thought the duty to the slave."[34]

Joseph Kimball, another invalid-abolitionist, also wanted to die in the field, fighting for the cause. Too frail to attend college, Kimball found in the antislavery crusade an opportunity to do good and ensure his personal redemption. "I feel every day that my disappointment was for the best," recalled Kimball about his thwarted college plans. "My days on earth will be few, I have much to do in a little space. Had I devoted my time to retired study, I might have passed away and left no prints, no memorial that I have ever lived. Now by the blessings of God on my efforts I may be of some benefit to mankind, may leave the world better than when I found it.... The vices and sorrows of the world may be somewhat tempered by my labors." To this end, Kimball became the editor of a New Hampshire anti-slavery journal and then an agent for the American Anti-Slavery Society. "The cries of the crushed slave," he wrote in his dairy, "are coming up to my ears for succor.... May I prove true to my responsibilities.... And when I die have the blessed assurance that I have not lived in vain." The very next entries record the growing severity of the pains in his side and the "general irritability" of his system.[35]

When fellow abolitionist Theodore Weld suggested that Kimball inves-tigate the impact of emancipation upon the British West Indies, he seized the opportunity. "My health requires that I should seek a warmer clime, and I hope in benefitting that, to benefit, also the cause of impartial free-dom." His companion was another consumptive, James A. Thome, a young man from Kentucky whose family had recently emancipated their slaves. "We were both in feeble health and fled together from the rigors of an American winter," Thome later reported. "We corresponded for the most part in sentiment and views, with just enough difference to afford occasion for friendly discussion." Kimball's own diary recorded every step of the journey, in a form especially suitable for publication. He went so far as to head each page with a subject—not trusting the judgment of a later editor. Kimball died in 1838 secure in the satisfaction that he had left "a print" behind.[36]

The short life of Charles Turner Torrey embodies the passion of the invalid-abolitionists. Before Torrey was four, both of his parents had died of consumption, and even before he became an antislavery agent, he himself had the symptoms of the disease. Still, he ignored his health in order to fur-ther the cause. In 1844, in the course of his agitation for the abolition of slavery, Torrey was apprehended, convicted of aiding escaping slaves, and sentenced to a six-year term in the Maryland Penitentiary. Although he knew that he would never live out the sentence, he would not ask for a par-don; better to die in jail and become a martyr for the cause. "If I am to suf-fer, it is a great consolation to know that it will not be in vain; that Provi-dence will use even my sufferings to overthrow, more speedily, the accursed system that enslaves and degrades so many millions of the poor of our land.

So in *that* I do, and I will rejoice." And Torrey, too, believed that his work on behalf of the slaves increased his own chances for salvation. "The chain that is riveted to my ankles will not hinder our Lord from communing with me. I suffer for his sake and in his cause, and he will not forsake me." On December 31, 1844, Charles Turner Torrey died of consumption in the Maryland Penitentiary.[37]

For all their bravery and determination to further religious and secular causes, invalids, including the most devout and zealous among them, were haunted by the fear they might lack the inner strength to face death alone. So although the voyage for health was essentially a solitary venture, invalids, particularly those who knew they were in the last stages of the disease, tried to plan a journey that included the company of friends and kin. But friends could not always be uprooted or might not live along the most accessible route.

Invalids who faced this predicament often selected a destination popular with other Christians, making a surrogate family of casual acquaintances. It was not the stigma of the disease that brought these people together, but rather a need to share the pain and burden of dying away from home. The effect, perhaps unintended, was to create a community of invalids.

On the island of St. Croix, for example, the invalids who gathered during the winter tried, albeit not always successfully, to approximate a New England town. They arrived in November and departed in May; they boarded in a handful of houses near the harbor and undertook for each other the social and religious obligations that otherwise would have fallen to family or minister. They visited and nursed each other, watched over and prayed with the dying, mourned at the funerals, and wrote to the family of the courage and serenity with which husband, brother, or son had faced his final trial.

Guidebooks and conversations with other invalids had prepared the men for the discomforts of travel and the Spartan nature of boardinghouse life. But nothing they had read or heard had prepared them for the obligations they would incur in their new communities. Visiting the sick and attending funerals, as they often discovered, weighed on them heavily and forced them all too often to contemplate their own impending death. Living on an island or in a southern city with other northern invalids was a bittersweet experience. Invalids tried to maintain the hope that the winter in the South would restore their health, but the daily sight of men who looked like walking skeletons and emitted "graveyard coughs" tempered their optimism. So, too, the startled looks on the faces of friends they met on the street were painful reminders that their appearance belied their expectation.

Abby Champion accompanied her brother, George, and his wife, Susannah, both of whom were suffering from consumption, to St. Croix in the winter of 1841. Her reports on the appearance of those who boarded in their house indicate just how cadaverous the invalids looked and how slim their prospects for recovery seemed. Among the boarders were Mr. and Mrs. Beckley of Philadelphia who came with their child. Mr. Beckley, Abby wrote to her mother, "looks very thin, had an attack of bleeding in the spring is very much troubled with a cough but suppresses it entirely." Other boarders were "Mr. Syrant from Rochester, who looks very ill, and is so in reality but does not own himself an invalid. Mr. Spencer from Syracuse, a married man without his wife, here for his throat and quite an amusing character." As the winter wore on, even those who appeared to improve for a time soon lost whatever progress they made. "Dr. Burroughs is gradually gaining," Abby reported. "He looks wretchedly and has not yet been able to ride or walk out, one part of his lungs is entirely inactive, yet he is very cheerful and will soon be a pleasant companion." But these expectations were not realized. Several weeks later she wrote: "Dr. Burroughs is in a very critical state and Miss Briggs thinks it is doubtful if he returns."[38]

The descriptions indicate that being part of community of invalids required a willingness to assume the most somber and difficult tasks. Many invalids were far closer to death than they acknowledged to family and friends and their presence placed a burden on the healthy. At the same time, kindness offered during sickness was a debt that a family could never fully repay. Eliza Smith was twenty-four when she accompanied her invalid father to St. Croix in the winter of 1823. On the boat Eliza met a former schoolmate, Mrs. Burlock, whose husband owned a plantation on the island; during Eliza's stay the Burlocks visited the Smiths regularly, always bringing packages of home-cooked food and also arranging for medical and ministerial visits. Eliza's father died two weeks after they arrived and the Burlocks' insisted that she spend the remainder of the winter with them. "Oh the sorrow of that hour cannot be described," Eliza recalled years later. "Alone, in a strange land so far from home! The kind Burlocks came at once to help and comfort me and made all the arrangements for the funeral. . . . That night Mr. Burlock took me to his house and was a father to me."[39]

But many invalids could not manage these responsibilities. Some were just too enervated to see or to help others. "I carried a number of letters of introduction to Spanish and American families," Henry Cleveland informed his friend Margaret Cushing shortly after he left Cuba. "But my health was so poor that I had no desire to visit them. When the evening came, I felt too tired to go out or make any effort what so ever." His lack of energy and strength turned his initial optimism to despair.[40]

A few invalids—really the exceptions—were determined not to preview their own death in the gaunt faces of others and so kept their distance from invalid communities. Jeffries Wyman tried to avoid "invalids with emaciated forms, sunken cheeks, hollow eyes & sepulchral coughs" by circumventing Jacksonville during his winters in Florida. These sights, he informed his brother Morrill, "make one feel sad in spite of himself. It must have anything but a cheerful effect on sick strangers, to see so many weary ones sinking into their graves." [41]

But Wyman remained the exception. Despite the pervasive daily reminders of the precariousness of their own predicament, most men preferred living among invalids to the pain of dying alone. In a way that is all too familiar to the AIDS community today, the routine included frequent encounters with death. During the first month of his visit to St. Croix, Jonathan Smith attended five funerals, all of American invalids. Smith recorded each death in fulsome detail in his diary, and perhaps to distance his own situation from theirs, he tried to draw lessons from each of them. Smith had been on the island only four days when an invalid, "a Mr. Miller—a young gentleman from New Orleans about 23 years of age," living in the same boardinghouse, died of consumption. Miller was rumored to be heir apparent of one of the "richest men in New Orleans," and yet he died without the comforts of family. His solitary death, Smith remarked, "furnished subjects for our most melancholy reflections. He breathed his last in the room opposite ours, with no one present to close his eyes but his nurse, a mulatto woman—far from his native country—with no friend to sympathize with him in the dread hour of dissolution, or render to him those kind offices that can only come acceptably from near and dear friends." In the absence of family, the other invalids accompanied his remains to the grave. "The Americans were all invited to attend the funeral, and most of them came."[42]

Eight days later a Mr. McCall, a twenty-year-old from New York, died. His passing, Smith maintained, represented "the sad admonition of the uncertainty of life." "A week before he called at our house. . . . His plump, round, rosy face indicative of perfect health. [He] came here very reluctantly, I understand, [at] the urgent solicitation of his parents who were alarmed at some slight indications of pulmonary affection." But apparently he was guilty of the "grossest imprudence." McCall, Smith reported, ignored the advice of friends and "exposed himself to the sun at *midday* and to the air at *midnight*. The consequence was, he was violently seized with inflammatory fever, and in four days breathed his last."[43]

Less than a week later, Smith recorded the death of a young woman, a Miss Seymour from Rochester, New York, who had arrived, as befit a woman, with her mother and her uncle. Miss Seymour, Smith contended, was the victim of "imprudent planning," for she, "never recovered from the effects of the voyage. . . . The fatigues of the passage are great, and unless there is strength enough in the constitution left to rally after it, a speedier termination of life is the consequence." Then, two weeks later two more deaths occurred, one, a man from Savannah, Georgia, the other a young woman from New Jersey. She suffered from an "absence of affection" from her family, forced to spend "her last days among strangers. . . . Poor lady she did not linger long."[44]

For invalids to die away from home was all too common. Dexter's biographical accounts of Yale graduates in this era are replete with men who died on a journey for health. There was Gail Fitch Wheeler, class of 1820, who became a lawyer in Bridgeport, Connecticut. In 1837 he took a voyage to Santa Cruz for his health but died on board ship. Joseph Kerr, Jr., class of 1820, was studying law when the symptoms of consumption became unmistakable; he took a journey South and died en route in June 1823. William Hollister Guernsey, class of 1844, was an ordained Congregational minister, but he held a pulpit for only two years. In the fall of 1849 the symptoms of consumption forced him to go to Savannah and the following spring he died. Joseph Hurlbut, class of 1849, was studying for the ministry at the Divinity School when the symptoms of consumption forced him to leave. He died in Paris in July 1855 on his voyage for health.[45]

For religious Protestants the thought of not ministering to a family member at the moment of death was a recurring nightmare. It was considered both a privilege and a duty to offer consolation to dying family members, to "watch" and guide them in their final hours and in this way learn their innermost wishes and execute them in the manner desired. Hence, those who could not accompany the invalids on their voyage wanted to be certain that they died in peace. When Thomas Day learned that his brother Jeremiah had repeated hemorrhages from his lungs and had been advised to go to Bermuda for the winter, he was irked that his beloved brother had been so foolish as to ruin his health from studying too long; he was even more disturbed at the thought of losing the privilege of consoling Jeremiah if he were to die away from home. "If you knew the alarming account we have had of your illness before you left," he wrote Jeremiah, "and the apprehensions we, all of us, entertained that your disorder had taken too deep a root to be removed by a change of climate, and that your eyes would be finally closed by foreign hands in a foreign country, you could judge what a Brother who never believed that the ardor or sincerity of affection consists in professions, must feel at the reception of your letter." But Jeremiah was one of the lucky ones. His symptoms disappeared after his voyage for health.[46]

Other family members raced against death. When word arrived that their husband, brother, or son was dying, they rushed to the bedside. John Hull Olmsted, Frederick's younger brother, was in Nice on a voyage for health with his wife, Mary, and small children when he died. As soon as Mary sent word of impending death to John's father, he booked passage on a steamer and left for France. He wrote to Frederick describing John's final hours. "He spoke with a great deal of feeling and heart felt thanks for all I had done for him through life. He said it seemed hard to be called to part with life at so early an age as 32 but that he had enjoyed in that time a great deal of life especially in the past 6 years since his marriage and in the mutual friendship and brotherly love that had existed always between you and him." Olmsted noted his own loss and Frederick's with sadness. "In his death I have lost not only a son but a very dear friend. You almost your only friend." During his final days John, using his father as amanuensis, composed a final letter to Fred. It contained his last wishes—wishes he knew his brother would honor. "It appears we are not to see one another any more— I have not many days, the doctor says. Well so be it since God wills it so. I have never known a better friendship than ours has been and there can't be a greater happiness than to think of that. . . . Keep something of mine—my watch or cane." The final line altered Fred's life. "Don't let Mary suffer while you are alive." Two years later Frederick Law Olmsted married Mary and raised his brother's children.[47]

Sarah Cleveland, the wife of Henry Cleveland, also won the race against death. When Henry Cleveland realized that his winter's voyage to Cuba had not improved his health, he decided to go to New Orleans by boat and then take a circuitous overland route to Boston. In New Orleans, Cleveland chanced to meet an old friend, Ralph Emerson, who was there on business. The two men set out together for St. Louis, but during the voyage Cleveland's condition suddenly worsened. What was to be for Emerson a pleasant trip with an old friend was rapidly turning into a deathwatch. They were forced to stop in St. Louis, and Emerson, unwilling to leave his friend, assumed the duties of a nurse and sent frequent bulletins to Henry's wife, Sarah, assuring her that although the end was near, "his patience and courage have been heroic."[48]

Sarah Cleveland was shocked when the first bulletin arrived. Like her husband, she had assumed that the voyage would restore his health, and she was unprepared for his death. Furious at being denied the privilege of caring for him and watching with him as he died, she quickly made arrangements to go to St. Louis and arrived in time for a deathbed farewell. "I shall never forget the infinite mercy permitted me in seeing him once more and in hearing him say such kind and blessed words as he did," she told her friend Catherine Norton. "That will live with me and strengthen me, I *believe* to do my duty. That I should have lost the last eight months! Is it not heartbreaking? I remember that I yielded to Henry's wishes and to the doctor's opinion in remaining at home yet this is a miserable consolation for the thousand remembrances I might now have had, had I been allowed to cheer and comfort him to the end."[49]

Sarah Cleveland lashed out at the physicians and by innuendo at her husband for not informing her how far his disease had progressed, and not allowing her to be there to carry out his last wishes. Underlying such angry outbursts was the fear that the invalid, particularly if he was a young and inexperienced pilgrim, might not have the courage to face death with resignation and, concomitantly, that there would be no Christian watchers to inform the family about the final hours. To be present was to know that the invalid had died in peace and with the expression of salvation on his countenance.

Other families were less fortunate. Not only did the invalid die away from home, but the families also had reason to believe that he had experienced despair during the final moments. Dr. Nathaniel Cheever II, like his father, died from consumption, but his family was convinced that, unlike his father, his death had not been tranquil. When Cheever sensed that death was near, he approached the only Protestants he knew in Cuba, the American consul and his wife. In accordance with his wishes, they immediately arranged for his passage to New York and even accompanied him. His brothers wanted to be with him as well, and so as soon as they heard of his departure, they set off to meet the ship when it arrived in its first port, Charleston. But Nathaniel died before they reached him. To lessen their despair, and manage their grief, his brothers published a biographical account of Nathaniel's short, frustrated life. They intended the book to serve invalids and families who were embarking on a "trying pilgrimage." It also contained warnings about invalids traveling alone. "The bitterest part of the sorrow of having him die away from home, after so many such long wanderings with him," they declared, "was that none of us could be permitted to be by his side—to walk with him down to the borders of the River of death—to mingle our prayers with his—to save him, if possible, from the bitterness of that indescribable depression of soul, which at one time he experienced . . . and to receive the utterance of his last aspirations of faith." Unable to rescue Nathaniel from "terror and despondency," they wanted to prevent other families from experiencing the same defeat. "It yields a lesson well marked in this biography," they concluded, "as to the importance of the presence of a friend, and the hazard to health, happiness and even piety, of permitting an invalid to launch upon a journey alone."[50]

This lesson was not one that most male invalids would accept. Despite the hazards that marked these journeys, thay dared to join religious and social values to medical precepts in novel and purposeful ways. Invalidism in this context did not mean taking to bed but initiating a search for health that required energy, determination, and a willngness to take risks.

PART II

THE FEMALE INVALID: THE NARRATIVE OF DEBORAH VINAL FISKE, 1806–44

5

Coming of Age

To understand the impact of consumption on the lives of ante-bellum New England women, one must leave the public arena and enter the more intimate world of the family. Although educated men expected to regain health on lengthy and often daring voyages, women from the same social class and background expected to restore their strength within the confines of the home. The highly variegated regimens men charted as they sailed the world in search of a cure narrowed into a single track for women. It was a track that stopped abruptly where the men's began—at the end of the town.

Women pursued curative regimens that were consonant with their values and domestic responsibilities. A few women did travel briefly and in the company of family members to tropical climates. A handful combined a journey for health with the imperatives of evangelical Protestantism; as wives of foreign missionaries, they joined the search for a cure to a commitment to convert the heathens. An occasional unmarried woman even went South to teach free blacks and illiterate whites. But most invalid women remained at home, functioning within a series of concentric circles of children, husband, kin, friends, and neighbors that defined the privileges and obligations of their gender.[1]

If the challenge confronting men was to fit personal ambition to the precepts of invalidism, for women, it was to carry out domestic aspirations and duties as they tried to regain health. Physicians tacitly acknowledged this tension not by subverting women's domestic obligations but by offering them different prescriptions. They told men to dare to leave home and allowed women to remain at the hearth.[2]

This prescription confined women invalids to the home and placed an extraordinary burden on their female relations and friends. The women came for lengthy visits to assist the invalids with child care and to provide emotional and spiritual support. They also would board the invalids' children when illness provoked an acute crisis. Not only was the care of children was the responsibility of all women.[3]

An examination of the death records of one town, Amherst, Massachusetts, offers a lesson in just how heavy the shared duty of child care was. In 1844 Amherst had 2,550 residents and in that year, the town clerk recorded 61 births and 51 deaths. Of the fifty-one, fourteen, or more than one out of four, were from consumption.

Deborah Fiske	38	married
Harriet Fowler	46	married
Sarah Robinson	58	widow
Isaac Orr	51	clergyman
Sophronia Alexander	38	married
Eunice Smith	42	married
Mary Ann Smith	28	married
Nabby Taylor	57	married
Nancy Chapman	81	single
Eliza Parsons	55	widow
Rebecca Edwards	38	married
Vesta Dickinson	25	married
Augusta Holden	9	girl (colored)
Louisa Finemore	11	girl (colored)

Although the ages of the victims ranged from nine to eighty-one, many were married women between the ages of twenty-seven and fifty. In Amherst as elsewhere, the death rate of females was greater than that of males.[4]

When these raw numbers are linked to the odd course of the disease and basic social data about the town, the obligations that female invalidism and maternal mortality conferred on a community vividly emerge. Since consumption was a disease that slowly wasted its victims, many of the women who died in 1844 would not have been able to manage the household chores and child-rearing tasks in the last years of their lives. Each would have required sustained assistance. If the invalid could not afford domestics, the sewing circle would repair the clothing, and friends and neighbors would supply meals and do the nursing. When the invalid became incapacitated, an unmarried aunt or sister moved into the household to care for the children. Even death did not abrogate the obligations. Few widowers could manage caring for the children by themselves, and if they did not remarry or were themselves invalids (and consumption often struck both husband

and wife), the orphan children would have to be placed—and again, the responsibility fell on kin and friends.[5]

Since male invalids followed so many different geographic and professional routes in their efforts to regain health, their diverse stories are best captured through the presentation of multiple narratives. Female invalids, on the other hand, tended to make a more uniform choice to remain within the domestic circle. Therefore, the most effective way to understand the intensity of their experiences and the impact their illness had on family, friends, and neighbors is to explore in depth the life history of one female invalid. The power of a vertical, as opposed to more horizontal approach, emerges from the narrative of illness of Deborah Vinal Fiske. Not that she was typical of all women invalids; she was wealthier and better educated than most. But her life history illuminates the interaction of chronic illness and social obligation, how the experience of illness shaped and was shaped by cultural norms.[6]

Deborah asked her husband, Nathan, to preserve an unusually large cache of letters, which she had self-consciously composed to instruct her children and grandchildren. Deborah emerges in these letters as a saintly woman—a self-portrait reenforced by the testimonials of female friends and ministers. If there were only these letters and eulogies to document her life, Deborah, like other pious New England women invalids, would have appeared too virtuous to be genuine. But a second cache of letters survives. These letters, which Deborah did not intend to preserve, reveal her pain and anger at living a life constrained by consumption, the debts she owed to the many women who helped her, and the burdens that invalidism and religion placed on her marriage. To bring these two selves together, to link the "official self" to the "hidden self," is to reconstruct the authentic experience of a female invalid. In Deborah's life we will see the way consumption affected women's education, marriage, child-rearing practices, female friendship, religious precepts, and relationships with doctors, and how it altered the social fabric of the community.[7]

Because Deborah believed that she had a hereditary predisposition to consumption and because she had suffered from bouts of respiratory ailments throughout childhood, every aspect of her life reflected the experiences of being an invalid. Deborah came from solid New England stock. Her parents traced their lineage back to the earliest seventeenth-century New England settlements on the South Shore of Boston. By the beginning of the nineteenth century they had through their frugal habits and commercial acumen become prosperous members of their communities. But the continuity that they represented stood in stark contrast to the instability and insecurity that consumption brought to Deborah's life.[8]

In 1805 David Vinal, a contractor, lumber dealer, and distiller, returned from Boston to his native Scituate to marry Deborah Waterman. On December 13, 1806, Deborah delivered a daughter whom they named after her. The baby thrived, but not the mother. Deborah Waterman Vinal became more enfeebled after her pregnancy and died from consumption at the age of twenty-nine before "little Debbie" celebrated her second birthday.[9] David Vinal was unprepared for the loss. A blunt and private man, mainly concerned about making shrewd investments and accumulating capital, he was daunted by his new responsibility and moved to discharge it quickly. "Little Debbie" went to board with willing relatives in nearby towns. David Vinal provided her material needs—in a lavish manner. He sent money not only for her maintenance and schooling but also for ponies and pianofortes. He gave her whatever affection he could muster; he visited regularly, took her for long horseback rides, and stayed for tea. But since he was uncomfortable under the watchful and often disapproving eyes of relatives, his visits were brief.[10]

Perhaps because her father so totally equated goodness with worldly success, Deborah searched throughout her childhood for evidence of her mother's virtues. The stories she heard from family members aroused a curiosity that was not satisfied. "I was sadly disappointed in being unable to obtain some of my mother's [letters]," she told a friend. "I have always felt that her letters would give me a more correct idea of her character than any descriptions of her friends." Her mother, however, eluded her daughter's considerable efforts to breathe life and nobility into her disembodied form.[11]

Although Deborah enjoyed the privileges that accrued to children of well-established Protestant New England families, she was a "wanderer" and a "pilgrim." Her mother's death from consumption turned her into an orphan, and the insecurity that it engendered marked her education, marriage, child-rearing practices, and religious preferences as profoundly as any genetic trait. Until the age of fourteen, Deborah shuttled back and forth between relatives in Marshfield and Newburyport. Her energy was absorbed in making herself a welcome guest in other people's homes. She quickly learned to conform to the high expectations of adults who boarded relatives in their homes: she was excessively neat, docile, obedient, and adept at performing those extra tasks that were tacitly expected of such children. The truisms that mothers teach children but do not expect them fully to obey—"never speak until spoken to" or "always be cheerful"—were imperatives that Deborah dared not violate. She took responsibility for lining up the chairs after dinner, making certain they did not accidentally touch the wall, and sweeping up the crumbs. Even when sick she was cheerful and grateful, finishing her chores, and folding her clothes. Whatever anger or resentment she might have felt, she repressed.[12]

When she was fourteen Deborah finally found a permanent and comfortable home with her Aunt Martha and Uncle Otis Vinal in Charlestown, Massachusetts. "I shall never forget your kindness and faithfulness in praying with and for me," she later wrote to her aunt, "but for such a mother that I could go to with perfect freedom, I don't know what would have become of me."[13] During these years Aunt Vinal, as Deborah called her, took in other orphan nieces. Soon after Deborah's arrival two cousins both named Martha (Martha Vinal Chickering and Martha Bowker Vinal) moved in. Their shared predicament as well as the maternal character of Aunt Vinal turned the three young women into sisters. The family circle was further extended to include three cousins, Ann, Ellen, and Adeline Scholfield, who lived in nearby Boston.[14]

The stability of the Vinal household turned the shy and timid Deborah into a sociable and gregarious young woman. But she could never totally escape the insecurity of her past or the fetters that disease imposed on her. Whenever Deborah left Aunt Vinal's home, she was bereft and lonely. She longed for her aunt's solicitude and the companionship of her cousins. "Aunt is a model of patience and of hospitality," Deborah maintained. "It is just like going home to a father's house."[15]

Consumption had not only deprived Deborah of a mother and a home but it also left her with a legacy of ill health. Deborah had small bones, a "narrow" chest, fair skin, and rosy cheeks, signs of an invalid constitution. Throughout childhood she was prone to prolonged sore throats, fevers, and coughs. David Vinal, knowing how closely Deborah resembled her mother, chose as her physician John Collins Warren, a professor at Harvard Medical School and one of the founders of the Massachusetts General Hospital. Given the prevalence of consumption in New England, many of Dr. Warren's patients were invalids like Deborah, requiring treatment at times of acute illness and advice on how to devise an appropriate life-style.[16] Dr. Warren visited Deborah at Aunt Vinal's and prescribed opiates to relieve pain or applied a blister or leeched her to remove an inflammation. He counseled her, as he did all his other patients, to exercise daily. "Exercise during the early period of life," he insisted, "should be regularly enforced . . . [and] when practicable, should take place in the open air."[17]

Deborah followed his prescriptions and at the age of seventeen felt strong enough to enroll in the Saugus Academy, a female seminary, that provided an unusually rigorous religious and secular curriculum and time for daily exercise.[18] The school, located in a meeting house in the center of the town, was headed by Reverend Joseph Emerson (the invalid minister who chose to become a headmaster rather than a farmer). It consisted of one large room for seventy students who ranged in age from thirteen to twenty-five. Deborah lived with thirteen other girls in a large boarding-house and found it an ordeal.[19] Still, she stayed there for two terms and then went to the Adams Academy in Londonderry, New Hampshire, to continue to study with her favorite teacher, Zilpah Polly Grant.[20] For all her discontent at being away from home, Deborah learned that she had a keen mind and strong religious sensibilities.[21]

Both Emerson and Grant modeled their schools on a well-ordered Christian family. Time for prayer was an immutable part of the daily routine, and students were expected to memorize long biblical passages. This method of rote learning was designed to "stress obedience and submission . . . to make the student aware of God's omnipotence and the need to obey."[22] Emerson had a deep respect for women's intellectual capabilities and wanted his students to be "accomplished readers, accomplished writers, accomplished grammarians, accomplished reasoners." The systematic course of study included philosophy and logic, advanced mathematics, and ancient as well as modern history.[23] But intellectual achievement was not to undermine women's domestic and religious duties or, as Emerson phrased it, their "subordinate and dependent station." Higher education was to enhance woman's sphere of influence. "Females should be qualified to fill their various important stations in the best possible manner," to be "benefactors and blessings to their parents . . . to their husbands, to their children, to their pupils, to their friends and associates, to the church of Christ, to their country, to the world."[24]

The female teachers, Zilpah Grant and Mary Lyon, were responsible for cultivating the religious sensibility of the students.[25] Through private conversations and personal example, the women encouraged the students to profess their faith and lead their lives according to Congregationalist strictures. "As to your conduct," Grant told them, "I do not wish to have many particular rules. Consult your own sense of propriety, your reason, your understanding and the Word of God. Make fervent supplications to Him who is able to lead you in the right way." Every student was expected to attend "public worship seasonably, solemnly and devoutly," and "to be instrumental of each other's salvation." For Grant and Lyon, the number who professed their faith was at least as important as the number who passed their courses.[26]

Since both Emerson and Grant were invalids, their daily routines and attitudes toward disease were as instructive and inspiring to Deborah as the biblical passages she committed to memory.[27] They stressed the importance of diet and dress every student had to spend several hours a day in "laborious exercise," preferably "some useful employment for charitable purposes."[28] They also taught the students that if sickness enfeebled the body, it empowered the soul. Deborah was convinced that "in the course of life we all take our turn in being sick and ministering to the sick and in this way we learn patience and submission."[29]

Deborah's education at both schools provided her with a code of conduct that guided her decisions as an adult. In 1825 she returned to Charlestown and began to attend the Park Street Church, one of Boston's most orthodox institutions, and taught Sunday school.[30] In 1827 Deborah, along with nine other young women, committed herself to the service of Christ and to the promotion of the "empire of truth."[31] At the same time, she adopted the identity of an invalid. "My health is very much better, though I am not as strong as I used to be," she wrote to a friend from school, "neither do I sleep as quietly, but these are trifles." Her hope was that she would be "permitted to spend an eternity, an existence without end, in the presence of God our Saviour, Angels and Saints." The precepts of evangelical Christianity did not eliminate the pains of chronic disease, but they did hold forth the reward of eternal salvation.[32]

The only portrait that remains of Deborah was painted in this period. Peeking out from under a proper white bonnet and heavy somber clothing is a thin, delicate-boned woman with brown curly hair, a narrow, pointed chin, and intense sparkling eyes. It suggests that beneath the thick and well-insulated layers of religious piety and decorum was not only a devout but also a charming young woman.

In 1828 Deborah met Reverend Nathan Welby Fiske, a professor of languages and rhetoric at Amherst College. He was a man with religious beliefs as strong as her own. Eight years older than Deborah, Nathan came from a subsistence farming family in Weston, Massachusetts, and his parents' lack of piety remained a point of humiliation for him. Despite the disinterest of his family, Nathan graduated from Dartmouth College and Andover Theological Seminary. He differed in every way from Deborah's father. Where David Vinal was blunt and pragmatic, Nathan was tentative and ethereal. He knew little about the world of business and cared less. His passion was to proselytize for Christ, either by preaching or by writing. Nathan delighted in translating classical texts to demonstrate the importance of divine revelation. He was, his colleague Edward Hitchcock maintained, "a diligent student and not well fitted to come in contact with men in the rough and tumble of life." Nathan lacked "a knowledge of common things" and had no interest in acquiring it.[33]

Nathan recorded his religious activities in a daily diary, examining their usefulness to God. Given his tendency to self-castigation, he found far more evidence of his failures than of his successes. Occasional entries report a religious ecstasy and a stirring of spirit, but they are buried among the chastisements and self-deprecations. This dark vision may have come from his inability to fulfill his chosen calling as an ordained minister of the gospel. Immediately after graduation Nathan went on a mission to Savannah, Georgia, to convert seamen, sick slaves, and illiterate whites. But despite his prodigious efforts—in the course of six months he preached almost one hundred sermons and made more than three hundred pastoral visits—he won few converts. He had neither the commanding personality nor the passionate rhetoric of the more successful evangelical preachers. His friend Heman Humphrey, the president of Amherst College, who wrote extensively on revivals, commented: "His voice was small, and his utterance, when he began and till he was roused, was rather laborious. It wanted that fullness, flexibility and strength." Nathan longed to preach like a "Whitfield, Chalmers or even a Paul," but his audience, he conceded, was "as indifferent as so many sheep." The experience convinced him that he was "wholly unsuited to the duties of a Foreign Missionary," and in 1824 he accepted a professorship at Amherst College.[34]

Nathan was comfortable with the school's mission to "promote Christian knowledge and piety" to young men of "hopeful piety and promising talents." As a faculty member, he remained in the mainstream of evangelical Christianity even though he lacked the stamina and charisma required of a gospel minister.[35] By teaching Hebrew and Greek to young men intending to proselytize for Christ, he promoted the goal of the crusade.[36]

Nathan and Deborah were introduced by Henry B. Hooker, a Congregational minister, who had recently married Deborah's cousin, Martha Chickering. Nathan admired Deborah's accomplishments and piety. When she agreed to marry him, he was ecstatic, having found a woman who was his "equal" and would become his "dearest friend." Deborah, in turn, respected Nathan's educational credentials, his facility in language, and his extensive knowledge of the Bible.[37] They both had a penchant for orderliness and a fixed daily routine. In a letter to Deborah Nathan set down his schedule in characteristic detail.

> I rise from the bed at 5 o'clock, kindle a grand fire in the stove, attend to some little cleanings and emptyings, wash, attend to devotions, and generally do a little studying or writing before college prayers. Then comes my walk to College, recitation, and breakfast at Mrs. Moore's. Then follows, necessary business in the village if there be any, and study until 11 o'clock, then recitation, dinner, then study, more or less as may happen till evening prayers and tea. Then lectures, faculty meetings or calls, then sometimes study, or reading, devotions and various preparations for retiring which takes place at 10 o'clock.

As Deborah checked her schedule, the only possible conflict was in the hour each of them had set for prayer. Nathan resolved it by proposing they pray separately. "For the hour of prayer 5 o'clock in the morning would be best for me but not for you. Take 2 o'clock p.m."[38]

In November 1828 Deborah and Nathan were married at the Park Street Church. The couple moved to Amherst, where the newly constructed college buildings were surrounded by large open fields and forests. To some it appeared as if a speck of civilization, a "city on a hill," had been plunked down in a clearing in an unlogged wilderness.[39] And the town, even by New England standards, was strict in its religious standards. "It is true," Lydia Maria Child, the New York author and reformer maintained, "the river is broad and clear, the hills majestic, and the whole outward aspect of nature most lovely. But oh! the narrowness, the bigotry of man. To think of hearing a whole family vie with each other, in telling of vessels that were wrecked, or shattered, or delayed on their passage, because they sailed on Sunday."[40]

The couple first boarded with a family, and the experience brought back unpleasant memories. Deborah's letters to Aunt Vinal once again became plaintive, even childish. In fact they are so at odds with Deborah's earnestness that one wonders whether she was finding Nathan too wooden and too clumsy. Living in a farming community required an agility that Nathan lacked. "As for keeping house we cannot get along without you," she wrote back to her father less than a month after she was married. "For Mr. Fiske, I dare say, is as ignorant as I am, though he is much more careful about saying so. You are older and wiser than both of us together and when you see us in danger of shipwrecking our establishment you can lift up a warning voice and we will alter our course."[41]

Whatever her domestic dissatisfactions, Deborah set about fulfilling the duties of the wife of a faculty member. She called on other faculty wives and soon became friends with Harriet Abbott, whose husband, Jacob, taught mathematics and natural philosophy. Sophia Humphrey, the president's wife, invited her to join the ladies prayer circle. Deborah hoped to work among the poor and bring them to Christ but was disappointed to learn that there were few destitute families in town. "I have been introduced to 2 poor black women, their names are Venus and Sukey, but Venus lives so far off I shall not be able to see her very often. . . . She is very poor and has a rheumatic fever which you know is very distressing, [and] she . . . gives no satisfactory evidence of piety."[42]

Deborah became pregnant during her first year of marriage. The couple, with the concurrence of David Vinal, decided to rent a cottage, although the price was high—$250 a year—for Nathan's salary of $800. David Vinal came to Amherst to appraise the property and tersely announced that it "taint fit to live in." But since it was the home Deborah wanted, he agreed to repair it and subsidize whatever part of the rent they could not afford.[43]

In June 1829 the couple moved to the cottage. Deborah hired a young woman who was "strong, healthy, active, and teachable" to help with the chores. The sight of her own furniture, including the bundles of infant clothing that she was accumulating, provided her with much satisfaction. When the baby arrived, she would have both a family and a home.[44]

Whatever expectations Deborah had for her marriage and her health were shattered with the birth of her first child, David Vinal Fiske, on September 11, 1829. The delivery left her so "fatigued and feverish" that Sophia Humphrey, who had been with her during the delivery, and Dr. Gridley, her physician in Amherst, persuaded her that it was "unsafe" to breast-feed or care for the infant. Sophia took in the child and Deborah wrote Aunt Vinal that she and the baby were doing "much better" since he was at the Humphreys and on a diet of cow's milk. But in less than a month the baby began to suffer a "bowel complaint." His condition rapidly deteriorated, and the day before he died Heman Humphrey baptized him at Deborah's bedside.[45] It fell to Nathan "to follow him to his short and narrow house." "Poor little sufferer," he wrote to Martha Hooker. "His course was full of pain, though brief. He is now where the God of holy love chooses he should be. . . . Pray for us that this affliction may work for our good, and produce in us the peaceable fruit of righteousness."[46]

Though the couple tried to accept God's judgment, they could not repress their grief, nor Nathan, his guilt. At night Deborah would sigh and contemplate the unused clothing she had so painstakingly sewn and the empty nursery fully furnished, while Nathan would recount once more the "fond hopes" he had had for little David. If he had lived, he told his wife, he would have been "an *Idol*." But Nathan was also convinced that David's death and Deborah's continuing illness were evidence of God's displeasure for his depravity. "I do pray my dear wife, that the punishment of my sins may fall on myself and not on those connected with me. It is distressing enough to my heart to think how much our little David suffered for his father's guilt, it is insupportable if his mother must have a portion too on my account."[47]

As the cold New England winter set in, Deborah pressured Nathan to let her return to Boston for a few weeks. Perhaps a change of climate, a Christmas celebration with her family, a personal consultation with Dr. Warren, and—although she would not say it—a period away from Nathan would relieve her symptoms and raise her spirits. Deborah promised to shop for furniture and wallpaper for the new house they had leased and to return with her father, who would supervise the renovations. Nathan reluctantly consented; to try to preserve some semblance of the order and "comforts" he so enjoyed, he took his meals with neighbors.[48]

For Nathan the separation was a period of soul-searching, penance, and regeneration. "Here I sit by a charming fire in your nursery in the rocking chair," he wrote to Deborah, "wishing for only two things, first that the fetters and bonds of my *sin* were broken and secondly that you were at my side. I do not doubt that this separation will, if we are permitted again to meet, strengthen our union."[49] Deborah was in no rush to return, however. She told him that she had to wait until Dr. Warren declared her sufficiently recovered. As the weeks dragged on, Nathan grew impatient but had to defer to the physician's authority. "The first of January is just two weeks from tomorrow," he wrote Deborah, "and just *two* weeks from *tonight* I expect to see you here, that is, if your physician approves it; nothing but Dr. W's opinion must keep you at Boston."[50] As the separation continued, Nathan, increasingly vexed, appealed to Deborah's sense of respectability. He described his forlorn appearance, which he attributed to his wife's absence. "Perhaps, I might say something about my *ragged* coat sleeves, they look a hundred times worse than when you left, and something about torn shirts, and rusty andirons, and cobwebs and the like, but it would neither make you wiser or better."[51]

Finally, in January, Deborah returned home, accompanied by her father. Although she was still coughing and tired quickly, she dutifully mended Nathan's torn clothing and intermittently began to attend the weekly meetings of her prayer circle. Within a month, Deborah became pregnant again. This second pregnancy was more difficult than the first; during the early months her physicians worried she would miscarry. Deborah remained "entirely motionless upon my bed for nearly ten days," and for the rest of the pregnancy, "I was very cautious about exercise to prevent a premature confinement."[52] On October 15, 1830, Helen Maria Fiske was born. The lively, energetic infant thrived, but the delivery left her mother weak. Lingering colds, sore throats, continual coughs and fevers continued to plague her and she still had them more than a year later, when she became pregnant a third time.[53] In October 1832 Humphrey Washburn Fiske was born. Deborah nursed him for almost a year, but it so drained her that she hired a nurse to care for Helen and two other servants to do the household chores.

In September 1833 Deborah, Helen, and Humphrey contracted whooping cough. Deborah remained in bed, while Nathan and a nurse cared for the children. Humphrey contracted diarrhea, which soon "exhausted his strength and produced an inflammation."[54] Within a few days he died. Although Helen and Deborah were still sick and coughing, the nurse unexpectedly left. Resorting to her network of friends and relatives, Deborah conducted an extensive search for a substitute; her father's generosity allowed her to offer more than the going rate in Amherst. But she was unable to locate anyone suitable, and with Dr. Gridley's concurrence, decided to take Helen to Boston to recuperate. She remained there several months but did not regain much strength. At Aunt Vinal's Helen was pampered and doted upon. Deborah, who worried that Helen was too stubborn and willful, decided to go home when Nathan found a nurse. In the spring of 1834, six months after her return, Deborah became pregnant for the last time. On Christmas 1834, a daughter, Ann Scholfield Fiske, was born. Shortly after Ann's birth the Fiskes moved to a larger cottage—Deborah's third and final home in Amherst.

The solidity of a well-furnished and comfortable home and the presence of Helen and Ann, two healthy young children, contrasted starkly with Deborah's own sense of vulnerability. Her continuing debilitation and fear of impending death convinced her that they would never realize the well-ordered household she and Nathan had planned—a home in which a mother and a father carried out the duties prescribed by their Maker. At any moment, a sudden and incapacitating attack of consumption could render her helpless and then make her children orphans. This understanding framed her relationships with her husband, her children, her physicians, and neighbors. It led her to subvert all other relationships and fulfill her maternal duties in a manner that was at once inspiring and terrifying.

6

Domestic Duties

Deborah's conviction that her daughters, Helen and Ann, would be orphans dictated her child-rearing practices. It led her to impose the most stringent standards upon herself and her daughters, which made family life intense, and ridden with crisis. Deborah was fastidious with her household servants, irritated when meals were not perfectly cooked or clothing was not washed and mended. But the standards she set for them were mild compared with those she set for her daughters. She insisted that they be extraordinarily neat, clean, obedient, and pious. Behavior was correct or incorrect, right or wrong. There were rewards for good conduct in both this life and the next and severe penalties for disobedience and impiety.

Deborah's unqualified insistence on proper comportment emanated in part from her deep religious convictions. Submission to authority was at one with submission to God. And only through spiritual resignation would one find peace and salvation. A profession of faith, she told a friend who had not yet given herself to God, "will assure to you a calmness of mind in the anticipation of sickness and other changes that nothing else can give. Thus far your barque has glided calmly and smoothly along but life is truly called a 'tempestuous sea,' and we must not expect to complete the voyage without many fogs and calms and high tides and rough winds to make the passage less pleasant than a sanguine light-hearted youth anticipates."[1]

When Deborah understood that she might not live to see her children grown, she added to this original vision an emphasis on a very tangible kind of eternal life. Deborah endured her burdens and remained cheerful by describing life after death in domestic terms—as the well-ordered family protected and guided by God in "his Home." This conception of heaven was not an exercise in maudlin sentimentality, but a deeply held conviction that enabled a young mother to bear the affliction of a fatal disease without succumbing to despair or becoming immobilized by self-pity. "The world is not our home, we are slow to believe it," she wrote Nathan, "and when those who we love are taken from us, it is to make us feel that we must follow. Let us aim at being with our little ones, a family in Heaven, and try cheerfully to do our duty and leave all results to God."[2]

The idea of a "family in heaven" was a literal one. Deborah expected her mother to be there to greet her. "Every relic of so dear a friend is precious," Deborah told Elisabeth Terry, in explaining her disappointment at never finding her mother's letters. "But more precious still is the thought that their spirits *still live*, and may be among the first to welcome us to the blessed home of the redeemed. God grant that they may not look in vain for us at the last great day."[3] When Deborah was "called," the two of them would await the arrival of the rest of the family.

It is not certain just how much Deborah's vision of eternal life was informed by the prospect of an early death, but there is no doubt of the powerful hold that the vision had on her child-rearing practices. To make certain that Helen and Ann shared her faith, even after she was gone, she made herself into a model they could emulate. "We realize but very faintly what a bearing our every day example may have upon the salvation of those about us," she told Hannah Terry.

> I often think of it in connection with my children, and fear that I shall not only fail in being a blessing to them, but be the means of their *eternal* ruin. All children, especially little children, look up to their mothers for precept and example, and whatever they see them regard as right or wrong, important or unimportant, they are apt to regard in the same way. This influence may not be manifested at once, but when they grow up the effect becomes visible in their character and opinions.[4]

Having spent so much of her childhood trying to reconstruct her own mother's character, Deborah wanted to make certain that although her daughters would not always have a mother physically present to guide them, her standards would govern their behavior.

She used her considerable skills at composition to create a person that her daughters could emulate. Her letters to her female friends and family members were intended ultimately to edify Ann and Helen. The friends were merely the temporary custodians of the letters: in accordance with Deborah's wishes, they saved all of them. After her death, Nathan collected the letters, arranged them in chronological order, bound them in wrappers and penciled the message: "To Ann and Helen: For your gratification and improvement; and I think you may hereafter derive pleasure from their perusal as well as benefit." On the packet of letters he arranged for Helen he noted: "The perusal may sometimes beguile a weary moment, and under the blessing of God may inspire you with a suitable emulation of your dear mother's many virtues. That you may be prepared to meet her among the redeemed is the constant prayer of your affectionate father."[5]

Thus, letters that may appear to be the exchanges of news between friends were really a series of carefully constructed lessons. Interspersed with family gossip was a deliberate and clearly etched portrait of a humble self-effacing Christian, whose dress, demeanor, and daily activities were meticulously recorded to define a woman's proper place and actions. The letters emphasized Deborah's determination to carry out her domestic duties and to submit to God's will. In these letters some aspects of a "hidden self" emerge, like weeds that confound the gardener's efforts to control them. One finds in Deborah's asides irritation at the demands of her husband and a delight in being pampered; one can see her anger and resentment at having her dreams shattered by a disease whose progress she and her physicians could not reverse. But taken as a whole, the letters are a series of instructions, a pedagogic exercise.[6]

Believing that she had a shorter time than other women to guide her children and desperately wanting to be united with them in heaven, Deborah was obsessed not only with their spiritual but also with their moral development. She read and reread every child-rearing book that was reviewed in the *Boston Recorder* and became piqued when the Amherst bookseller did not have them in stock within a month of publication. Among the favorites she took along to Charlestown were Lydia Child's *The Mother's Book* and John S. C. Abbott's *The Mother at Home*, both of which extolled the value of a well-ordered family. The authors shared her conservative outlook on child rearing, her narrow definition of woman's place, and her insistence that moral lessons suffuse everyday life. With days and months rather than years to impart the necessary instruction to her children, Deborah turned spontaneous interactions between mothers and children into a didactic interchange. Instead of teaching children values as situations arose, Deborah set aside time daily for moral instruction and contrived opportunities to teach. Thus, a game, a letter, a visit from friends all became grist for her moral mill, occasions to promote obedience, neatness, or piety.

This style influenced Deborah's relationship with Helen, her older daughter, in particular. Deborah was deeply attached to Helen. "If it were proper to spend much time upstairs alone," Deborah wrote to her during one of their first long separations, "I should have written to you almost every day since I left home, for everything I see that is new or pretty, and everything I hear of that would interest a little girl makes me think of you." Helen was bright, even precocious, but strong willed with a tendency to disobedience—the type of child most in need of careful instruction. "Ann does not require the vigilance Helen does," Deborah maintained. "She is honest, artless, and affectionate—telling the whole truth right out and [telling] everybody how well she loves them, while Miss Helen has no idea of 'liking all those folks' nor telling the whole of everything."[7]

Helen became the center of attention when Deborah took her to Charlestown in 1833. With aunts and cousins all amusing and pampering her, Helen turned "peevish," and Deborah could not control her. Whatever the benefits to health of remaining in Charlestown, she decided to return to Amherst. "I want to get home," she wrote Nathan. "My friends are very kind but home is the best place for me and for *Helen*. Helen has become quite *wild*, but it is not strange, she has been noticed and indulged so much."[8]

Deborah tried to keep Helen by her side and within her sight when they were at home. They read Bible stories together, and Deborah taught Helen, whose manual dexterity was not impressive, how to sew and embroider. While Deborah was proud of Helen's intellectual accomplishments, she frequently fretted that her daughter was "much more fond of her books than her needle."[9] Sewing, whether plain or fancy, was an important skill in New England. Every girl learned "plain sewing," to repair and mend the family clothing neatly; an accomplished young lady learned "fancy sewing," intricate designs to be displayed on her household linens. Sewing was also a social skill. At the Amherst sewing circle the faculty wives mended the worn garments of the "indigent and pious" college students and the worthy but poor families in the town. It was not an idle comment when Deborah told Helen: "I am very glad to hear that you have done some [needle] work, you can make something for your baby when the patch work is all sewed. You have a little cousin Deborah Vinal who sews very neatly. She says you must come and see her next winter." Indeed, sewing proficiently was even more important for a child who would become an orphan. Relatives expected children who boarded with them to take on chores—including sewing. If Helen could perform well, she would be a more welcome guest in other people's houses.[10]

Helen followed her mother's commands when Deborah was at home. But when Deborah was on one of her periodic recuperative trips to Aunt Vinal's, she would get reports that Helen was restless, fretful, and neglecting her lessons. Accordingly, Deborah stressed in her letters the penalties for disobedience. The sight of ragged children aimlessly wandering the streets of Boston and intoxicated men and women begging for alms particularly alarmed Deborah and made her even more determined to teach Helen the importance of obedience.[11] Seeing these unsupervised children and drunks as she rode through the city, Deborah, unlike reform-minded Bostonians, did not fear so much for the "future of the republic" as for the future of her children. To Deborah the social space between the vagrant children and her Helen was narrow. Families could reduce the finacial dislocations caused by the early death of a parent through a careful conservation of property, but Deborah's own experience taught her that willful character, sloppy habits, or lack of piety were no less perilous for an orphan. No sooner would Deborah return to Aunt Vinal's than she would write Helen a letter filled with cautionary tales.

These tales read like excerpts from one of the "advice to mothers" books that Deborah read rather than like the lessons that the wife of a college professor would be imparting to a five year old, who, for all her petulance, was writing the Hebrew alphabet, memorizing biblical passages, and learning history and geography. But Deborah feared that all Helen's intellectual accomplishments would prove useless—might even be detrimental—unless they were combined with a willingness to obey. "Yesterday," she wrote,

> I saw a poor woman who was so intoxicated that she could not walk, carried in a cart to the house of correction. The house of correction is a large building where people who are intemperate and lazy are shut up and made to work, and not allowed to have any rum or brandy to drink; it is very wicked to drink rum and brandy, and every little girl should learn to love *work* while very young; you must remember that you are *five* years old and that if you try, there are a great many little things you can do to be useful.[12]

The sobriety that pervaded this advice reflected her fears: the disobedient orphan might be expelled from the homes of kin and be forced to become an asylum inmate.

As Deborah watched what happened to other children whose mothers had consumption, she became more frantic. Mrs. Bent, the wife of a Congregational minister in town, was near death but had not made plans for her children. "A sister of Mrs. Bent's and her husband were here last week and took Henry with them," Deborah wrote to her cousin Martha Hooker.

> Two of the other boys have been returned to Mrs. B. because the family in which they were staying could not keep them any longer. One of them she has sent to a cousin of hers in Sunderland. But it is high time some permanent arrangement was made for the children and I have thought somebody ought to write to some of Mr. Bent's or Mrs. Bent's brothers

and sisters . . . to have them come and take the children and divide them
among them. There is *no* probability that anybody here will adopt any of
them, and it will only make the people feel like doing less for Mrs. Bent if
all her children are here and staying round in families where it is inconve-
nient to have them.

Deborah was determined to make certain that Helen and Ann would not be
in this predicament.[13]

Death was also a topic of discussion between Deborah and her daughters. Some of Deborah's cautionary tales drew on a deathbed scene. The
details differed, but the message never varied: to face death with tranquillity
required a submissive will and a humble spirit. In traditional New England
fashion, Deborah had to prepare her daughters for their own death and
more immediately for their mother's. "When death occurs in the family,
use the opportunity to make the child familiar with it," Lydia Child
advised. "Tell him, the brother or sister, or parent, the loved one is gone to
God; and that the good are far happier with the holy angels, than they
could have been on earth; and that if we are good we shall in a little while
go to them in heaven."[14] Child's advice accorded with Deborah's own vision
and was incorporated into her stories. "The other day I saw little Mary
Lothrop's mother," Deborah wrote to Helen. "She wept when Mary was
mentioned to think how much and how patiently she suffered and that she
would never see her again in this world. Little Mary's papa is very sick, his
physician thinks he cannot live but a short time. He is willing to die for he
loves the Saviour very much and is happy when he thinks of going to
heaven to live with him and little Mary."[15]

Deborah also made certain that the magazines Helen read contained the
same morals. When she was five, Helen received a subscription from Aunt
Vinal for the *Youth's Companion*, the children's supplement to the *Boston
Recorder*. In every issue there was at least one obituary notice of a child,
which described the circumstances of death, recounted the piety of the
family and the child, and emphasized the need for even small children to
prepare for death by professing their faith. As Deborah became more concerned that Helen might not fully understand the importance of these messages, she became even more ingenious at providing moral instruction.
Deborah secretly wrote and submitted articles to *Youth's Companion*. Written under a pseudonym, they were similar in style and content to those of
the other contributors. Their distinguishing feature was their central protagonist: a nine-year-old girl (just Helen's age) who could not sit still during Bible lessons, who interrupted with irrelevant questions, and who was
sloppily dressed when visitors arrived, her hair in a tangle and her sleeves
torn. In these stories, the fictionalized Helen, like her real-life counterpart,

had not yet fully comprehended the importance of the lessons her mother so patiently impressed upon her.

The intensity of Deborah's efforts all pointed to the same goal. Whatever else happened, Helen had to be a welcome guest in other people's homes. Deborah did not doubt that her aunt and cousins would provide a place for her daughter, but she also knew they would not tolerate Helen's willfulness for very long. To remain in their homes, Helen would have to respect their authority and not contradict their wishes.

In 1835 Nathan decided to take Helen with him on a trip to Boston; Helen was to remain with Aunt Vinal while he preached in the nearby towns. Deborah, remembering all too clearly Helen's disastrous visit two years earlier, saw this stay as a pedagogic opportunity. In her talks to Helen before she left and in the frequent letters she wrote, Deborah stressed the necessity of obeying her aunt. "*Be very obedient and pleasant and obliging wherever you go.* It will make me very happy if Papa can write that Helen is a good girl and making her friends no unnecessary trouble." Since she knew just how hard the assignment was for Helen, she reminded her that the willfulness she demonstrated in her own home would not be tolerated by relatives. "I hope you are very happy among your kind friends, and that you try everyday to make them as little trouble as possible. Remember that it is a great deal for them to put you to bed every night and help dress you every morning and prepare your food and answer your questions. . . .You can do many things *at the time to repay* their attentions. You can dust chairs, and take the lamps down from the chambers, and carry away dishes, and several other things." Deborah knew from her own childhood that it was even more important *not* to have annoying habits. "There are some things you must be careful to avoid doing, and I shall print them on separate lines that you may notice every one.

Never talk when others present are speaking.
Never occupy the rocking chair or the easiest chair in a room when any
     older person is present.
Never turn your head away in silence when anyone asks you a question.
Never speak of hating things or people.
Never say you do not love that is placed before you.
Never eat after all at the table are done but yourself.
Never get down upon the floor.
Never leave chairs out of place or push them up against the paper and
     paint when you set them away."[16]

Deborah turned the visit into a trial run for Helen, having her learn in advance the lessons she would need later on.

Deborah worried less about Ann, for her younger daughter seemed as compliant and obedient as Helen was restless and independent. Ann would sit patiently beside her mother. "Ann has just trotted up to my elbow and tells me to tell cousin Ellen that she hopes she will get well very soon," Deborah wrote to her cousin. "Ann often says mornings, 'I do wish Ma I could cough for you,' and as she cannot do that, she makes it up by bringing shawls or nightclothes or something to throw over me till I stop."[17] Deborah's disease so dominated family life that Ann, while still a toddler, already understood its portent for her own future. "My Ann's wish very often expressed, that my cough and hoarse voice were things she could take in her hands and carry off and bury up in the ground so *deep* they could *never* get out."[18]

Deborah also imparted to Helen and Ann a very conventional definition of a woman's proper place drawn from her seminary education, her orphaned childhood, her rigid religious creed, and her own invalidism. Deborah taught them that women had been given by nature and religion a very special, albeit subordinate, status. It was proper for women to leave the home to form benevolent societies, to uplift the children of the poor, and to give moral and religious instruction to intemperate men and women. But these activities were not to cross over into the male sphere. "Isn't it really sickening to think of these *female* anti slavery societies, *female* petitions to congress and *female* lecturers," Deborah wrote a friend. "Some editor in speaking of such ladies called them our 'female *brethren*' a very good title for them when they exchange their slippers for gentlemen's boots."[19]

Even a woman as traditional as Deborah occasionally longed to break out in new ways. She had a literary bent, and whenever her disease was in remission and she felt stronger, she fantasized about writing a book, albeit a very domestic one. Her primary audience would be invalid women who were frustrated as she was at being too enfeebled to run an efficient household. "I have some hope of making discoveries," she told Ellen Scholfield, "that will be of great advantage to housekeepers and invalids. I will not specify them here but if you see a work advertised with the title, 'good news to hard workers,' you may *suspect* that you know the author, and I advise you to buy a copy, but the worst of it is, good news of this sort I fear will come too late to do us much good."

On occasion Deborah even expressed annoyance at the constraints domesticity placed on her life. "I feel as if I must *run* to keep up with the house," she complained to Martha Hooker,

and yet what do I accomplish? . . . It does make me feel dreadfully sometimes to see and think how . . . *my life* is slipping away and I am doing nothing but taking care of my family. I know this is my *proper business*, but then, some do so much *good besides.* Sometimes I think I will try to write something for the benefit of *little* children in the *Youth's Companion* and make a business of it. . . . This world is full of misery, I do nothing to alleviate and of sin I do nothing to check.[20]

Her friends and husband knew nothing of Deborah's pseudonymous contributions to *Youth's Companion*, which, to her surprise and delight, Nathaniel Willis, its editor, published. When her cousin Martha Hooker learned through her husband that Deborah had sent the stories, she confronted her and Deborah reluctantly confessed. "The truth is just this. I have never been in the habit of writing anything but familiar letters about family matters or nothing at all and it is all I am fit for. Since I have seen how much can be written to please and do good to children I have regretted that somebody did not teach me how before I had become too old to learn, for I have time that I might just as well as not spend in this way if I only could write anything useful and attractive." She also justified her writing as necessary for Helen's instruction. "I think sometimes I might just as well catch a blue jay and lecture it as to talk to my Helen. Before I can get the last word out of a most pathetic exhortation she will be hopping off to the window upon one foot asking as she hops away if I will let her go out now in the new building to have a real frolic."[21]

It was Deborah's father's generosity that allowed her to do all that she did. A bevy of domestics made it possible for Deborah to remain at home, visit friends, attend sewing circles and prayer meetings, and even write articles. When Ann was born in 1834, Deborah had an inflammation of the lungs. To keep the household running, she employed two domestics and a nurse. "I have only *three* to help me," she reported. "My little girl goes to school and helps mornings and evenings—Miss Leonard, my nurse, sews and knits and bakes and washes, and Maria, the large girl does the remainder. And I 'see to things' and 'putter about' as Aunt Vinal calls it."[22]

Deborah supplied room and board for any single female relative who would help out. Nathan's unmarried sister, Maria, came during crises, and a cousin Jane could be cajoled into service. If a hitherto unknown relative turned up, Deborah also accepted her assistance. "Mr. Fiske has a maiden cousin about fifty years old," she informed Martha Hooker, "a Miss Stearns who is visiting me this term; she has no real home and stays around among friends and assists them. She is making up all the patch work and doing all the plain sewing I can muster. It is very fortunate for such a slim woman as I am to have sewing company." Deborah knew well that the situation of these single women enabled her to keep her household running. "I really think *useful* single people may be called the salt of the earth," she mused. "What would become of us if everybody was married? I am sure all the invalid wives would soon be sold for rags." And

Deborah for all her burdens did not want to change places with these women. "I think single ladies are more to be pitied for their loneliness in going about from place to place than those who are married for their cares and domestic perplexities."[23]

Deborah had a pecking order in hiring domestic help. Her first choice was white Protestant women; her second young black girls; and lowest on her list were the Irish. Over the course of her illness she descended the ladder. Sharing the biases of her generation, she thought the Irish were ignorant and lazy; worse yet, they were Catholic. "I have a prejudice against the Irish," she readily confessed, that "makes it impossible for me to place *much* confidence in any of them." Even when the women worked hard, Deborah was not pleased. One woman was "affectionate and kind, *apparently* willing to work in the kitchen, and not *aspiring* to anything else, neater than most domestics, a good cook in many respects, and gets done in the course of the week all I want her to do." But Deborah complained about her temper. She was "*very passionate*, but when the explosion is over she is 'so sorry and so mortified that she should *spoke* so to such a good mistress,' that we make right up and are as good as pie."[24]

Deborah frequently had to turn to family and friends to help her engage suitable domestics. "I must find some help, or keep house alone, or quit and *board out*, which *end* I hope not to come to at present," she frantically wrote to her cousin Martha Hooker. "Tho' my health is so feeble I am wholly unfit for taking care of children and doing housework in addition. Can you find me a girl in Lanesboro? I will give more wages than she could get there if that would be an inducement." When these strategies did not work she asked her father to go to the office of the *Intelligence*, where the unemployed Irish immigrants waited for prospective employment, and find "a girl" who was willing not only "to sweep, do chamber work, sew some, and wait on me if I need it," but also to live in Amherst. The fact that he always located "a girl" is indicative of how few options these immigrant women had.[25]

On one occasion Deborah accompanied her father to the employment office. The sight of ragged, unemployed women begging for work disturbed her.

Such an assembly I never saw together, old and young, from ten years of age to fifty. The office is rather a large room, in the middle sits a judge-like looking old gentleman with a book, pen, and ink at a table to record the names of the applicants, and there were two rows of benches all round the room, on these benches, round the door and in the passageway were as many as fifty girls and women, some of them trying to get your attention by every possible way, and others sitting looking like firm believers in *fate*, independent of any personal exertion. I walked all round studying every face and forehead, and then went back to a girl in the passageway whose countenance pleased me as I went in. There was such a crowd and so much chattering I could not talk much with her, but she promised to call and see me this afternoon. The rain may prevent her, and she may not choose to come, but I was quite taken with her looks.[26]

But picking a woman from on the basis of her look was a long way from carefully selecting a domestic from a poor but pious, farming family in Amherst. Here as elsewhere, illness forced Deborah to make compromises that healthy women in similar economic circumstances avoided.

As Deborah's illness progressed, even these compromises were not enough. In 1841, when another acute attack debilitated her further, Deborah knew that she would have to "quit" housekeeping at least until some semblance of strength returned. She sent Ann, now age seven, to board with Miss Nelson, a neighbor and schoolteacher, and Helen, now age eleven, to board with Deacon Dickinson in South Hadley. Deborah still fretted about Helen's habits and made this occasion for reinforcing the need for obedience. "Now you are *Miss* Helen Fiske," she wrote shortly after Helen left home, "*boarding out* in Hadley, you will speak when you are spoken to, and write when you are written to, or else you will prove yourself quite below your station and honors." Instead of lists of rules, Deborah used the device of a dream to remind her daughter of the importance of good habits. Deborah told Helen she had dreamed about her for two nights.

> The dreams were too indistinct to be worth telling but I will tell you what they were *not*. I did *not* dream that any of your things were out of place, nor that your cape and collar and ruffle were put away to work themselves if they would, nor that your hair looked as if it had been out in a hurricane . . . nor that your finger nails had all been dipped in the ink bottle. *None* of these things have I *dreamed* . . . for I have great confidence that *you* will take my place in the care of Helen Maria Fiske, and see that she does all the things that I have been in the habit of doing for her, or reminding her of doing; see that you will fill the office well, for she is a little girl I love dearly, and would not have her spoiled or neglected for all your scoured money and a dollar bill besides.[27]

The abiding concern that Deborah displayed for her daughters' welfare did not mark her relationship to Nathan. Their marriage was filled with frustration, disappointment, anger, and remorse. As with any unhappy marriage, the causes for dissatisfaction were numerous. Deborah's preoccupation with her health and her periodic absences strained the relationship. She was physically incapable of fulfilling the needs of the household in general and those of her husband in particular, which disturbed her. But at the same time, Deborah chafed at gender responsiblities and was not above using illness as a pretext for avoiding them. She paid obeisance to female submission, but she had ambitions, literary and social, that competed with it. And she was ultimately disappointed in Nathan. For all his religious and educational commitments, which she truly admired, he was not the man her father was. In 1835, after Ann was born, Deborah and Nathan began to lead separate lives in the same household. Deborah tried to meet her domestic obligations, but her illness often left her too weak and prompted her periodically to visit with Aunt Vinal; Nathan was left to manage the household along with his professional obligations. The correspondence between them reveals the darker and far more troubled part of Deborah's invalid life. These were the very letters that she had intended not be preserved.[28]

In 1836, when Helen was five and Ann two, Deborah went to Charlestown for a recuperative visit, and all the strains that the disease had placed on the marriage erupted. Nathan had to supervise the three domestics and oversee the care of the children. Knowing that the assignment was difficult and accepting that child care was her responsibility, not his, Deborah was apprehensive and somewhat apologetic even before she left home. "*Be sure* to write often," she asked him as soon as she arrived at Aunt Vinal's, "and if the children are sick, don't hesitate to let me know the *whole* truth. Nothing can be more trying than the apprehension of being deceived, or kept in ignorance about the family."[29]

Within a week of Deborah's departure, Helen, whose behavior was always the barometer for reading the level of stress within the family, missed her mother and expressed it by disobeying the domestics and refusing to carry out the assignments Deborah had left behind. To try to bridge the separation and reduce her loneliness, Helen dictated a letter to Nathan, who sent it off to Deborah. "Tell Ma I have begun to read Joshua today and have redeemed a number of my books and that I want to see her so much I sometimes get almost ready to cry." Helen did have a few good deeds to describe, and some evidence that she had been "a good girl," but the centerpiece of her letter was a report on how naughty her sister had been. She "was noisy tonight at supper and got hold of Ma's Bible and tore out two leaves—she [Ma] won't feel so bad, if she knows who did it."[30] Nathan's own news was no more comforting. Although Deborah had meticulously tried to organize the household in advance, the arrangements unraveled soon after her departure and the children had become unruly. "As to [Helen's] sewing," he reported, "there seems to be some difficulty in the matter; it does not get on very well; and my time has been so much occupied, or rather broken into pieces, that I have been able to give but little attention to her reading. The Latin all vanished the third day; however, I only took it up to amuse or rather employ her while she was so mopish that I thought it best to keep her in the study rather than leave her below." Even Ann, who was generally placid, had became "exceedingly tyrannical," and he warned Deborah: "Unless you buy or borrow a new stock of decision and independence you may calculate on being a slave on your return."[31]

Nathan's report heightened Deborah's anxiety and her guilt. In fact, there was really no news that did not upset her. If Nathan wrote that the children were misbehaving, she became peevish; if he did not tell her about the children at all, she became apprehensive. If he informed her that the help was discontented and that he spent hours trying to keep the relatives who had been pressed into household service from going home, she began to doubt that she would ever have enough strength to return and resume her responsibilities.

Deborah was thus caught between these intense and conflicting emotions. "I feel perplexed whenever I think of home," she told Nathan. "I am in a strait betwixt half a dozen, whenever I think of the children. I want to see them, and yet fear the care of them and want to keep house again and yet know I have no strength for anything. I feel the worse for any exercise that is fatiguing, still I am as well as I could expect to be so soon after such a prostrating sickness."[32] Out of frustration, Deborah would criticize Nathan for not empathizing more fully with her or managing more adeptly. "How can *I* step into the perplexities that *you* with all your philosophy and firmness can hardly bear. You know when I am at home, I have the place that you occupy in my absence." Not only would she have to placate and motivate the help ("see all Jane's downcast looks, Aroline's maneuverings and listen to all cousin Sarah's lamentations as you do now"), but to oversee the cooking. "This I dare say you think need not be anything, but it comes three times a day and you know if anything is burnt or smoked or not half-done, how badly you feel and how badly I feel." Daunted by the prospect of managing the household in her invalid state, Deborah warned Nathan that if he did not untangle the "snarl," the family might have to board out. "I hate to think of breaking up housekeeping, it makes so much work and is attended with so much inconvenience of every sort." She asked him to try to negotiate among the help. "If Jane can be induced to stay till after Commencement I think I have reason to hope that by that time I may be able to take my place again."[33]

Nathan, unable to control the domestics, decided to send Ann to board with a neighbor, Mrs. Parsons. When he told Deborah that Ann was thriving, it raised her doubts about her own competence as a mother. "I am not surprised that Ann does so well," she responded. "I have always noticed that Mrs. Parsons has perfect control over her children; we had better let her take Helen I think. I have no talent of this sort either natural or

acquired and it sometimes seems mysterious that when there is nothing in
the world that I can not do better this should have been my employment."
Deborah then reproached herself for undertaking marriage and child rearing, certain that her children would have fared better with a mother who
had the wherewithal to be firm and consistent. "I feel that I have wasted
my time and ruined my health in a fruitless attempt to perform the duties
of a wife and mother. As much as I love Ann and wish to see her I shall
almost dread to take her home for fear she will be sick or grow ugly in my
hands."[34]

With Ann settled with the neighbors, Nathan had more time to spend
on his translations and was enjoying a kind of bachelor status, which Deborah interpreted as evidence of the extent to which her illness had thwarted
his ambitions.

> I was glad to learn . . . that you are having so good a chance to study and
> enjoy it so much, it is the best opportunity you have had this long while.
> Cousin Sarah *almost wept* to think you should be so glad to be alone, but
> Maria said if anybody cried it ought to be me because I must go back to
> break up your enjoyment of solitude. . . . I presume you will get a huge
> pile of volumes upon Moral and Intellectual philosophy and be married
> to them before my return, and I give my cheerful consent.

She concluded her letter on a note of eceptional ambivalence. "But no tears
will find their way upon my face, for this I can assure you I am enjoying as
much as most people [being] independent of you, and I am glad to have you
happy independent of me."[35]

For all her self-abnegation and misgivings, Deborah, in fact, was rel-
ishing her visit to Aunt Vinal. At the center of attention, her every whim
was satisfied. "You have no occasion to be anxious about my situation,"
she wrote to Nathan. "I have the best of care in the family, the best of
medical advice, the opportunity to ride as much as I please, due to the
kindest of fathers with nothing to do but anticipate and supply every
want." At Aunt Vinal's as at home, Deborah remained fettered to her
invalidism. On many days she was too weak to leave the house, and
throughout the visit, she consulted physicians. But when she had some
strength, she would spend the day riding about in an open carriage and
visiting friends. In the course of a week she might make calls in Boston,
Cambridge, Roxbury, and Newton. Her cousin Martha Hooker came up
from Falmouth, and the two of them spent an afternoon shopping for
shawls and gifts. Visiting with childhood friends and being catered to by
her aunt and her father made Deborah want to remain longer within this
protective environment. Ascribing her own wishes to her father, she
wrote Nathan: "I would however *jump* at the chance of living in Boston or

very near Boston, so as to be near my father *where he can be happy*. It is so dull for him in Amherst that he cannot endure it. Boston is the place for a man of his habits and tastes, he seems very cheerful for him, and don't like to hear me say anything about going back."[36] She even contrasted her father's generosity to Nathan's meager salary, reminding her husband that she was "so miserably calculated to live upon a small income." Perhaps a more successful provider would have found a way to earn a living in Boston, so that Deborah could have had the ministrations of family and friends far more often.[37]

Having remained at Aunt Vinal's as long as a respectable mother and wife could, she was overcome by sadness as she prepared to return to Amherst. "I have enjoyed every hour of my visit and think being entirely free from care has been of decided advantage to my health. Were it not for remembering you and Helen and little Ann, it would not seem as if I were married. I've seen a great many old friends and so forcibly reminded of many pleasant scenes that I passed through more than *seven* years *ago* that it seems as if they occurred but *yesterday*."[38] The reminiscences of her childhood also reminded Deborah that although she was only thirty, she felt ages older as she confronted an early death. "I can hardly believe myself to be the same person that I was ten years ago," she confessed to Nathan. "In short, my sun has set and the rest of the way through this vale of tears, I expect to grope through thick darkness. My harp is hung upon the willows and will never be taken down but to play. I would not live always but I ask not to stay where storm after storm rises dark over my way." But the choice was not hers. "I know God can prolong my life just as long as He pleases, and will, as long as He has anything for me to do."[39]

From October 1836 until she died in February 1844, Deborah and Nathan lived in their own demarcated spaces, coping separately with the trials of chronic illness and their own disappointments. Nathan occupied a peripheral place in the household. He remained most of the day in his study, and when he entered the family circle at formal moments of meals and prayers, added a gloomy and somber note that reflected his recurring fear that the death of his two infant sons and Deborah's illness were "messages from God," signs of "divine displeasure."[40] His diary entries pleaded: "Oh most merciful God, let not the disease which thy wisdom has brought upon her be suffered to fix its seat upon her vitals. In thy hands are all the springs of life. Bless the means for her recovery and graciously spare her to me and this family, to her lonely father and her friends."[41]

Deborah dominated the sitting room and maintained a demeanor of calculated cheerfulness. From this position, she instructed the children, supervised the washing, ironing, and cleaning, hosted the sewing circle, and chatted with visitors. Her vision of a domestic reunion in heaven comforted her. "Let us aim at being with our little ones," she reminded Nathan and herself, "a family in Heaven, and try cheerfully to do our duty and leave all results to God." Nevertheless, the situation at home continued to deteriorate. As Deborah's disease became more incapacitating, Nathan began to evince the symptoms that marked the first stage of consumption. Deborah's long-standing anxieties about her children's future deepened.[42]

7

Deborah and Her Doctors

Over the course of her illness, Deborah, like many other educated New England invalid women, had a regular relationship with a number of physicians. Although she relied on doctors in Amherst to prescribe remedies for a cough or pain, her most important associations were with physicians in Boston. She wrote to them regularly, describing her ailments in cogent detail, requesting both specific medications to relieve one or another complaint and general advice on how to pursue a cure. Her frequent trips to Boston to stay with Aunt Vinal also afforded opportunities for consultations and examinations with them. But as important as the physicians were, Deborah was also part of circle of female invalids who compared their symptoms and discussed the advice and prescriptions they received from their doctors. They even went so far as to read medical textbooks, pooling their knowledge so as to understand their illness better. Thus, Deborah, like many of her friends, was a wary and sophisticated consumer of medicine, questioning her doctors, changing them when she was dissatisfied with her own progress or their answers, and adapting their recommendations to her own circumstances.

The relationship between women invalids with consumption and their physicians, as they described it in their letters, was a fluid and negotiated one. On the one hand, the women sought advice and relief; on the other, they were unwilling to allow medical regimens to override social and religious values. These negotiations produced a reciprocal relationship in which physicians modified their prescriptions to fit with and reenforce women's social and domestic duties. Moreover, there appeared to be an empathy between the women and their doctors. The physicians were acutely aware of the women's preferences—that the invalids wanted to remain with their children and placed domestic duties above any particular

curative regimen. Medical advice and medical prescriptions became subservient to social and religious duties.[1]

Deborah's attitudes towards her physicians over the fifteen years of her
illness changed as her symptoms and her personal circumstances changed.
The balance that was struck in the first stages of her disease altered as her
illness became chronic and then again as it became terminal. Her first and
perhaps most important association was with Dr. John Collins Warren. Her
father had first engaged him to treat Deborah during her childhood, and
she continued to consult him even after she moved to Amherst. Thus, when
her "old complaints" left her weak and enervated immediately following
the death of her infant son in 1829, she solicited Dr. Warren's advice and
counsel. Too weak to travel to Boston and confident that he knew her constitution thoroughly, she anticipated that he would be able to dispense
appropriate medications and guidance on the basis of a verbal report. She
wrote to her father asking him to serve as intermediary, for Dr. Warren
"can tell much better than any other physician what is best for me, and Mr.
Fiske is desirous that I should be doing something for my lungs."[2]

Anticipating that her father would be "alarmed" both at the "sight of my
penmanship" and at her request that he consult Dr. Warren, Deborah
assured him that despite her fatigue and cough, her lungs were "much less
affected than they have been many times, but still there is some irritation
that it would be well to attend to in season." She carefully set down her
symptoms and outlined her routine: "What I wish to have Dr. Warren
know, is the time of my confinement . . . about ten days after, I took a cold
in my head and had a sore throat with it, and since that cold left me I have
been troubled with hoarseness morning and evening and a *slight* difficulty
of breathing. It sometimes occasions an inclination to cough, but I can generally suppress it without much effort." She went on to report that her
appetite was good and her diet simple—wheat breads, apples, coffee, boiled
rice, and a little beef. She also wanted her father to tell the doctor that "I
ride out; and have walked out since I last wrote but only a short distance."
Also "I have a good deal of milk . . . and I wish to know Dr. Warren's opinion about the length of time I must keep it." She asked her father to consult
Dr. Warren immediately and if he did not have the time, to have Aunt
Vinal do it. She expected a prescription for "bark or something to
strengthen me faster as I gain strength, slowly." And she directed the
courier with whom she sent the letter to await a return letter (containing
Dr. Warren's responses) and a package (of his medications).[3]

The confidence that marked Deborah's posture toward Dr. Warren, her
very ability to pen a phrase like "what I wish to have Dr. Warren know,"
reflected not merely the fact that she had seen him over many years but also
her expectation that he would always tailor his prescriptions to her domes-

tic and religious commitments—she was determined that illness not subvert them. Indeed, both of them had no problem in elevating social duty over medical knowledge even if it might shorten her life.

One of the most salient examples of this ranking of values concerned the advisability of pregnancy for women with possible consumption or with consumption itself. Physicians in this era believed that repeated pregnancies were dangerous for those with the disease. During the pregnancy itself, the woman might appear to be free of symptoms or even experience some improvement. As Dr. James Thacher explained in a widely read medical text: "When women are affected with consumptive complaints previous to a state of pregnancy, the symptoms are generally suspended, or so disguised during that period, that both the patient and friends are unconscious of any impending danger." But soon after delivery, the symptoms reemerged with a new tenacity. Or as Dr. Thacher put it: "Shortly after parturition, the disease resumes a more rapid progress, and soon terminates in death."[4] This knowledge accepted, neither Dr. Warren in particular nor other physicians more generally counseled female patients to avoid pregnancies. Bearing children was a woman's duty, and medicine had no business in abrogating it. Thus, when Deborah became pregnant, as she did four times, she was not contravening doctor's advice or acting out of ignorance. After all, her own mother had died not very long after giving birth to her, and a number of her consumptive neighbors had died in the aftermath of delivery. Rather, Deborah made calculated choices, and her physicians did not challenge them.[5]

Deborah's daily regimen affords yet another example of how medical advice was made to conform to domestic duty. Unlike male invalids of her social class and background, Deborah did not undertake a long voyage for health; instead, throughout her adult life she took her cure at home. She scheduled her outdoor exercise around her domestic chores and joined it whenever possible to other social and religious duties; thus, she rode on horseback to visit friends or to make calls. As one might expect, the daily obligation to exercise became oppressive, and Deborah often found excuses to put it off. "A violent wind prevents me from taking a good ride on horseback this afternoon," she let Martha Hooker know, "so I treat myself with a call upon you to make up for the privation."[6]

As Deborah's symptoms became more severe, she started to question the accuracy of Dr. Warren's opinions even as she continued to consult him. In 1833, after Humphrey's death, she went to Aunt Vinal's to recuperate and immediately went to Dr. Warren for a consultation. Although Dr. Warren made "his inquiries and prohibitions and prescriptions," as she wrote Nathan, he was not "alarmed." But this time, Deborah did not find his words of comfort convincing. Her strength depleted from months of coughs and fevers and her spirits depressed by the death of her child, she frankly did not believe him when he told her, "You have some fever brought on by a cold but I think with careful treatment it will be thrown off in a day of two." She dutifully took the prescribed medications (mostly opiates) and was grateful for a comfortable night's sleep. But in the morning she still had her hacking cough and pains in her shoulder and chest. As she told Nathan, for all Dr. Warren's optimism, she was convinced that she would "always be a burden for someone to carry."[7]

This skepticism notwithstanding, she continued to consult Dr. Warren over the course of her stay in Charlestown. Each time he reported that her lungs were free of disease, and each time Deborah complained to Nathan that she was not getting any better, that the pains in the side could only be partially relieved by the application of blisters, the cough was so deep that it caused aches in her shoulders, and was so persistent that it prevented her "from doing scarcely any work." As the weeks passed, she became the more convinced of the gravity of her condition. "It is best you should know the truth," she told Nathan, "and that neither myself or friends should be cherishing sanguine hopes of my recovery—there is *no danger* in *this;* but in the opposite delusion there is."[8]

Before making a final decision to return to Amherst in the fall of 1833, Deborah had a consultation with Dr. Warren. She told him that she preferred to go back to Amherst; the Boston climate was not helping, and, besides, Helen, her three-year-old daughter, had become almost impossible to control. Dr. Warren went along with her sentiments, telling her that in September the climate in Amherst was as beneficial as Boston's and that her distress over Helen might be delaying her recovery. The only thing he did insist upon was that she arrange to have adequate domestic help.

Although Deborah stated her preference clearly and firmly to Dr. Warren, one cannot help but wonder whether he agreed too readily. Nowhere in the many letters that Deborah wrote is there any mention of Dr. Warren, or any other physician for that matter, telling her to travel for health, to go South immediately, to take a voyage that might well represent her one chance at life. The advice that physicians delivered to male invalids, often as a command, was not offered to their female patients. Not that physicians prohibited women from traveling for health, but women had to take the initiative. If they did not, physicians did not raise or encourage it. To be sure, it is by no means apparent that Deborah would have complied with an order to go South. As someone who had read medical textbooks, she undoubtedly knew that travel for health was the recommended intervention; but her eagerness to keep her children within the familial and community net (as befit her overwhelming concern for their future as orphans and her determination to guide them to profess their faith to ensure a heavenly reunion) more than outweighed this prospect. In Debo-

rah's value system, religious conviction took precedence over medical prescription.

Deborah's return to Amherst in 1833 ushered in a new stage in her illness, in her relationships with doctors, and in her relationship to other
invalids. Her primary concerns now had less to do with the prospect of a
cure and more with relief of pain, and still more particularly, in knowing
just how long she had to live.

Following professional prescriptions, Deborah often took opium to
relieve her racking coughs and had frequent recourse to leeches, blisters,
and poultices to purge the inflammations. Given the duration and the
severity of her symptoms, she learned to apply these treatments herself, to
the point of raising her own leeches. She became so skilled in all these tasks
as to become the butt of family humor. "And to everybody about home,"
Deborah wrote Ann Scholfield, her cousin and fellow invalid, "Mr. Fiske
always says, 'You had better look out for my wife skins people alive.' And if
my father is present he begins to rub one of his limbs and adds, 'You had
better not let her spread any blisters or make any mustard poultices for
you.' And since these external applications being my chief hobbies, my
chance for playing the physician is all up."[9]

In fact, Deborah and her circle of invalid friends came very close to playing physician, sharing with each other information about remedies for pain.
Their descriptions were at once intimate and specific, going well beyond
casual gossip to a level of explicit and precise physiological and medical
detail that only an invalid searching for guidance, or a doctor, would want
to know. "I am very desirous of hearing whether you are benefitted by Dr.
Gregerson's prescriptions," she wrote Ann Scholfield, who was then suffering a bout of extreme pain. "Your disease is one which I don't pretend to
understand so you will escape any old woman 'certain cures,' but I have had
it myself, as some spleeny invalids always declare if you describe to them
fifty diseases. But seriously, two or three years ago I used to have very
severe attacks of what Dr. Gridley called a *neuralgic affection*, it was generally in my left side, and always came on *suddenly* and while it lasted it was
next to impossible for me to draw a long breath. How unlike this was to the
searing pain in your limbs, but perhaps there is just this difference between
neuralgia and neuralgic *affection*." The aim of the communication was thoroughly practical. As Deborah told Ann: "All these medical technicals are
like so much Greek to me, and I am willing they should remain so unless I
could make such knowledge a means of relief to somebody."[10]

Deborah self-consciously solicited this level of information. "Do write to
me very soon and be particular in telling me about your health," she told
one of her friends. "I have felt encouraged that you were getting better
from Martha's letters. She wrote that you said you were growing fleshy; and
I thought that a good symptom, tell me exactly how well you are, what you

are able to do etc. etc." In the course of correspondence, these women invalids were informing each other about the prognosis that came with symptoms so that they would each know what to expect next. "I was surprised to hear that your *lungs* were troublesome," Deborah wrote to Martha Hooker. "It was something so new for you. If you could not take a long breath you have learned how to pity me." And she then informed Martha that "my health has been remarkably good this winter, the release I had from all the care in my visit to Boston in the autumn was of great advantage to me. I have not had *but one* attack of that difficulty in breathing and spasmodic pain in my left side this winter and that was brought on by fatigue, the first time we were left without help. It yielded readily to a blister and since then I have been able to go out and work at home."[11]

Deborah was perfectly comfortable offering medical advice to friends. Moreover she was not afraid to contradict physicians' findings. These interchanges demonstrate that the women were not passive or unwilling to confront their physicians; their considerable knowledge about the disease gave them the confidence to question a diagnosis or a prognosis. "I can hardly *believe* that Ellen is so comfortable," Deborah volunteered to Ann Scholfield. "Is it not possible that her *lungs* are not really diseased and that her physicians have been mistaken? Perhaps she has had what I have been told is my difficulty, the *chronic bronchitis*—some sort of obstruction or inflammation in the passages that lead to the lobes of the lungs. This may be cured, and should this prove to be the cause of Ellen's feeble health and be removed, many will rejoice beside herself, I am sure I shall most heartily."[12]

These women resolutely tried to comprehend the origins and course of their disease even if it required "delving into things" and trespassing in the physicians' domain. The women accepted formal medical learning and were not attracted to alternative therapies (whether in the form of folk medicine or water cures). What troubled them most was the uncertainty inherent in having such a capricious and unpredictable illness. "I am a firm believer in the opinion discarded by many, that lung diseases are curable," Mary Bennett wrote to Deborah.

It is stated by the *Boston Medical Journal* that cases have occurred in this vicinity of persons who have exhibited strong marks of consumption, who have recovered and after the lapse of years have died of some other disease and on a postmortem examination the scars discernable upon the lungs, showed that tubercles of a large size once existed there and which, owing to some cause, were happily removed. Probably such cases are not very common. But enough have transpired that none need despair but [too] few that none ought to presume [a cure]. But the impression which is sometimes received that it is incurable may in some instances render it more difficult of cure.

And Mary also reminded Deborah: "I was reading the other day in B. B. Edwards book of self-taught men the account of R. Baxter, who though attacked at the early age of sixteen with cough, spitting blood, lived to the advanced age of seventy-five. His oft repeated sicknesses quickened him in being good and doing good. Most of his writings were penned under the impression that he was about to die. Would that all similarly afflicted might be thus benefitted."[13]

Deborah shared their frustrations and fervently wished to understand her illness in material terms. "We are indeed a complicated piece of mechanism," she wrote to Ann Scholfield. "And I sometimes think physicians might as well prescribe for watches that are out of order by looking at them, feeling of them, and harking to their ticking, as to prescribe for us without *seeing* the parts that are diseased." Would that she had a magical device that would enable her to peer inside the body. "It is a foolish wish because a vain one, but I *do* wish I could take a peep into Adeline's windpipe, Ellen's lungs and mine, and your *joints* that *ache*. But what good would it do? Like a thousand other gratified wishes, the result would bring nothing but vexation. The *pain* I shouldn't find in your poor knees. No dust that would explain Adeline's wheezing, nor apple cores or bits of flannel that would account for my cough or Ellen's."[14]

The very prevalence of consumption made for a large circle of invalid correspondents. Four out of the five cousins with whom Deborah kept in close contact had the disease. Although pulmonary consumption was the most common form, some women suffered from spinal tuberculosis, which was often manifested by rheumatic aches and pains, while others had tuberculosis of the bone, liver, or kidney. None of these differences were lost on the correspondents. "Cousin Ellen you will wish to hear," Deborah informed Martha Hooker,

> went out to Newtown to board last Thursday. Ann went with her for company and [to] nurse but Ann herself is very unwell, suffering more than she has done this long while with neuralgia. It is now in her arms as well as other limbs. Her anxiety for Ellen is so great that it is evidently making her sick, and some of Ellen's symptoms are alarming and *some* of them are better, and I cannot help hoping that she may be comfortable again. These pulmonary invalids come to life again so many times.[15]

The women's letters often offered both medical information and psychological support, an exchange not only of symptoms but also of anxieties. "You may have heard of the dangerous illness with which I was attacked three weeks after your husband was here," Mary Bennett informed Deborah.

> The day previous I was out on a begging excursion for Mt. Holyoke [and] felt no unusual fatigue on account of my walk, but after sleeping well dur-

ing the night, [I] began at an early hour in the morning to expectorate blood quite freely for six days. Then it ceased and I have since been rapidly gaining to the surprise of my friends and physicians and am now quite comfortable though feeble. [I] have been able to attend Church four and a half days and to assume my labors in the Sabbath school. . . . My health has been so precarious of late that it seems as if one foot stood upon life, the other upon death.

Mary then assured Deborah that she was prepared to die. "Of one thing there is a certainty that I am in the hands of Him who does all things well and knows infinitely better than his short sighted creatures what is best for them."[16]

As Deborah's symptoms grew more severe and as her own knowledge of consumption increased, she became even less deferential to the opinions of physicians. As her disease entered its final, terminal stage, her letters cast doubt on a second widely held assumption about physician-patient relationships—the physician's apparent reluctance to tell patients the truth. It has been assumed that physicians in the nineteenth century carried so inflated a sense of wisdom and authority that they unilaterally chose to withhold from their patients a grim diagnosis, preferring instead to act in what they presumed to be the patient's best interest. The statements of Dr. Oliver Wendell Holmes become the case in point. Historians frequently quote his address to the graduating class of Bellevue Medical School in 1871: "Your patient has no more right to all the truth you know," Dr. Holmes informed them, "than he has to all the medicine in your saddlebags. . . . He should get only just so much as is good for him."[17] Deborah's experience demonstrates that a more complex code of communication existed between physician and patient. Physicians were ready to tell patients the "truth" in the last stages of the disease, when they knew death was imminent and their patients had religious duties to perform. Once again, medical authority deferred to social and religious values. In truth telling as in decisions about pregnancy, duty came first.

In the summer of 1836 Deborah went to Charlestown. Because Dr. Warren was in Europe, she was examined by his assistant, Dr. Leach. He listened to her lungs and gave an optimistic report that "my lungs are not diseased," as she reported to Nathan. "But my opinion is that the left lobe is in some way affected by this cough."[18] Rather than wait for Dr. Warren to return, she decided to take advantage of his absence and consult another physician. To avoid insulting Dr. Warren, or for that matter Dr. Leach, she made Nathan into the intermediary. "I *wish you* would write to Dr. Leach about it, *thanking him* for his very *kind and faithful attention* to me and then telling him, since my lungs have been so variously affected within three years you would be glad to have me avail myself of this opportunity for [another] consultation. Adeline Scholfield tells me it is the custom to request the attending physician to invite the one to be consulted."[19]

Nathan did as requested, and Deborah saw Dr. James Jackson, a colleague and close friend of Dr. Warren's who also taught at Harvard Medical School. His examination yielded an opinion that differed very little from Warren's. "This forenoon I had a visit from Dr. Jackson (Dr. Leach seemed glad to consult with him)," she informed Nathan. "He examined my lungs and said his opinion was that they are not diseased, though possibly there might be disease which his ear could not detect."[20] This last concession may have been Jackson's way of preparing his patient for bad news in the near future, or it may have come from Deborah's plying him with questions. In all events, Deborah found him more forthcoming and helpful than Dr. Warren and from then onward, she saw only Dr. Jackson on her trips to Boston.

Dr. Jackson struck the same balance as Dr. Warren insofar as Deborah's domestic obligations were concerned, letting her determine the course of action. When Deborah asked him when she would be able to return to Amherst, he told her that "at this season of the year, it will make no difference whether I am in this vicinity or farther west. But in relation to going home, he says if I can *feel easy* away I ought not to return to any care before September." Left to make her own decision, she told Nathan that "if I find that I am not *gaining* by staying away, I shall be starting for home. If I was well *enough* I would come tomorrow . . . but I feel as if there would be no chance for my recovery to come home in such weakness and commence taking care of the family and the children. . . . I find it at times difficult to be patient, I am anxious to get well, and get well *quick*."[21]

In 1841 Deborah was constantly hoarse and could speak only in a whisper, which she knew was a classic symptom of the second stage of consumption. But seemingly Dr. Jackson disagreed, insisting that "this hoarseness has nothing to do with my lungs, but is a weakness . . . of a certain little spot about the opening of the windpipe. He said it was an obstinate difficulty to remove and gave me no encouragement that my voice would ever be strong and natural, but it is not immediately dangerous. . . . So you see Dr. Jackson calculates to have me live some time longer . . . but I know after all . . . he cannot promise me very long life—the number of my years are not with him."[22] Like other physicians, Jackson too reserved the prescription of travel for male patients. "He thinks going to a warmer climate," Deborah informed Nathan, "would be of no service and says I must accustom myself to a variety of temperatures."[23]

The explanations that Dr. Jackson and her other physicians gave on the source of her complaints clearly dissatisfied Deborah and she informed Ann Scholfield that she thought the doctors were as baffled as she. They might offer lengthy and detailed explanations, but she knew they had a very limited understanding of the physiology of the disease. "Nothing is left for me but a sense of hopeless ignorance—the most uncomfortable of all senses, but one from which we suffer much less than those who are always delving into unsearchable things."[24]

It was only when Deborah was in the very last stages of the disease, six months before she died, that Dr. Jackson indicated, and even then less than directly, the seriousness of her condition and the nearness of death. "As to my old topic health, I cannot say much in its praise," Deborah wrote Nathan in July 1843.

> Dr. Jackson tells me, and he says he is *honest*, that I have no immediate cause for anxiety, that the present irritation about my lungs is owing to the influenza and he thinks I shall be able to throw it off with no injury in the end but some loss of strength. I am under his care and see him every second or third day; I am better in *some* respects, I sleep nights, have less noise in my throat, and can lie with my head low and do not cough quite so much; he says I cannot expect to get better at once, nor ever be well, because my lungs are undoubtedly diseased, more so now than when I was in Boston last, still he says, I may with care, keep my head above water for some time.[25]

The critical phrase here is "because my lungs are undoubtedly diseased"—that is, her days were limited. Although she had "some time," she could not expect to "ever be well." In effect, Deborah and her doctors had been sharing a code. So long as she was not in the terminal stage of the disease, her physicians informed her that she had one or another infection but her lungs were unaffected. They did so not so much from complete ignorance—they had charted the course of the disease by the presence and severity of a number of symptoms and some of them could hear the progress it was making in the lungs—but because of their determination to keep hope alive. As they saw it, the medical profession had the duty to give comfort. But at the same time, physicians were themselves uncertain about the specific course of the disease as it affected a given patient. If they shied away from "the truth," it was also because they did not have a single, unambiguous truth to tell. The disease itself was so erratic that physicians had again and again witnessed cadaverous invalids come back to life. Why give a diagnosis of a mortal disease if the patient might live for another ten years? "Your lungs are diseased" was thus a signal that the physician had no remedies left, that the invalid had to make her preparations, although no one could say how many days she had remaining.[26]

Dr. Warren's response to Grace Webster, the wife of Daniel Webster, who had been his patient for many years and whose husband he deeply respected, exemplifies how this dynamic worked. In 1828 Grace Webster was dying from pulmonary consumption. Unwilling to rely on the remedies of other physicians and wanting the solace and skills of Dr. Warren, she begged her husband to have the physician come to New York and minister to her at the bedside. Dr. Warren refused and wrote to Grace Webster what he must have told countless patients orally as he sat by their beds. First, he told her that he did not have any more remedies to offer (at least none that could not be prescribed by a colleague in New York). Second, and more important, it was time for her to prepare to die. In a style that seemed to more appropriate to a minister than to a physician, he urged her "to submit and be content." "I speak now of the comfort of that holy and blessed revelation of the divine with power and goodness which opens its arms to the afflicted and offers the most delightful consolations to all who are willing to receive them." He concluded the letter with a benediction. "Farewell madam. May the author of our lives shed his blessing on you."[27] It was time for the doctor to leave the bedside to family, friends, and minister.

8

Intensive Care

Women called upon family and friends to assist them during their illness and sustain them as death neared. Deborah received considerable support from a network of female friends that included former schoolmates, neighbors, relatives, and kin scattered through New England. As her relationship with Nathan became distant and formal, her domestic duties more burdensome, and her symptoms more incapacitating, she turned to them for aid and comfort. In letters, as in conversations, the women shared the vexations of rearing children, the drudgery of household chores, and the frustrations that accrued from not having the strength to fulfill these duties. Mingled among Deborah's detailed bulletins on her health and requests for medical knowledge and advice were self-deprecating comments about the problems of managing a household and being an invalid. Disappointments and fears do appear in these letters, but they are far lighter in tone and more humorous than anything in her correspondence with Nathan. In her letters to friends, unlike in her other activities, she was able to distance herself from the constraints of the disease.[1]

Composing intimate letters to her friends required time and the right frame of mind. On many an afternoon or evening, Deborah would sit at her desk with several sharp quill pens and spend a few hours crafting a letter. Just as she chose the time, so she chose the mood. "Well Miss Martha," she concluded a lengthy letter to her cousin, "I have had a good time this afternoon. My imagination placed you before me in a neat dress with agreeable manners and in a sociable mood. I shall be quite inclined to visit you again very soon."[2] For Deborah, as for her friends, letters were substitute visits, and she made them appear as part of a conversation.

When Deborah was too weak to attend a prayer meeting or the sewing circle, she spent the afternoon writing and reminiscing about past gatherings and noting the way her invalidism precluded her involvement. "The weather without the least regard to our dear, good, old, Sewing Circle which meets at Mrs. Humphrey's this afternoon," she wrote to Elisabeth Terry, "is too unpleasant for such a slim carcass as I am to go out. Helen says 'what a pity Ma, for very likely you would be chosen *President*, if there.' How sorry I must be to miss such an honor." Deborah then mentioned the many sewing circles she and Elisabeth had attended, recalling the pleasure they had had, all the while teasing about the circles' grandiose aims. Deriding the group eased her disappointment. She was not only too weak to be president but even too frail to participate. "I wonder if you remember those general assemblies of old coats and pantaloons and what ludicrous consultations were often held respecting the legs and arms and *bodies* that were missing."[3]

Deborah frequently wrote letters to dispel her gloomy mood. She opened with the wretchedness of her condition, but by the end of the paragraph her tone changed, and hope replaced despair. "I wish you were in Amherst that they [my eyes] might behold you for one thing," she wrote to Martha Hooker,

and I wish you could behold me, not because I am handsome, but so you might pity the poor thing creeping about in an old pink gown with an awful sore blister upon her throat and chest, coughing every fifteen minutes, and wheezing the whole time. It is a sober fact that I really *feel dreadfully*, but don't you go feeling dreadfully on my account till you hear again, for perhaps I shall be bright as a button by the time Mr. Jenkins [the stage driver] will reach Falmouth.[4]

Deborah did not delude her friends about the severity of her symptoms, but buoyed herself by making it appear that her persistent ailments at times abated. "As to work I am able to sew a good deal," she wrote to Martha Hooker, "oversee baking and other housekeeping matters just like any body, only I am careful not to lift the heavy ends of things. And when anything extra is on foot, such as house cleaning, or company, I take a *little nap* of two or *three hours* in the afternoon, after which I feel as bright as in the morning. As to going out—if I get started for calls nothing but dinner time or tea time brings me home." The number of days that Deborah was strong enough to visit friends or carry out household chores were few and far between.[5]

With her friends Deborah confessed the limitations of her strength; with Nathan she was aware of its ominous implications for their future. Not strong enough to do the washing and ironing, she sat wrapped in her shawls by the fire, supervised the tasks, and wrote about it. "Washing day—that worst of all days in the whole year; had Job wished this day blotted out instead of the one upon which he was born, millions would have approved the wish or at least said, 'I don't wonder at it.'" If she was too frail even to supervise household tasks, she consoled herself by writing to her cousin Ellen. "If as well as usual, I should be in the kitchen this forenoon, but this not being the case, instead of the splashing of suds, I hear no noise but the noise of the good fire; instead of wash tubs and *heaps* of clothes *not* clean I see this nice paper and your note and letter."[6] Or as she wrote to Martha Hooker: "I am not worth a cent for working except to 'see to things.' . . . Anything that requires *shoulder* strength is beyond me entirely."[7]

As her disease progressed and her symptoms became more pronounced, going out and socializing became more difficult, at times even embarrassing. In 1841 her voice became so hoarse she could speak only in a whisper. She used black humor to report this distressing symptom to her cousin. "I am as well as a year ago, *excepting* my *voice* which is weak and hoarse—it makes every one say who don't know that it is a permanent difficulty, 'what a bad cold you have.'" But this effort at levity could not diminish the seriousness of the symptom. "I can walk all over the village and make calls by the dozen excepting upon deaf people, I can't scream if the house should take fire."[8] Self-mockery appeared so often in Deborah's letters to other invalids that it can be understood as a strategy the women used to manage quite severe disabilities.

Deborah, like many women, believed old friends were the best friends, but invalidism and a need for comfort and guidance led her to develop a late and very close relationship with another invalid, Harriet Webster Fowler. Harriet was one of the four daughters of the erudite and pious lexicographer Noah Webster.[9] Although her siblings and parents were healthy, Harriet's adult life was marked by consumption. Her first husband, Edward Henry Cobb, whose family had amassed considerable wealth from the China trade, died of consumption in 1818, two years after their marriage. Harriet returned to her father's home and in 1825 married again, this time to William Chauncey Fowler, a Congregational minister who became a professor at Middlebury College. The couple had four children, all of whom survived infancy. Each pregnancy and birth, however left Harriet more enervated. In 1836 both Harriet and William were suffering persistent respiratory ailments; on the advice of their physicians, they traveled South together for the winter. (Harriet's sister, Eliza Jones, came to care for the children.) The journey restored William's health but not Harriet's. Soon after they returned, William received and accepted an offer to teach at Amherst, hoping that the move would improve Harriet's health.

One year later, in February 1839, Harriet had her first hemorrhage. She related the incident to her sister, Eliza, begging her not to inform their parents.

> At length I began to cough and the first mouthful I knew from the look and feeling was blood. . . . It was a very cold night, the family had retired, and I had one light and could not blow one if I tried. But I concluded to lay still and try what perfect quiet could do—[I] swallowed two mouthfuls of blood and became convinced that if I could keep from further coughing I should be able to wait till morning without disturbing anyone. As soon as morning arrived, I looked at the contents of my cup. Alas my fears were realized.

Convinced that she would suffer an early death, Harriet resolved to face it submissively and humbly. "Oh, I need much of the temper of Christ to exercise the *passive* virtues in a light manner," she wrote Eliza. I "feel disqualified for almost all active duties, combing my hair, writing a letter is wearisome to me. To feel that I must be a feeble wife and faithless mother, an inefficient Christian when I see much to be done, is painful to me. I try to cultivate a cheerful spirit, to subdue every internal discontent and my prayer is *Thy will be done*. Oh I would say it from the *very* heart. I never renounce the light in myself and do I suffer all the will of my heavenly Father."[10] Once again, invalidism undercut the trinity of women's duties. For Harriet as for Deborah, the dilemma was to find a way to be a strong wife, faithful mother, and pious Christian.

Around shared physical pains, domestic responsibilities, and spiritual resolve, Deborah and Harriet formed an exclusive friendship. On many afternoons they read their favorite biblical passages to each other, and when their voices permitted, sang hymns. They relished the privacy and intimacy of these visits and were sad when they were too sick to get together. "I am as sorry as I *can* be that the weather and a cold in my head won't let me come, for I want to have a real good chat with you," Deborah wrote to Harriet. "Just such as *two* can have together with no more." Alone, they did not have to conceal their worries with a cheerful smile. "But I won't detain you with any more scribbling," Deborah continued, "for the tears are just ready to drop from my eyes and I am afraid I should say something that would set you crying. That's the way, you know, first the speaker and then the audience."[11] With their husbands and children the women had to remain cheerful; with each other they could openly express their sadness at their predicament without seeing it as evidence of weakness or resentment.

In the notes, really substitute visits, Deborah often made it appear as if she were talking to Harriet in the parlor. "Don't go off quite yet, for you must hear about your sausages, mince pie, and dear little rice pies," she wrote to Harriet. "In the first place the sausages [you sent] made my family a grand breakfast and my eldest Irishee fixed them finely. In the next place, your good mince pie came right in for a Sabbath day dinner saving other cooking and being a treat."[12] As satisfying as real visits were, they were also often disturbing, particularly as symptoms worsened and appearances changed. "My health is much better except this ugly cough which tries me in this cold weather," Harriet noted. "I wish to see you and yet dread to call lest I excite *you* to cough or in some way agitate or worry you." A note, they both knew, shielded the other from the pain of witnessing her friend so sick—a portent of her own future.[13]

In their correspondence, Harriet and Deborah commiserated at having to relieve a cough by frequent spitting—a disgusting gesture they associated with the ignorant and unrefined. "How is your cough?" Deborah asked Harriet. "Mine sounds now very much like yours—deep and hoarse, and I am obliged to keep an *old cup* and expectorate, no matter if the governor himself is disturbed by it." Only another invalid could appreciate the humiliation of having to stoop to such undignified conduct.[14]

In 1843 both Harriet and Deborah became acutely ill; to add a touch of cheer they exchanged gifts along with notes. On a blustery winter day Harriet sent her maid, Laura, with a basket of food for the Fiske family. Deborah never allowed Laura to return without a note and treats for Harriet's children. Deborah's maid, Mary, went into the larder and found the herring that David Vinal had sent, or an apple pie she had baked, and packed it into the basket. Meanwhile, Deborah wrote a humorously chiding one-page reply. "I'll tell you what I think of you, my dear, good, naughty friend, and that is you have enjoyed your full share of the blessedness of giving and have no right to give anything more away for at least five years." And knowing from her own experience just how physically exhausting it was for someone in the final stage of consumption even to oversee baking, she added an appreciation. "You don't know how I felt to see Laura coming in with such a load but I am too sleepy to try to tell you."[15] The gifts signaled their mutual affection and concern, which had the effect of raising their spirits during the long periods of confinement.

Deborah admired Harriet's spunkiness and her determination to remain active. "Mrs. Fowler has been very unwell," she informed a mutual friend. "She is better now, but her cough is *dreadful* and it seems as if it must wear her out before long, but she is so *resolute* and so bent upon knitting, sewing, having company and *everything* that people in health engage in that I don't know but she will live *because she will*."[16] Deborah wanted to follow her lead.

The two friends openly discussed the nearness of death. In 1843 Deborah took Ann with her on what turned out to be her final trip to Aunt Vinal. There she took a turn for the worse, contracting "the influenza" as she called it. Deborah returned to Amherst quite weak and frail. When Harriet heard the news, she immediately sent a note. "I learn that you . . . complain of increasing debility. It grieves me much to think *it must be so*. I grieve when I think that I shall never again see your elastic step tripping up my yard to give me a morning greeting. Your cheerful words and pleasant smiles made an impression upon my heart which *can never be forgotten*." Harriet implored Deborah to allow her to do something to make her last days more comfortable. "Is there nothing that I can do for you—nothing that I can get for you that you could relish?" she asked her friend.[17]

Deborah tried to allay Harriet's fears by reminding her of the mysterious nature of their disease. "The influenza was a bad job for me", she wrote to Harriet, "but I have gained the last fortnight, and I have come to life again so many times I don't know but I shall again." The phrase "come to life again" was especially apt. Consumption had so often brought the women to the brink of death, when somehow or other some semblance of health returned. Even as they continued to decline, they could not be certain that there would not be one more remission.[18]

In the shadow death, the women spoke confidently about the prospect of eternal salvation. "I send you a bunch of poor grapes," Harriet wrote, "thinking you may like them for a change. These perishing fruits which quench our feverish throat in sickness are very tasteful but I cannot but remind you of that blessed Saviour to whom you are going, who will pluck for you the *fruit of the tree of life*. Give you health of body, and health of soul and you will never again say, 'I am sick.' *Trust in Him* my friend, He will surely appear for your relief." In the eternal home, the pains of consumption would be obliterated. "Believe me, my dear Mrs. Fiske," Harriet wrote to Deborah, "I love you and think of you every hour in the day and often do my desires ascend to Heaven that the arms of everlasting love be under you, around you, giving you strength to bear every pain and every weakness with quiet submission."[19] As Deborah and Harriet envisioned it, not only would they meet each other there, but eventually their husbands and children would join them, too. In their heavenly abode the broken shards of a half-finished life would be so carefully glued together that the scars of consumption, orphanhood, and death would no longer be visible.

Deborah and Harriet met for the last time on Friday afternoon, February 16, 1844, four days before Deborah's death. Both knew that this visit would be their last. As she waited for Harriet, Deborah sat in a low stuffed chair close to the airtight stove, a present from her father. As its heat penetrated the mounds of well-stuffed pillows and the layers of shawls and flan-

nels that she now required to support her bony frame, she knew that neither the warmth of the stove nor the bright rays of the sun filtering through
the frosty windows could alleviate the chills and fever. Her face took on a
rosy hue, but it only momentarily diverted attention from her sunken
cheeks and hollow eyes. When Deborah spoke, the ravages of illness were
more apparent. Her voice was barely a whisper, and her cough, she maintained, sounded like "a troublesome *concert* on all sorts of out of tune
keys."[20]

Although Deborah's disease had persisted for fifteen years, an untoward
event had suddenly sapped her strength. On a clear day in December,
Nathan took her for a ride in the carriage, but the horse became startled,
and she was thrown to the ground. Deborah injured her left side. A month
later she was still suffering from numbness and pain in her arm and admitted that "I have not felt like the same person since." She had also begun to
lose weight more rapidly. At seventy-nine pounds, her appearance, she
admitted, was "shadow-like."[21]

As her condition became more desperate, she turned to her family to be
with her. In January 1844, after much forethought and some hesitation, she
had asked her elderly Aunt Vinal to leave her husband and take a stagecoach ride of several days across the state—in snowy weather. "I have a
great desire to see you and have had all through my sickness, but supposed I
must not think of it owing to the exposure there would be for you in taking
a journey at this season of the year." Deborah wanted her aunt's spiritual
equilibrium to guide her during her last days. "I have been *overwhelmed
with remorse* in reviewing my past life, so selfish, frivolous, prayerless and
thoughtless," she wrote to her aunt. "It makes a *mountain* of guilt that
reaches the *heavens*, and my only hope of being saved from its most *righteous* punishment is in the infinite mercy of God manifested through a sanc-
tified Saviour." Deborah recalled how her aunt had welcomed her into her
home and remembered the nights that she had nursed her and tolerated her
"stumping up and down stairs enough to take all the paint off," all the while
teaching her to control her temper and then to submit to God's authority in
a profession of faith.[22]

No sooner did Aunt Vinal receive Deborah's letter than she set out for
Amherst and became so absorbed in the daily life of the family that she
neglected to write her husband, Otis, who was impatiently awaiting her
return. When Otis objected to her being away so long, she answered
bluntly: "I have hardly thought of you since I have been here, my heart
and thoughts have been so occupied with the present scene." She could
not give him an exact date for her return, she tersely explained, for Deborah "says she almost began life with me and she hopes she'll end it with
me." And Martha Vinal had no intentions of disregarding Deborah's
wish.[23]

As Deborah watched her aunt mending the children's stockings, she knew that Aunt Vinal would provide the continuity between Deborah's own childhood and her daughters' future. And as she thought about Helen, now thirteen, whom she had also summoned from boarding school to be with her, this maternal solicitude seemed even more critical. Deborah had hoped that Helen would profess her faith at school that winter, but despite the prodding of her parents and the persuasion of her teachers, Helen had not yet found her way. As concerned as Deborah was about Helen, she was confident that Ann, who remained a docile nine year old with a large circle of friends, would adjust to living in other people's homes and also profess her faith.[24]

Deborah had asked her father to come to Amherst, too, but his presence proved to be disquieting for her. Despite her insistence, her father had never professed his faith; not believing in eternal life, he anxiously clung to his dying daughter. Although Deborah had written him a graphic account of the changes in her appearance, he became so distraught at the sight of her "thin face and tottering steps" that she worried that her letter had unintentionally given him a "false impression."[25] As the other members of the family sat in the sitting room, he occupied himself with repairing the home. The noise of his hammer echoed through the house, reminding Deborah of his preoccupation with material concerns. After Martha Vinal arrived, David absented himself even more frequently from the circle and at night when Deborah retired and the children were put to bed, he would go to his sister-in-law's room to talk. "Poor brother D., it would grieve you to see him," Martha told her husband. "It seem as tho' his heart has been broken. It is a great trial to Deborah that he isn't willing to give her up. He has been with me all this evening in my chamber and [his] feelings got beyond control."[26]

Nathan was also frequently absent from the circle. A recent Amherst ruling required that the faculty remain in their college studies all day, and anyway, much to his consternation, his study at home had been appropriated to accommodate all the new arrivals. Deborah knew that although the decision was practical, the room had been his sanctuary. Worse yet, his college study was poorly heated and sparsely furnished. All winter he had coughs and hoarseness that both he and Deborah believed were becoming more obdurate. A makeshift study had been set up in the corner of the sitting room, but it was a reminder of just how completely disease had disassembled the household. Deborah was pleased that during the final stage of her illness, Nathan had unexpectedly experienced a revival of his faith. Although Nathan rarely slept soundly at nights, it was the "jingle" of her medicine bottles that kept him on the edge of wakefulness, not his perplexities and doubts.[27]

Although Deborah appreciated Nathan's concern and ministrations, she turned to Aunt Vinal and her female friends for solace. With them she shared the hope of finding eternal salvation. "My earthly house is *failing*," she told Aunt Vinal, "and while we are at home in the body, we are absent from the Lord, and I do hope through the *infinite mercy* of God that when my earthly house of this tabernacle is dissolved, my soul will find a home in a house not made with hands, eternal in the heavens." She would soon pass home into the eternal abode of a welcoming and beloved Saviour who would grant her peace and rest.[28]

Although Deborah knew that the disease was finally "wearing her out," she was not willing to take up Aunt Vinal's suggestion to make one last heroic effort to prolong her life and travel to the West Indies for the winter. Deborah knew that the journey was considered health giving, but she rejected the prescription—she wanted to die at home. "I dare say Aunt Vinal is wishing me in the West Indies," she wrote to her cousin Ann Scholfield, "but I would not *for all the world* be anywhere but just *at home* with all my family about me, situated precisely as I am for I have every comfort and convenience that any one could desire and as to friends they are so kind it absolutely makes me *cry* to receive so many favors."[29] With this decision, Deborah gained a new confidence. She found that as her physical stamina decreased, her spirit became more resolute.

In January 1844 she had also written to Harriet, candidly informing her of how feeble she had become. "I am so weak and need a great deal done," Deborah admitted. "I cannot get up alone or rise in bed to cough. . . . Frail and wasted as my poor body is, it takes a great deal to wear it out." Deborah asked Harriet to "pray" for her "that I may have a *special* sense of the presence of God such as I have never had in health. (I do not deserve it I know.) But it would be worth worlds to me to have some token of acceptance which would make me *feel* that I am really *adopted* into God's dear family."[30]

Although Deborah very much wanted a last visit, she was startled by Harriet's appearance. As Deborah looked at Harriet's thin and wasted body, and heard her rapid breathing, it was as if a mirror had suddenly and cruelly been placed before her. When she stood to embrace her she heard herself saying, "Why how quick you breathe! Perhaps you will follow me next winter, and I shall be the first to welcome you." Without regard to the others in the room, the two women began to discuss their impending deaths, mixing statements of confidence of their salvation with periodic concerns about their piety. The meeting did not last long—neither woman had the stamina. But before Harriet left, Deborah took her aside and gave her a "token of her affection and another affectionate farewell." William Fowler was stunned by changes in his wife's appearance as the women said their final goodbye. "They had looked together at heaven, now opening to receive them, and when she came out to me, the light of heaven was on her face, though a tear trembled in her eye."[31]

Over the next four days Deborah energetically finished all her remaining earthly business, calling in all her friends to say goodbye and handing each of them a gift. Even during the last night of her illness she was still summoning special watchers, the men and women she wanted to pray and sing with her as she waited for her final call. "Mrs. Fiske's last days and weeks were very peaceful," Sabra Snell reported to her sister Louisa. "I was told that she disposed of nearly all her things, gave or left something for the neighbors, and wrote notes to her friends and cousins." Deborah carried out these final acts with "as much judgment and composure as if she had been in perfect health and setting out upon a long journey." On February 19, 1844, with neither a "struggle nor a groan," Deborah died.[32]

On April 2, 1844, less than two months later, the members of the First Congregational Church of Amherst filed into the meeting house to attend the funeral of Harriet Webster Fowler. They came to offer consolation to her family and to hear once more how Harriet, although invalided by consumption, had submitted humbly and found eternal peace. Heman Humphrey, the spiritual leader of the congregation, delivered the sermon. It was for him, as for the congregation, the second time in less than two months that he had to bear witness to the faith of a pious woman and teach "the great practical lesson" that such lives exemplified.[33]

Deborah Fiske was very much on Humphrey's mind as he wrote his eulogy for Harriet Fowler. The two women had taken so much strength from each other that their deaths, like their illness, seemed linked. Out of his deep respect for both women, he had spent weeks preparing the funeral orations. For Harriet Fowler, as for Deborah Fiske, Humphrey eulogized with the biblical phrase, "The woman who feareth God she shall be praised." For Deborah, Humphrey had written a lengthy and more abstract disquisition, the type of sermon she enjoyed; it only obliquely joined her virtues to the text. Harriet requested a shorter oration. Humphrey was uneasy with this constraint. He worried that he would "do but very imperfect justice to what her acquaintances know to have been some of the finest traits in her character." Nevertheless, Humphrey constructed a sermon for each of them that recounted their virtues and reminded the congregation how the trials of disease could energize invalids and blur the boundaries between earthly probation and eternal life.[34]

As Humphrey prepared his sermon, he recognized that his audience needed a reaffirmation of faith to transcend the repeated afflictions brought by consumption. Although his congregation was God-fearing, those who had not yet professed their faith could surely experience anger or spiritual doubts in the face of what they saw: the melancholy William Fowler, the distraught Nathan Fiske, and the anguished and bewildered children who clung to them.

To Humphrey's eye the children of both women were floundering. Helen Fiske had not been able to contain her rage as her mother's coffin was lowered into the ground. Instead of being subdued by her mother's tranquillity, she rebelled. Almost two months later she still refused to find solace through the acceptance of God's will. Emily Fowler, Harriet's oldest daughter, was also disconsolate. The day of her mother's death, she angrily wrote to her Aunt Eliza: "Absorbed in the present, I dare not look forward to the future. I cannot realize that she is gone never to come again. That no more words of counsel and affection will ever fall from her lips, that I am motherless for life."[35]

The powerful and highly evocative oration that Humphrey delivered for Harriet explored the seemingly paradoxical connection between bodily frailty and spiritual strength. Harriet had been an invalid for the last nine years of her life, Humphrey reminded the congregation. "By this I do not mean, that during any great part of that time, she was confined to her chamber, for she was generally able to oversee the affairs of her family and to enjoy the society of her friends." And even as her health failed, "she visited, as her strength would allow and beyond her strength, the widow and the fatherless in their afflictions. . . . How she could accomplish so much in any emergency, particularly after she became an invalid, was a mystery to her friends."[36] Humphrey resolved the paradox by linking her fading body to her emboldened faith.

Humphrey had witnessed the remarkable change in both women. As their corporeal forms began to resemble "empty vessels," their souls appeared driven by an irrepressible inner spirit. With a determination that was equal to the rapaciousness of the disease, they fulfilled their domestic and religious obligations. "With a composure which was astonishing to herself," he told the congregation, Harriet, like Deborah, "gave her parting counsel to her family and the friends about her, and directed letters and messages to such as were absent. . . . So great was her confidence and 'boldness in coming to the throne of grace,' that she said on one occasion, a day or two before her death, 'I fear I am not enough awed by the greatness and majesty of God as I am about to enter His presence.'"[37]

Humphrey concluded his sermon by evoking the friendship between Harriet and Deborah. He assured the congregation that Harriet Fowler would be admitted to the community of saints and that Deborah Fiske would be waiting for her. "And who of the shining ones met her in the vestibule of heaven?" he rhetorically asked. "A friend of a kindred spirit, whom she tenderly loved, and who was daily expected to be called home said to her a few weeks ago as she bade her farewell, 'I think you will come to me next year, and I will be the first to welcome you.'" Surely, some who followed Harriet's coffin to the graveyard and watched as the mourners shoveled the wet earth over it envisioned Harriet and Deborah standing together. And perhaps, as Humphrey intended, the vision gave them energy as well as solace in the face of consumption.[38]

PART III

HEALTH SEEKERS IN THE WEST, 1840–90

9

Come West and Live

THERE ARE FEW CONSTANTS IN THE HISTORY OF DISEASE—OR IN THE history of the sick. Epidemics have an ebb and flow that undermines predictions and resists explanation. Surprises recur, despite the increased sophistication of investigators, physicians, epidemiologists, and historians of medicine. AIDS is one case in point, belying the confidence with which physicians announced in the 1970s the end of the era of deadly infectious disease.[1] Tuberculosis is another.

By all accounts, the scourge of consumption in the United States, and in England as well, declined over the period 1850–90. The disease that in the 1830s had been responsible for one out of every four deaths was by the 1880s reported as the cause of only one out of eight.[2] There is little certainty as to why the decrease occurred. Perhaps a kind of natural selection took place: those who survived the earlier epidemics had a genetic resistance to the disease and passed it on to their progeny. Or perhaps an improved standard of living, including better ventilated housing and more nutritious diets, deserves the credit. Whatever the cause, the third generation of an American-born family more frequently escaped the fate of the first two.[3]

The epidemiological changes are far more apparent in retrospect than they were to contemporaries. In the period 1850 to 1890, consumption still crossed lines of social class, education, and sex. And it still forced those men and women who evinced its symptoms to alter their life patterns in dramatic fashion. The experiences of those who contracted the disease in this era did not altogether recapitulate those of the earlier New England invalids. Indeed, the term invalid does not capture the essence of their self-definition. They are better understood as health seekers, committed to travel to a salutary climate, where they could follow a health-giving routine, but the search was for a new place to live, not just to take a cure.

In ways that are quite remarkable, the biographies of health seekers are integral to the history of the westward movement. Beginning slowly in the 1840s and then gathering momentum in the 1870s and 1880s, men and women with the symptoms of consumption moved to the mountains and deserts of the West. By 1900 fully one-quarter of the migrants to California and one-third of the newcomers to Colorado had come in search of health. Indeed, every western state owed some degree of its growth to these itinerant health seekers. Although they settled everywhere in this vast region, the pattern of migration was not haphazard. Health seekers tended to congregate in locations that real estate developers, railroad agents, physicians, and other health seekers promoted as especially salubrious. And what was true for health seekers generally was even more true for physicians. In 1915 for example, the Denver Colorado Medical Society surveyed its members and found that four-fifths of them had come for their health.[4]

While practically every state west of the Mississippi had communities founded and developed for and by health seekers, Colorado, southern California, Texas, New Mexico, and Arizona, all situated on the dry and arid plateau of the Southwest, received the largest influx. More than half of the residents of Pasadena, California; Colorado Springs and Denver, Colorado; El Paso, Texas; Albuquerque, New Mexico; and Tucson, Arizona, reported to a 1913 public health survey that either they or a parent, grandparent, or sibling had emigrated in search of a cure for consumption. In communities like Sierra Madre, California; Silver City, New Mexico; and San Angelo, Texas, almost every one of the founding families had come for reasons of health. "Were all the consumptives to leave," the investigator commented, "Silver City would become a mere spot in the desert." In 1913 consumption still shaped the morbidity and mortality statistics of these communities. El Paso reported that four thousand of its forty-seven thousand residents were consumptive. Of the sixty-three deaths in the town in 1913, forty-eight were of consumptive men and women who had come in search of health.[5]

None of this is to imply that everyone with the disease went West. Despite the size of the migration, there were still large numbers of men and women who lacked the financial resources or physical strength to make the move. The poor among them, particularly those in the last stages of the disease, entered new facilities set up for the chronically ill or took a bed in one of the hospitals for "poor consumptives." The number of institutions and the people they served are reminders that although mortality from the disease declined, consumption continued to claim large numbers.[6]

*   *   *

To understand the underlying causes of this vast migration for health, one begins with the widespread and deeply held fantasies that Americans and Europeans shared about the West as Eden.[7] Its air was so "pure," its atmosphere so "wholesome," its climate so "reinvigorating" that diseases like consumption, which afflicted the residents of eastern states, were practically unknown there. The fantasies were fed by a variety of anecdotes, some coming from adventurers, others from health seekers, and still others from physicians. They appeared first in the 1840s and 1850s. Twenty to thirty years later, when the transportation network to the West was completed, the influence of these stories on the lives of the sick became all the greater.[8]

The anecdotes of regeneration that so appealed to health seekers are inseparable from the other myths that proliferated about the West. They all proclaimed in an exaggerated language the boundlessness of resources, embroidering and embellishing the facts to diminish the terror and deprivation of migration and to heighten its appeal to cautious or timid travelers. Those in search of fortune and those in search of health both saw the West as an "El Dorado," an "earthly paradise," where past failure (commercial or constitutional) would be transformed into future success (wealth and health). At the core of each tale was the discovery of a new life through an encounter with the natural bounty of the new land.[9]

Thus, George Ruxton, an English sportsman who had hunted big game in Africa, spent the winter of 1847 hunting in the Rocky Mountains. What he found most intriguing were the opportunities not for kill but for life. The "rapid consumption" of two of his companions, as he reported in the widely read English *Blackwood's Magazine*, was completely cured during their stay in the Rockies. "Their medical advisers had given up all hope of seeing them restored to health," but their sojourn in the mountains returned them in "robust health and spirits"—an experience, he insisted, that was not unique. "It is an extraordinary fact that the air of the [Rocky] mountains has a wonderfully restorative effect upon constitutions enfeebled by pulmonary disease. . . . I could mention a hundred instances where persons whose cases have been pronounced by eminent practitioners as perfectly hopeless have been restored to comparative sound health by a sojourn in the pure and bracing air of the Rocky Mountains and are now alive to testify to the effects of the reinvigorating climate." Ruxton concluded that the time he had spent in the mountains provided some of the "very happiest moments of my life."[10]

The autobiographical accounts of the first health seekers to go West testified even more enthusiastically to the region's curative powers. Josiah Gregg related in his very popular *Commerce of the Prairies*, published in 1844, how an excursion with a merchant caravan along the Santa Fe trail cured his consumption. "For some months preceding the year 1831," he wrote, "my health had been declining under a complication of chronic diseases, which defied every plan of treatment that the sagacity and science of my medical friends could devise. . . . In this hopeless condition, my physicians advised me to take a trip across the Prairies and, in the change of air and habits which such an adventure would involve to seek that health which their science had failed to bestow."[11] The experience was so restorative that whenever Gregg's debilitating cough returned—four times over the next decade—he joined another expedition. "You will doubtless be surprised to learn that I am again 'on the wing' for Santa Fe," he wrote to a friend in 1845, "a mere tour for health."[12]

Gregg's solution to his predicament was to incorporate the routine of repeated voyages for health into his career by taking his turn as an explorer, surveyor, merchant, and author. In *Commerce of the Prairies* he laid out the best travel routes, the most notable Indian customs, and his favorite locations. None surpassed New Mexico. "Nowhere . . . can a purer or more wholesome atmosphere be found. Bilious diseases—that great scourge of the Valley of the Mississippi are here almost unknown."[13]

Just as Ruxton celebrated Colorado, and Gregg, New Mexico, still others sang the praises of southern California. When one prospective settler, John Bidwell, asked a local trapper if fevers existed in the region, he was told: "There was but one man in California that had ever had a chill there, and it was a matter of so much wonderment to the people of Monterey that they went eighteen miles into the country to see him shake." Bidwell did not seem at all skeptical about this Paul Bunyan–like tale.[14] The tallest of the tall tales was of a man, at least 250 years old, who had to leave the region in order to die. But when he was brought back for burial, "the energies of life were immediately restored to his inanimate corpse! Herculean strength was imparted to his frame, and bursting the prison-walls of death, he appeared . . . reinvested with all the vigor and beauty of early manhood."[15]

Not only the western climate but also its manner of life was deemed health giving. Assuming the local dress, diet, and routine—riding a horse all day, eating buffalo meat roasted over an open fire, and sleeping under the stars were all thought to reinvigorate even the most delicate and frail. In 1843 Matt Field, a reporter for the New Orleans *Picayune*, joined an expedition into the Rocky Mountains to cure his consumption. "I will prove to you personally," he wrote to his editor, "and all doctors unequivocally, when I get home, that consumptives must . . . jump into the dresses of deerskin, and trot off to the mountains. We are the fattest, greasiest, set of truant rogues your liveliest imagination can call up to view."[16]

At least part of the faith in the rehabilitative potential of the natural life-style drew on a romantic image of the Indian. The long history identifying the primitive with the healthy took on fresh meaning in the West. However compelling the opposition of cannibal and Christian, there was the competing frame of the natural versus the enervated, the pure versus the corrupt. Just as civilization bred madness, so it bred disease; to escape civilization was to find a cure. Thus, despite the fact that westward travelers were both frightened and repelled by the heathen customs of the tribes—their "nomadic habits," "lecherous imaginings," brutality and dissipation—they were at the same time convinced that the Indian life-style offered protection from the illnesses that plagued white men. It was commonly reported by the first soldiers who went west that Indians had fewer "diseases and morbid affections . . . than that of civilized men. Rheumatism is rare, and gout appears to be unknown. No cases of phthisis or jaundice fell under our observation."[17] The first health seekers confirmed these reports. The Indians "are subject to few diseases," David Burnet wrote back, and "exhibit many instances of remarkable longevity." A physician who traveled to Colorado in 1860 found Indian habits "disgusting," but noted that "among all the Indian tribes inhabiting this tableau, tubercular consumption is almost unknown."[18]

The health of Native Americans was attributed not to their hereditary makeup (or, as later observers might suggest, to their isolation from European and American diseases) but to their manner of life. George Catlin, a young artist who went west in the 1830s to capture on canvas the habits and customs of the tribes, observed: "I do not believe that the differences [in their health] are constitutional or anything more than the results of different circumstances and a different education." To confirm his point, Catlin cited the exceptional health of the trappers or mountain men who "have lived exactly upon the Indians' system, continually exposed to the open air, and the privations peculiar to that mode of life." But as soon as the mountain men returned to "a confined and dissipated life," their health would "fall to pieces."[19] Similarly, fur-trading companies often commented upon the unusual healthfulness of their employees. "Among our partisans in the mountains," one of them remarked, "sickness and natural death are almost unknown." In the first four years of their company, commented another, we have not "lost a single man by death except those who came to their end prematurely by being either shot or drowned."[20]

Even those who disapproved of the dissolute and immoral habits of hunters and traders conceded the good health of both. They were repelled by white men dressed in fringed buckskin suits decorated with porcupine quills, knives and pistols dangling from their belts. They sneered at mountain men whose hair was unkempt, beards ragged, and clothing filled with lice. They denounced as savage those who had so little respect for law and order that at the least provocation they would maim or kill those who offended them. And they had nothing but disdain for hunting trips that became the occasion for drunken revels, in which the men gambled away their earnings. But all that notwithstanding, they agreed that these renegades from civilization were vigorous and unusually healthy.[21]

The letters between the Sublette brothers, among the most famous of the Rocky Mountain hunters and guides during the 1840s, attest to the power of the belief that life-style could counter constitutional infirmities. The brothers suffered from consumption (their "family foe"); and they believed they were still alive only because of the many months they spent in the mountains and the deserts of the West. "I am traveling after the buffalo with my cart and lodge with three mules, five horses and two Spaniards," Andrew Sublette wrote from along the Arkansas River in 1845. "I am not making much but enjoying good health which is more than I can do in the states. . . . Come and see me I am fat, ragged and saucy." Andrew "looks better than I ever saw him and has gotten entirely well of his cough," his cousin Margaret Hereford wrote to her mother-in-law from California, "and says he never expects to return to the States as he knows he could not have health there."[22]

The anecdotes were generally about men, but there were hints that women's health, too, would benefit from a natural life-style. George Catlin, for example, was astonished by the Native American women; although they were "obliged to lead lives of severe toil and drudgery," he found them "exceedingly healthy and robust, giving easy birth and strong constitutions to their children." Indeed, he wondered whether following their example might restore the health of "pale-faced" women. "If from their childhood, our mothers had, like the Indian women, carried loads like beasts of burden—and those over the longest journeys, and highest mountains—had swum the broadest rivers—and galloped about for months and even years of their lives, *astride* of their horses' backs," not only they but their children would be stronger and healthier.[23]

Women who traveled West also noted the health and strength of Native American women, especially when measured against their own. Susan Magoffin gave birth to a baby while on the trail to Santa Fe. She was in severe pain for hours, required large doses of sedatives, and remained bedridden for days after the infant arrived. But a Native American woman who gave birth at the very same time had taken her baby to bathe in the river a half hour after its arrival. "Never could I have believed such a thing, if I had not been here. . . . It is truly astonishing to see what customs will do."[24]

In the 1840s some women did go West as health seekers, not joining hunting expeditions but as members of the large caravans of covered wagons. Many years later, Catherine Haun recalled her voyage in 1849: "My health was not good. Four of my sisters having died, while young, of consumption and I had reason to be apprehensive on that score. The physician advised an entire change of climate . . . [and] finally approved of our contemplated trip across the plains in a 'prairie schooner' for . . . an out of door life was advocated as a cure for this disease. In my case, as in that of many others, my health was restored long before the end of our journey."[25] Others like Margaret Hereford gave positive reports on the benefits of an overland voyage to California. "This must be a healthy climate," she wrote to her mother-in-law, "or it may be that hard work agrees with me, for I do all my own washing and ironing. . . . So you see . . . I am blessed in that respect, for I regained my health and strength."[26]

As more and more invalids went West, the number of narratives proliferated, and so did the belief that health would come to all who journeyed across the plains. In Mark Twain's *Roughing It*, the anecdotes of rejuvenation achieved their ultimate acknowledgment, becoming the stuff of parody. "Three months of camp life on Lake Tahoe," recounted Twain, "would restore an Egyptian mummy to his pristine vigor. . . . The air up there in the clouds is very pure and fine, bracing and delicious. And why shouldn't it be?—it is the same the angels breathe." Drawing on the anecdotes of others he declared: "I know a man who went there to die but he made a failure of it. He was a skeleton when he came and could barely stand. . . . Three months later he was sleeping out of doors regularly, eating all he could hold, three times a day, and chasing game over mountains three thousand feet high for recreation. And he was a skeleton no longer, but weighed part of a ton. This is no fancy sketch but the truth. His disease was consumption. I confidently recommend his experience to other skeletons." But Twain's hyperbole paid full tribute to the myth—and the consumptive could well be forgiven for taking it quite literally.[27]

The fantasies of the West as a health-giving Eden shaped the approach of medical treatises, particularly those emanating from the West itself. These texts appeared to give a scientific grounding to the fantasies, popularizing and legitimating them still further. In the process, an American brand of medicine emerged, distinct from the traditions of Europe and seemingly capable of curing consumption. The most influential of these medical texts that inspired invalids to become health seekers and gave a peculiarly New World stamp to the treatment of consumption was Daniel Drake's *Systematic Treatise, Historical, Etiological, and Practical, on the Principal Diseases of the Interior Valley of North America*.[28]

Published in 1850, Drake's text brought together the observations of physicians, explorers, and early health seekers, added statistics about the cures, and in this way promoted both the idea of a local pursuit of medical knowledge and a regional theory of therapeutics. Drake mingled seemingly objective data on climate (hours of sunshine and numbers of cures) with popular anecdotes (the dying coming to life in California). The book brought fame to its author and gave a new direction to those seeking health.[29]

Drake was Cincinnati's foremost physician in the 1840s and according to the English visitor Harriet Martineau, the "complete and favorable specimen of a westerner." Apparently indistinguishable in dress and speech from "any farmer on his way to market," he was "ill at ease in more formal eastern dress, etiquette, and . . . rules of grammar." His sentences, Martineau noted, *"take whatever form fate may determine but they bear the rich burden of truth hard won by experience."*[30]

Drake's upbringing and education fit with Martineau's comments. Raised in a log cabin in Kentucky, educated locally and sporadically, his medical training was essentially empirical. Drake apprenticed to a Cincinnati physician (whom he later described as incompetent), attended some lectures at the Medical College in Philadelphia, and eventually (many years after he began practice) received a diploma. But he did not see either his lack of formal education or his reliance on experience over theory as liabilities. He had a naïve and innocent passion about nature, convinced that a boy learned more by rambling in the woods than sitting for long hours in the classroom. In his own case, expeditions through the wilderness had trained him to become "an acute and vigilant observer . . . the pathless wilderness may be a schoolbook, and nature is the institution . . . whose works of taste and genius constitute an important part of your college course." Drake, an autodidact and self-made professional, was convinced that intuition was still more important than systematic education.[31]

Drake believed that the conditions of frontier living and an encounter with a natural life-style regenerated men's bodies even as it purified their souls. Watching men discover the seemingly inexhaustible resources of the frontier, seeing the city of Cincinnati grow from a small hamlet to a thriving city in the course of twenty years, convinced him that "the inhabitants of this region are obviously destined to an unrivalled excellence in agriculture, manufacture and internal commerce; in literature and the arts; in public virtue and in national strength."[32]

This prophetic vision of the frontier as a place of national renewal influenced Drake's practice of medicine. He devoted great energy to establishing westernl medical institutions and journals. More, he incorporated his vision of the promise of nature in general into his system of therapeutics, citing as documentation the anecdotes of the explorers and travelers who had ventured into the southwestern plateau. He believed the traveler's tales of regeneration, for he was already convinced of the power of the climate and a natural life-style to restore the sick and dying. Thus, *A Systematic Treatise*, his most ambitious book, published at the height of his career, endorsed and publicized traveling west and living in the wilderness like a hunter.

The organizing theme of his text, like so many other western medical treatises, was "medical topography," that is, the therapeutic influences that a region "may be presumed to exercise as an influence either directly or indirectly on health." Evidence came from personal observation, with no apologies offered for so empirical an approach. To gather information for the book, Drake traveled to towns and hamlets, recording in detail data on climate and collecting information from local physicians on morbidity and mortality. His travels reinforced what he already knew, that most of the areas of the Mississippi Valley were woefully unhealthy and that victims of its deleterious environment should be strongly advised to go farther west.[33]

In Drake's section on therapy, all pretense of marshaling scientific data disappears, as he unabashedly set forth his fervent belief in the power of climate and life-style to cure the sick. In a style hardly to be distinguished from travelers' accounts, Drake recommended long overland voyages for even the most frail and sickly. He insisted that these trips would be good for almost all invalids suffering from consumption, "from the earliest predisposition to that in which the patient has merely the ability to keep in his saddle through the day."[34]

"In the voiceless solitudes of the desert," Drake counseled, invalids were to "pitch their tents and plunge into rustication." The dry arid climate of the plains would be a wonderful antidote to the feverish atmosphere of the valley. A natural, spartan life-style would add to the restorative potential of the regimen. Conceding that "these journeys abound in exposures, fatigues and privations . . . it is on them that the benefit chiefly depends. Take them away, and a journey over the desert to the Rocky Mountains would be scarcely more efficacious than the fashionable voyage to Europe." Eating simple food, drinking only water, and exercising all day was guaranteed to make the delicate more robust. Even the scenery was therapeutic, for "the traveler's mind and eye are constantly exercised on objects which stand in contrast with those he has left behind."[35]

Drake openly admitted that his enthusiasm for this therapy came from poring over the reports of explorers in the West, including Lewis and Clark, Zebulon Pike, Stephen Long, George Catlin, John Fremont, and Josiah Gregg; it was not drawn from the classic medical textbooks of European physicians. This was western American medicine at its most provincial—and its most optimistic.

More pessimistic, or perhaps realistic, reports did exist, but they found their way into print far less frequently. Occasionally a tale was recounted of a man who found death, not life, in the West. One invalid, for example, "on the way to the mountains for the recovery of his health, with a frame reduced by the ravages of that fell destroyer, consumption," died in the course of the journey. Others reported similar events. "Last night, a Mr. Phelps, who had left his home to try the health restoring climate of the Rocky Mountains, died. Being in the last stage of consumption, he had hoped that the pure air of the prairies might ameliorate his disease." Or from another account: "A short distance from our place of encampment, I observed a newly made grave . . . and in examining the wooden head board, I found it to be the last resting place of George W. Tindal . . . who had died of consumption."[36]

These admissions of failure did not undercut the more general confidence in the efficacy of the western cure. Drake simply ignored or dismissed data that refuted his claims. When a resident of Mackinac Island, a favorite stopping place for trappers, told Drake that he had encountered two of them with consumption, the doctor insisted they had chronic bronchitis and were not "examples of true phthisis." When they hunted along the lakes, they were healthy, "but when they came to winter in huts and eat fresh meat, they were subject to catarrhal affections." In Drake's West, and in the West that attracted these first health seekers, consumption had no place.[37]

Even the most powerful myth requires practical assistance to be realized on a grand scale. Beginning in the 1870s the completion of the transcontinental railroad and concomitantly the appearance of a throng of town promoters gave an entirely new force to the idea of the West as therapeutic. The railroad builders and the entrepreneurs turned a trickle of health seekers moving westward into a torrent. Earlier, as one traveler reported, "a venturesome invalid had to brave the fatigues and hardship of a long stage drive over back roads." Now, "a great army of health seekers" was fanning out over the vast plateau between the Mississippi and California. "I never sat in a south or west bound train in Texas," W. H. Taylor told the readers of *Harper's New Monthly Magazine*, "that I did not note some consumptive who journeyed toward the dry plains with hope and good prospect of regaining his lost heritage of health."[38]

In the 1870s and increasingly thereafter, the dependability of railroad service made the hardships of a long overland voyage across the plains a relic of pioneer days. Civilization in the guise of relatively swift and punctual transportation transformed almost every aspect of the migration. The continent seemed smaller, and the region, less primitive. This shrinking of space along with the rapid construction of towns along the route made the health seekers into passengers. Spared the deprivations and risks of an overland voyage, they could look out the windows of their train compartments and see buffalo grazing, and they ate the meat cooked in the dining car ovens. (A few passengers did "hunt," that is, shoot the animals from the train windows.) In far less time than Daniel Drake imagined, the overland voyage had become indistinguishable from a "fashionable trip to Europe."

The very comfort of the journey meant that the health seekers were deprived of its rehabilitative benefits: It made little sense to travel by Conestoga wagon when several trains made the trip daily, cutting through the farms that fanned out on both sides of the track. But crossing the plains in a snug compartment detached them from a "natural" life-style. A few hardy souls tried to replicate the earlier adventures, but the result was inevitably a quaint imitation of life in a bygone era.

In June 1871, just a year after the railroad reached Denver, a party of invalids decided to take an old-fashioned overland journey from Leavenworth, Kansas, to the Colorado Territory. They aimed to recapture the essence of the older regimen while still enjoying the amenities that were now available along the route. Thus, they purchased two open-seated carriages and a covered wagon and mules, and they hired several drivers. In keeping with the spirit of the trip, the men wore wide-brimmed hats, buckskin suits, and "revolvers . . . slung at their belts." The women dressed in "dark flannel dresses and ankle length bloomers." But convinced that there was "no use acting like savages even though we are going to a savage country," each night they turned a cot into a dinner table and substituted butter, eggs, and milk purchased at the farmhouses along the way for the buffalo meat their predecessors had roasted over campfires. So too, they deliberately planned a route that paralleled the railroad line, both for "safety" ("We have orders for an escort if in danger") and for convenience. This way the railroad conductors could supply them with mail and daily newspapers, which kept them "from feeling quite out of this world." So much for "living like an Indian."[39]

Somehow the advantages that were to accrue from camping out and living the natural life had to be gained in other ways. It was the town promoters and western developers who quickly and effectively framed the alternative. In the particular climatic conditions of their own town lay the cure. They spared no effort to convince health seekers that buying a lot in their development was the best way to restore health. Their tales of remarkable cures made the unbelievable appear prosaic, and almost every subdivision issued its own accounts. "Let a man travel for six weeks in western Texas," declared one promoter, "and if he is not cured of whatever ailment he has, it will be because there is no blood in him." A San Antonio enthusiast claimed that its climate "has cured thousands affected with consumption and pulmonary complaints. . . . Its death rate is less, compared to its population, than any city in the world."[40]

No town's history better illustrates the impact of boosterism on health seekers then Colorado Springs. In 1869 the future town was nothing more than a barren, semiarid plot of several thousand acres. By 1879 it had three thousand residents and was heralded as a most desirable destination for consumptives. Colorado Springs did not have a better climate or better scenery than other locations. Rather, it had two very effective promoters— General William Jackson Palmer, who had gained national prominence in the Civil War, and Dr. William A. Bell, an English geologist who acquired his medical title when he filled the vacant post of physician on a surveying expedition. Together they made the town into one of the biggest winners in the lottery of western land speculation and development. They did it by aggressively pursuing a new idea—a town that catered to affluent health seekers.[41]

Having thus defined their market quite precisely, Palmer and Bell planned the settlement accordingly. It would have "all the refinements and amenities of eastern civilization" but, at the same time, enable the residents to spend their days riding, hunting, and fishing and their nights sleeping out under the stars. Living in the midst of one of the roughest mountain ranges in a territory that was still filled with Indians, health seekers would enjoy all the comforts of home and the "pure air" and outdoor life of the West.[42]

The idea of trying to domesticate the natural was initially Palmer's. Awed by the physical beauty of Colorado and bored with army life, Palmer resigned his commission at the close of the Civil War and set out to make his fortune. His service as a Union captain, then colonel, and eventually general had taught him a good deal about transportation, setting up camps, and maintaining order and discipline among the troops. It had also brought him in contact with the right people; drawing on his connections, he was able to win introductions to members of the board of directors of the Union Pacific Railroad. He persuaded them that they needed a representative with energy and knowledge to conduct surveying expeditions in the West and oversee the actual construction of the roadbed. "Young men without money can only make a fortune by connecting themselves with capitalists," he wrote his uncle right after the end of the war, and "the best place to invest capital is in the West." Over the next several years he conducted a series of surveys for the Union Pacific in the Southwest. Next he was given responsibility for managing the construction of the track to Denver and made a director of the company. It was then that he devised the plan that made his fortune.[43]

The grandiose scheme was born in the wilderness. As Palmer recounted (and no doubt embellished) the tale, it occurred one moonlit night while he was camping at the base of Pike's Peak (a short distance from the future Colorado Springs). Although he had been there several times before, on this particular night he was awakened "by the round moon looking steadily into my face"; and as he stared at the "magnificent" mountain "towering" above, he saw in this "wild government land" a sign of his own destiny.

These majestic mountains, Palmer was convinced, could alter men's constitutions, making the angry bucolic, the stormy calm, and, most important, the invalid healthy. Here he would build a town that would prosper by attracting well-to-do health seekers.[44]

This vision guided him as he set out to transform the barren region into a settlement, in his terms a "famous resort," with a "castle" surrounded by "fountains and lakes, and lovely drives and horse-back trails through groves." He would design and stock a park with antelope, black-tailed deer, even provide a range for buffalo. And as the final flourish to this extravaganza, he would hire Indians to come to the town in native costume and "recall more vividly the wild prairie life."[45]

Palmer was both a pragmatist and an impresario, a military commander who had moved squadrons like chess pieces and a dreamer who spent hours painting his reveries on the largest possible canvas, carefully highlighting the most flamboyant details and obscuring the less appealing aspects. The project imagined, Palmer began to plan its execution. First, he would have to raise the capital to purchase the land and underwrite the cost of building a track from Denver to it. Then he would have to lay out the town and attract the right settlers.

Daunting as this all seemed, many others were trying to do the same thing. Palmer had several advantages, however, not least of which was his selection of a location in Colorado, a territory that enjoyed more than its fair share of encomiums as a remarkably health-giving climate. Although most of the territory's promotional literature was self-serving, it was none the less impressive in its claims. "Doctors are not in demand," wrote the Denver Board of Trade in its 1868 report. "The climate is too healthy."[46] A visiting physician concurred. "Discard drugs and doctors, and leave the crowded cities," he advised consumptives, "forsake sea coasts and watering places—the common grave yards of consumptives—and spend a season at Pike's Peak—not necessarily in searching for gold—but, in chasing deer, antelope and bear, and living upon their flesh . . . whose fats consumed in this elevated mountains home are worth all . . . the Cod Liver Oil in the world." The Kansas Pacific Railroad with a terminus in Colorado also touted the region's virtues: "Many [who] have tried Minnesota, the West Indies, California and sea voyages, in vain, become sound and well by a sojourn in Colorado."[47]

Bayard Taylor, whose travel accounts were especially popular, summed up the popular enthusiasm by proclaiming that "Colorado will soon be recognized as our Switzerland."[48] A. A. Hayes, a fellow of the Royal Geographical Society of London, for his part encouraged European consumptives to forgo Nice and Cannes and head for Colorado. "Wandering in this region you may meet an acquaintance, remembered in New York or Boston as a thin, pale man, of whom people used to speak as 'poor fellow' and to whom each winter was a new terror. You will hardly recognize him in the brown-bearded horseman who has come in thirty miles that morning, and will think nothing of riding out again before night."[49]

Palmer and Bell recognized that there was no shortage of aspiring dreary towns, but they were convinced that their enterprise would succeed because it would attract a new crowd—not prospectors for gold but the already prosperous in search of health and pleasure. The men divided their chores. As Palmer met with investors and politicians, Bell headed back to England to sell lots to those who came from families with long histories of consumption and who would be eager, by virtue of it being not only exotic but also safe, to take up residence in the American West. With remarkable speed, both men accomplished their tasks.[50] Palmer arranged for a spur of the Denver and Rio Grande Railroad to go up to Colorado Springs and Bell imported the special narrow gauge track for the roadbed. Their subscriptions sold quickly on both sides of the Atlantic to a select clientele. Palmer was committed to sell lots only to those of "good moral character," who were to enjoy "all the comforts and refinements appertaining to Eastern civilization."[51]

In the winter of 1871, just after the Rio Grande Railroad began carrying passengers from Denver to Colorado Springs, the town received two influential guests, Charles Kingsley, the noted evangelist, and his daughter Rose. The visit was not serendipitous. Maurice Kingsley, Charles's son, was an investor in the town, and the two came to visit him and have a western adventure. Rose's published account of the journey described in detail the primitiveness of the setting and its allure. In a lengthy section on the "resources and progress" of Colorado, she unabashedly promoted not only the territory but also more specifically Colorado Springs. To be sure, the town Rose saw was more a blueprint than reality. The streets had been laid out but there were only twelve houses, hastily constructed shanties and tents, and few of the promised amenities. But to Rose the natural beauty of the setting and the opportunity to explore the canyons and the mountains more than compensated for the primitiveness. "The climate," she told her readers, "is bracing and healthy, and so dry, that even in winter, one does not feel the cold nearly so severely as at a higher temperature and lower altitude. For invalids suffering from asthma or consumption, if the latter disease is not too advanced, the air works wonders." To back up her assertions she added the required anecdote: "One invalid whom I happened to know came out in the summer of 1871 apparently dying of consumption, obliged to be moved in an invalid carriage. In the spring of 1872 we wished him good sport as he started on foot for a week's shooting and camping in the mountains!" This firsthand report by a young woman from a noted English family had a certain credibility—it was just the type of promotional literature the founders desired, for it would attract temperate, church-going families.[52]

By 1873 Colorado Springs had two thousand residents, three hundred homes, four churches (all Protestant), two schools, six grocery stores, a hardware store, two tailor shops, and a photographer's studio—but no saloons. Its streets were wide and tree-lined. Palmer had hired a British landscape architect to design the parks and plant the trees in formal English style. The editor of the local newspaper was also British, and he chose a typically English typescript and layout for the paper.[53]

Palmer went so far as to found a college, modeled on Amherst, and hired a New England Congregational minister, the Reverend Edward Tenney, as its president. Tenney, a consumptive, arrived in 1876. Within two years his health had markedly improved and he became one of the town's vocal boosters: his enthusiasm for the restorative powers of Colorado Springs knew no bounds. To share his good fortune—to give "hope to thousands of invalids . . . in eastern states"—and to encourage them to migrate, Tenney wrote *Colorado and Homes in the New West*, a book that went through two printings in its first three years. He informed his many readers that "one-third of the population of the plains in Colorado are reconstructed invalids" and that it was the Colorado climate that was responsible for their recovery. "Damp nights and incipient consumption are needless. Those who live upon the Atlantic sea-board in a climate that is killing them by inches, can get out of it upon any Tuesday afternoon and find themselves upon Saturday in a dry and sunny country. . . . Multitudes of people in the valley of the Mississippi are slowly dying within two days' ride of perfect health. Invalids die in Colorado only because they seek the remedy too late."[54] With endorsements like this, it is no wonder that Colorado Springs flourished.

Innumerable settlements in southern California also thrived, particularly those along the San Gabriel and San Bernadino mountains. Reports of the remarkable California climate had been filtering back East for at least twenty years, but it was not until the completion of the transcontinental railroad that the army of health seekers arrived. "Men go [West] not to buy land but to buy lungs," observed the editor of one southern California newspaper. But the railroads and the town promoters left nothing to chance in their search for profits. The railroads published thousands of brochures touting the benefits of the region, usually putting health first. And they worked closely with tour operators such as Raymond Excursions, which brought visitors and potential settlers from Boston to Los Angeles.[55] Where the railroads left off, guidebooks began. One of the most widely read was Benjamin Truman's *Semi-tropical California*. Truman insisted:

"The facts are that no one can take up a long residence . . . having predisposed tendencies to consumption, or in the early stages of the disease, who is not immediately relieved, while many pronounce themselves cured."[56]

Over the course of the 1880s and 1890s, the entire southern sector of the state became a "sanitarium belt," dotted with communities, resorts, hotels, and boardinghouses, some more makeshift than others, but all hoping to attract invalids, especially consumptives. San Diego, Santa Barbara, Los Angeles, and Pasadena were among the most successful recruiters, in part because of their climatic advantages, in part because a considerable number of their promoters were themselves consumptive. Alonzo Horton, also known as "the Father of San Diego," arrived there in 1867, before the railroad was completed, and when six months later his chronic cough had disappeared, he knew he had found a mecca for health seekers. He promoted San Diego as the fitting place to take a cure and set about constructing housing for the invalids who arrived daily.[57]

Los Angeles and Pasadena, nestled and shielded from the damp ocean breezes by the mountain range, became the most sought after locale for consumptives. Nathaniel Carter was typical of its developers, a consumptive who had come out in 1871 from Lowell, Massachusetts, convinced that he had less than a year to live. His regeneration never ceased to amaze him, and he spent the remainder of his life promoting the miraculous climate of Southern California. In 1872, brimming with pride at his own physical transformation, Carter contacted the Southern Pacific Railroad Company, and sold it on the idea of organizing transcontinental excursions for invalids. Carter proposed to return East to sign up the passengers, and, to persuade the skeptical, he had business cards printed up with two photographs of himself, "before" and "after" coming West. Within a few years business boomed to the point that Carter became known as the "famous excursionist." In 1882 he used his considerable profits to purchase land in the San Gabriel Valley, a tract known as Sierra Madre, and in the style of William Palmer, he laid out a community designed to attract wealthy consumptives.[58]

The town of Pasadena prospered around another health seeker's revelation. In 1873 a resolute but physically frail D. M. Berry arrived in southern California as a scout for a group of consumptives from Indiana. He was charged with buying fertile land in a salutary location. His choice, however shrewd in retrospect, was the result of one night spent on a ranch just northeast of what became Pasadena. Berry, who suffered from severe respiratory ailments, was never able to sleep soundly—his lungs were so impaired that he would wake and have to remain sitting in a chair until morning. On this particular night, however, he slept soundly and awoke the next morning feeling refreshed and revived. As he maintained when he told the story—over and over again—he "struck his chest and exclaimed, 'Do you know, sir, that last night is the first night in three years that I have remained in bed all night?'" Berry had found his site.[59]

The Indiana Colony, as Pasadena was first called, was composed primarily of midwesterners who had come "to sunny California to benefit the health of some member of the family." By 1886 the colony had grown into a small city, and the boasts of its cured consumptives had become the subject of satire. "I thought I came here to die," went one of them. "Alas! When I left home I had but one lung and it almost gone. I couldn't speak above a whisper, and had no appetite. I have been two weeks in Pasadena, have three lungs, can roar like a descending avalanche, ate three mules for breakfast, and am going to try it for another week."[60]

California developers also promised health seekers boundless and highly profitable opportunities for outdoor living. In the nearby mountains they could hunt, camp, and fish, while in the valleys, even the most delicate among them could become citrus growers. The San Gabriel Valley was an ideal climate for the crop, and it was a type of agriculture unusually well suited for those with modest strength and a modicum of capital. For a dollar the health seeker could purchase enough seeds for five acres of trees, and within ten years, the trees would each be bearing about a thousand oranges. It cost more to purchase and transplant seedlings, but in either case, the time required and the financial investment were low. It took just a few hours a day to water, feed, and prune the trees, and all the while the health seekers could raise vegetables and barley on the fertile land that surrounded the orchards. The prospects seemed so attractive that an 1883 guidebook entitled *California for Fruit Growers and Consumptives* encouraged everyone, including lawyers and doctors, to enjoy "a life of out door luxury associated with good health." Still others, with less capital to invest, purchased aviaries and became beekeepers, drove a stagecoach (thus keeping out of doors and exercising) or became postmen (for the same reasons). One had only to set up a routine of outdoor activity in the right climate, and consumption—surely in its first stages and perhaps even in its later ones—would be cured.[61]

10

The Physician as
Living Proof

However persuasive the publications of western promoters and travelers, it was the personal testimonials and professional publications of a particular group of physicians that legitimated the idea of the West as curative. These physicians, themselves health seekers, became the most vocal and adamant proponents of its restorative powers. Citing their own cases to stimulate the migration of others, they were the "living proof" of the possibility of a cure, the embodiment of the slogan—Come West and Live.

These physicians developed an idiosyncratic style of practice that incorporated their faith in the power of climate and an outdoor life to cure consumption. They emphasized the benefits of their particular place of residence: its pure air, long hours of sunshine, uniform temperatures, and, if they were in Colorado, high dry altitude. At the same time, they stressed the importance of a daily regimen of exercise, again framing it in personal terms. In fact, they often promoted the benefits of outdoor living by dressing in the garb of frontiersmen and boasting of their prowess in hunting.

As health seekers themselves, the physicians dispensed to other consumptives the highly specific prescriptions they had followed. A large part of their practice was devoted to initiating others into life in the West; they filled their medical tracts not with formulas and dosages but with paeans to the curative powers of nature as experienced through climbs in the Rockies and trips through its canyons. Together they would ride and hike, their saddlebags packed with camping gear rather than the traditional purgatives and opiates.[1]

The autobiographical accounts of western physicians typically opened with descriptions of early disappointments, especially how debilitating disease had thwarted careers and lent premonitions of premature death. But rather than succumbing to fate, they came West and aggressively fought their disease. Good luck had played some role, of course—they chanced upon the right climate. But now others could learn from their own success.

So persuaded were the health-seeking physicians of the efficacy of their prescriptions that they not only ardently promoted their particular regions but were also highly intolerant of anyone who doubted their claims. They were usually on the offensive, boldly giving advice to would-be health seekers and to the medical profession at large. They published prolifically in medical journals, joining anecdotes of regeneration with statistics on rainfall, temperature, and hours of sunshine. Subjective experience was conflated with quasi-scientific data, all to the point of illustrating the curative power of the climate and outdoor life.

With the prospect for success so apparent, the physicians were ready to blame the victim of consumption for failure. The health seekers who did not thrive had come West too late or lacked the will and courage to follow the proper routine. They stayed indoors too much or were unwilling to find a suitable outdoor occupation—or most flagrantly, returned East. Unwavering in their optimism, physicians cloaked their advice in moral injunctions. They replaced once vague instructions to travel West with specific orders on where to go and what to do. They represented themselves as models for emulation. It was not the treatment but the doctor that was heroic.[2]

The career of Dr. Samuel Edwin Solly, one of the most prominent physicians of Colorado Springs, exemplifies this phenomenon. Born and educated in England, Solly contracted consumption in 1863 at the age of eighteen. He interrupted his studies and went to stay in an "old country squire's place . . . riding his horses and drinking good port wine until I felt better." Then, like other European invalids, Solly traveled to Egypt, the French Riviera, and Switzerland. He regained sufficient health to return to school, carrying what would be a lifelong belief in the importance of "open-air exercise." He was healthy enough to get his medical diploma in 1867 from the Royal College of Physicians but shortly thereafter suffered a severe relapse. He recovered, only to have the symptoms of consumption reappear a few years later. In 1874, desperate to find a cure, Solly accepted an invitation from Palmer and Bell to visit Colorado Springs. He spent his days hunting and hiking and sleeping in the open air at Manitou, a few miles outside the center of town. Within a year Solly pronounced himself cured.[3]

He immediately began promoting the health-giving qualities of the site. His 1875 pamphlet, *Manitou, . . . Its Mineral Waters and Climate*, recounted his own progress and incorporated into the celebration of the Rockies the claims that such well-known European physicians as Hermann Weber were making for the Alps. "The greater dryness of mountain air acts beneficially in phthisis," he declared, "the air being rarefied, the *sun* which is always more constantly visible in mountainous districts has a *much greater influence* and enables the enfeebled invalid to spend several hours, almost daily, in the sunshine with very great advantage." Manitou, he insisted, had even more advantages than alpine villages. The town was so perfectly sheltered from winds and storms that "even on the shortest days of winter, there are at least six hours of warm sunshine." This combination of dry air and sunshine "*almost uninterruptedly and with sufficient power* . . . enable even the enfeebled invalid to enjoy outdoor exercise, without an additional wrap." And opportunities for outdoor exercise came in great variety. In summer there were "camping tours through the mountains with the attractions of fly fishing. . . . In the winter, the country around abounding in all varieties of game, invites the sportsman to harden his constitution by healthy exercise and exposure." In all, Solly justified "the high reputation that Colorado enjoys for the cure of phthisis." The climate and regimen would prolong the lives even of invalids who "had come out here as a *dernier resort*."[4]

Solly's pamphlet moved easily between medical tract and promotional literature. In addition to all its other virtues, the town was a "fashionable watering place," with several mineral springs, and it boasted "unusually luxurious accommodations." Not only was the wilderness vast and beautiful, but health seekers had access to "amusements" such as "bowling alleys, billiard saloons, croquet grounds and concert theatricals." Manitou, at least as Solly described it, was not a frontier outpost or even a primitive imitation of a European resort, but a spa that could appeal to the most demanding invalids.[5]

Solly's pamphlet attracted attention in the United States and England and was reviewed in the prestigious British medical journal *Lancet*, by none other than Hermann Weber. Just as Solly used Weber's observations to support his own findings, Weber, in turn, cited Solly's claims to confirm his clinical observations. Weber recounted how two young American consumptives had consulted him after failing to find a cure in either the European Alps or various seaside resorts; he recommended that they try Colorado, "of which I then had only heard as a new mountain region with a good climate." The results were astonishing, for several years later, when Weber examined them again, he found no trace of disease.[6]

As Manitou grew, so did Solly's practice. Within a decade he had become the most prominent physician in Colorado Springs, the doctor that health seekers sought out as soon as they arrived. To embellish his reputation and to keep a steady supply of migrants coming to the area, Solly accepted a commission from the county medical society and in 1883 published a second and still more elaborate pamphlet, *The Health Resorts of Colorado*

Springs. "Nine years ago," he observed in his preface, "I resigned the practice of medicine in England to try the influence of the Colorado climate upon my health, with satisfactory results, and the opinions and statements here advanced are founded upon my experience and observation as a practitioner of medicine in this locality."[7] Extolling the potency of the climate and the endless opportunities for outdoor exercise, Solly now also emphasized the importance of medical supervision. New arrivals should seek the services of a "resident physician" to instruct them in how to gain most from the region. Health seekers had to take care not to exercise too strenuously or follow the wrong diet. The general prescription to Go West was now shading into Go West and consult a knowledgeable physician/guide.[8]

Charles Denison was another physician who pronounced himself cured in Colorado. When he was twenty-six and beginning the practice of medicine in Chicago, he contracted consumption. Believing he faced imminent death, he decided in 1873 to go to Denver. The results were startling: "I took a journey and lived out of doors three or four months . . . sleeping on the ground . . . and getting so brown and strong that my friends did not know me when I returned." He gained weight and strength (riding forty miles a day) and was soon writing about his "personal experience" for the *Chicago Medical Examiner.* Denison urged health seekers to come to Colorado; like Solly, he, too, issued a series of more precise recommendations. "The change of residence from lowlands to this airy region," he informed his colleagues, "is of such a nature that an accurate knowledge of the character and varying influences of this climate is of special importance." Consumptives were to acclimate very slowly to the Rocky Mountains, for too fast an entry increased the possibility of hemorrhages. "The effect of the sudden rise coming though Kansas seemed quite decided to one who had, nearly a year before, a pulmonary hemorrhage, followed by chronic pneumonia." Drawing on this newly found expertise, Denison urged his colleagues in Chicago to send their consumptive patients to Denver—and to him. "A residence in this bracing climate has a peculiarly reviving influence on most phthisical patients who come here quite early in the progress of their disease."[9]

In short order, Denison was presenting papers at international medical conventions on the benefits to consumptives of residence in the Rocky Mountains. And in 1880, just seven years after he had arrived in Denver, he published his widely read book, *Rocky Mountain Health Resorts.* He, too, cited the findings of European physicians on the advantages of the Alps, buttressed them with anecdotes about his own cases, and added some physiological data to clinch the argument. By the time he was through, the Alps could hardly compete with the Rockies as a site for cure. "The most favorable climatic qualities, the coolness . . . and dryness of the air, the amount of sunshine and atmospheric electricity, are increasingly found with increasing elevation and distance from the sea; *the localization of the ideal climate* we have been seeking is rendered easy in the Rocky Mountain plains and foothills between the altitudes of four to eight thousand feet." Denison was confident that the dreaded disease had now become manageable: "Consumption has stages remediable by climate, and that the disease is more effectually arrested by that means than by any other, are very generally acknowledged. . . . There is a prolongation of life, health and happiness . . . for thousands of those who are destined, by inheritance, or acquired tendency, to die of consumption where they now live."[10]

Climate and atmosphere were not enough, however. The consumptive had to follow the proper regimen as set out by physicians. Left to themselves, health seekers might sit all day on a porch, thereby jeopardizing their recovery. In an earlier, more rugged era, it had not been so vital to emphasize this point. But now, the comforts of civilization, as exemplified by the railroad, required that the routine be planned. The model was the outdoors man—"There is no healthier life in the West"—and he instructed the health seeker to assemble the basic supplies (plates, pots, mattresses, and tents) and special clothing (warm flannels and buffalo robes), to hire a guide and spend their days "sketching, botanizing, geologizing, fishing or hunting, but always recuperating."[11]

The western physicians eagerly served as guides, leading camping and hunting trips for health seekers. It was a particularly attractive assignment because physicians could simultaneously sustain their practices and protect their own health. As Dr. Charles Gardiner of Colorado Springs, himself a former consumptive, recalled: "I had a sort of riding class which met every afternoon and rode over to Manitou, had some soda water, and rode back. . . . I saw to it that the consumptive had a gentle horse and we took it easy. . . . Once or twice some one would cough up some blood, and then we would hunt up a hack and send him home, the pony led behind, and . . . the rest of us continued on our merry way."[12]

Exercise was so important that physicians even offered advice on how to carry it out when confined to home. Denison devised a series of "artificial rules" for those too weak to go outdoors. "*Live as much as possible in the open air,*" he advised. Do "gymnastic work . . . with the windows open."[13] They also designed and endorsed special camping equipment for very frail invalids. Gardiner spent ten years developing a "sanatory tent" for consumptives, self-consciously modeled on the tepees of the Ute Indians who lived near Colorado Springs.[14]

With the stakes for both cure and profit so high, a fierce competition broke out among physicians promoting the special attributes of their own community. Each amassed meteorological data to demonstrate the advantages of the climate and boasted of the number of health seekers who had found a cure there. Indeed, the process fed on itself, for each time a physician cured his own consumption, he became an advocate for the particular location.

Take the case of Dr. Boyd Cornick. Practicing in a small Illinois town, he contracted consumption and in 1890 left for the Southwest to restore his health. He avoided Colorado, convinced that the colder climate and high altitude would not suit his constitution, and settled on West Texas (having heard stories of numerous cures). Almost immediately after his arrival, he began to gain weight and strength. "The Texas air I think beats any fattening compound I have tried for the last ten years," Cornick wrote to his wife. He also regaled her with tales of cures from other physicians he met there. The most compelling story was of an eastern physician. "They brought him here a dozen years ago on a shutter, not expecting him to live. Now he is hearty and well, has had no lung symptoms for eleven years, is interested in several business enterprises, is a successful land speculator and a candidate for the legislature. So you see what is liable to happen to me if I just stay in Texas long enough." He told her, too, about Dr. J. B. Taylor, a health officer from New York City, who came as a hacking consumptive, but now was "the picture of ruddy health and very emphatic in his insistence that Colorado won't do at all while Texas is the greatest health resort for consumption on the globe. . . . All his patients whom he formerly sent to Colorado died or had to leave on account of the high altitude." Taylor now also owned a 300,000-acre ranch.[15]

Cornick became an avid partisan of West Texas—"that this is a great country, my own experience and observation prove"—and set out to find the right town in which to build a practice. The search turned out to be a more frustrating task than curing his disease. Although nearby Fredericksburg and Kerrville were popular with health seekers, Cornick rejected both for each already had two physicians. Since "there is hardly any sickness . . . it seems like a fine country for a sick doctor, but for a well doctor the most profitable employment is undoubtedly land speculation." He then toured the region. At first, the "dryness" of El Paso enticed him, but he thought the altitude too low; he breathed freely in the "air of Sherwood," but the town was too remote for raising a family. Finally, when a retiring physician offered to sell him his practice in San Angelo, an elevated and dry town not too far from the military post of Fort Concho, Cornick decided to settle there.[16]

Cornick spelled out the virtues of the region to his consumptive friend Dr. Carl Schwalb in Colorado. Schwalb responded with accolades for Colorado. "I am pleased to learn that you are improving fast, and that you find the Texas climate so perfect," Schwalb wrote. "I find Colorado no less so; it answers all my expectations." The men exchanged meteorological data and anecdotes, which reinforced each in his commitment to his own particular region. "You seem afraid of Colorado's winters," Schwalb chided Cornick. "Yet there are plenty of physicians here, and Dr. Denison . . . a great authority on climate, is one of them that came here in the same condition as you and I, which I know because he told me himself when I consulted him last August. His looks do not betray the least sign of consumption, he rather looks stout; and his practice is large, his charges also ($10 for an examination)." The men agreed to disagree; Cornick in Texas, Schwalb in Colorado.[17]

The regional competition over cures filled the pages of medical journals in the closing decades of the nineteenth century, with biography constituting proof. Cornick contested the claims of Drs. Solly and Denison for Colorado in an 1893 article in the *Journal of the American Medical Association*. He insisted that a dry climate with a slight elevation (identical to that of San Angelo) was far more beneficial to consumptives than a high altitude. "When the progress of pulmonary phthisis is arrested at a high altitude," Cornick argued, "this fortunate result is in no degree attributable to, but occurs in spite of the altitude." He cited as evidence his own experience and that of his cured patients.[18] By the same token, Dr. Mark Rodgers celebrated the curative climate of Tucson. Practicing in Philadelphia, he had suffered from a persistent cough and experienced two hemorrhages from the lungs. Within a year of going to Tucson, Rodgers had gained twenty-six pounds and pronounced himself cured.[19]

The testimonials of physicians led to endorsements for almost every conceivable set of climatic conditions. Warm moist air, dry cold air, warm dry air—all were promoted as curative. If the location was known to have damp mornings, the physician focused on the hours of sunshine and the purity of the air. So San Diego's doctors insisted that the "coast fogs" need not interfere with outdoor activities. "The fog bank usually rolls in about night-fall and disappears a few hours after sunrise. . . . There may be two or three days on which the fog will be more persistent, and a fine mist may last until 12:30 . . . but this only perhaps a half dozen days out of the year."[20]

The shared belief in the efficacy of climate and sharp rivalry among regions lead to the formation of the American Climatological Association (ACA) in 1883. Its mission was to serve as both scientific clearinghouse and travel agency. The association wanted to encourage "the study of climatology and the diseases of the respiratory organs," and then make its findings available to "the general profession for every-day use." Frederick Knight, a Boston physician, explained its aim at the opening meeting. He warned that to "revive and further a knowledge of climatology," without providing practical information on the network of resorts for health seekers, "can accomplish comparatively little." Knight urged members to supply not only precise meteorological data on their favored locations but detailed information on "ways of travel and the accommodations . . . after arrival." He also noted that while American communities were fiercely competitive, they had a common interest in improving the position of the United States as against Europe. "I hope that our health resorts may gradually approximate those of Europe in comfort and luxury," he concluded, "so that our patients will no longer look forward to a visit to those of Europe with pleasure, and to a visit to our own as a kind of banishment to be endured for the sake of health."[21]

The plea notwithstanding, the ACA meetings were marked by more discord than unity. Let a physician exalt the efficacy of the climate of southern California, and the others would immediately impugn the claims. Meanwhile, as physicians and health seekers reported cures in climates as diverse as San Diego, Colorado Springs, and El Paso, it became harder to make the case for one particular region as the ideal place for all consumptives. As a result, physicians began to emphasize routine over climate. New York's prominent physician Dr. Austin Flint expressed this view in his widely read textbook, *The Principles and Practices of Medicine*. "I would rank exercise and out-of-door life far above any known remedies for the cure of the disease. There are grounds for believing that the advantage of a change of climate mainly consists of its being subsidiary to a change of habits as regards exercise and out-of-door life." While such advice reduced the import of any single location, it did enhance the authority of the physician: *where* the health seeker went was becoming less important than the physician he consulted.[22]

The regional competition also focused greater attention on the quality of the housing arrangements. Knight began his discussion of "the selection of a climate" with a disclaimer. "I wish it to be distinctly understood," he declared in the *Boston Medical and Surgical Journal*, "that I am giving simply my own convictions . . . based upon twenty years experience, and that I do not claim that the principles which guide me are by any means universally accepted by climatologists." Accordingly, "if I designate any special places for residence, it is because they offer some accommodation and are well known, but of course it will be understood that there are scores of similarly situated regions which would answer just as well as far as climatic conditions are concerned."[23]

Perhaps most important, the squabbles over the ideal climate and the growing importance of the physician enabled many communities, whatever their climate, to present themselves as curative locales. Accordingly, eastern physicians, who had first sent invalids South and then later sent health seekers West, now began to consider keeping them closer to home. They probably knew some consumptives who had been cured without traveling and an even greater number who had migrated and not been cured. It seemed, then, altogether appropriate to begin to challenge the claims of others as they put forward their own. By 1885 regions that had once been considered positively dangerous for consumptives, specifically the Adirondacks, now joined the roster of recommended places.

One set of claims came from Dr. Dio Lewis of Boston. Although not an invalid himself, Lewis had spent years traveling with his wife in search of a curative climate, which earned him the authority to pronounce on treatment. After spending a winter in California, Lewis grew impatient with the endless anecdotes of cure, most particularly because the region had little effect on Mrs. Lewis's health. Convinced that the tales were self-serving, Lewis insisted that New England had much to recommend it. "Hundred of persons in California," he declared, "suffering from various forms of chronic invalidism, have found in the New England climate a vitalizing sanitarium. . . . I can fill this volume with the recital of cases . . . of sick persons residing in California who were cured by camping out." And "camping can be as well managed in New England as in California."[24]

The most influential voice for the Adirondacks came from Alfred Loomis, a prominent New York physician who found his cure there. A contemporary of Solly and Denison, Loomis also came from a family with a long history of consumption. ("I am the only representative of my own family," Loomis noted in 1889. "All my relatives have died of phthisis—father, mother, sisters, and brothers.") His own battle with the disease began in 1867 right after his appointment as lecturer in physical diagnosis at the Columbia College of Physicians and Surgeons. Although convinced that he "would not survive beyond thirty," he went to the Adirondack wilderness to try to restore his health. "Before the summer months had passed, I came out . . . free from cough, with an increase in weight of about twenty pounds, with greater physical vigor than I had known for years." Within six months, he reported, I "overcame my [hereditary] tendency" and assumed the lectureship at Columbia.[25]

Even as his practice expanded and his health remained robust, Loomis returned to the Adirondack woods every summer—"I very naturally became an enthusiast in regard to them." In 1879 he delivered a paper to the Medical Society of the State of New York encouraging colleagues to send consumptives to the region. It was not an easy sell for its climate was neither mild, uniform, nor dry. The rainfall averaged fifty-five inches a year, and even its staunchest supporters conceded that it had only two seasons, winter and July. But Loomis maintained that the total amount of rainfall was less critical than the porousness of the area's "sieve-like" soil. Because it soaked up the rain, the dampness did not linger in the air. Still more important, it was not the "hot or cold air, damp or dry air, but *pure* air which is necessary to diseased lungs." Finally, the Adirondacks, during both winter and summer, afforded opportunity for exercise and a "camp or tent life in the open air. . . . The very surroundings infuse new life into the feeble body, and one daily grows stronger and stronger and feels better, scarcely able to tell how or why." By 1879 fourteen of Loomis's patients had wintered in the Adirondacks, and some of them had been cured.[26]

One of the very first invalids that Loomis persuaded to go to the Adirondacks for the winter was Dr. Edward Livingston Trudeau, destined to become the most renowned figure in the history of tuberculosis in the United States. Loomis frequently cited Trudeau's stay in promoting the region to health seekers, and it was his referrals that enabled Trudeau to open and maintain a practice in the Adirondacks. Indeed, Trudeau made the Adirondacks almost as desirable a destination for consumptives as Denver or Pasadena.

Trudeau's tale of resurrection duplicated the accounts of his western counterparts. He, too, was the living proof of the efficacy of his cure, the difference being that he lived an outdoor life in New York rather than in Colorado or California. Later, in the period 1900–1920, Trudeau would become the most noted advocate for sanatoriums and an institutional method of care and cure. But in this earlier period, he was as enthusiastic about the therapeutic benefits of climate and outdoor life as any of the physician-health seekers.*

Trudeau believed he had inherited his passion for outdoor living, hunting, and camping from his father, Dr. James Trudeau, who had abandoned both his medical practice and his family (shortly after the birth of Edward) to join the westward expeditions of John James Audubon and John Fremont. Edward's image of his father came from a large oil painting in which he appeared dressed in a buckskin suit that was supposedly a gift from the Osage Indians with whom he had lived for two years. James Trudeau appeared a dashing and commanding figure, brimming with prowess and confidence, a man as much at home in a tepee as in a hospital. Fluent in French and English as well as the language of the Osages, he seemed to the son who never knew him at once urbane and virile, cosmopolitan and rustic. Edward always presumed that his own legacy from his father included not only a "passion for the wild out of doors existence" but a "strong leaning toward medicine," and around these two elements he built his life.[27]

If he ever had any hesitations about becoming a doctor, the death of his older brother from consumption in 1867, when Edward was nineteen years

*Although many people use the terms sanitarium and sanatorium interchangeably, they had quite separate meanings in the nineteenth century. A sanitarium was a health resort; a sanatorium was a medical institution established for the treatment of tuberculosis. It is this latter usage that will be followed in this study.

old, swept them aside. He enrolled at the Columbia College of Physicians and Surgeons, but was not a strong student. He was not well prepared academically, and the lectures, which he considered overly didactic, bored him. Nevertheless, he persevered, graduated in 1871, and shortly afterward married Lotte Baere, a clergyman's daughter. The next year, he suddenly began to suffer from fevers and inertia and, upon examination, learned that he too had consumption, "that most fatal of diseases." He and his wife immediately went to Aiken, South Carolina: "I had been told to live out of doors and ride on horseback." Two months later, more feverish and emaciated than when he left, he returned to New York. A friend, Lou Livingston, suggested that the two of them go up to the Adirondacks. Trudeau agreed, and in June 1873, leaving his wife and two small children home, he went to spend several months in that "rough inaccessible region . . . [and] most inclement and trying climate." "If I had but a short time to live," he later wrote, "I yearned for surroundings that appealed to me, and it seemed to meet a longing I had for rest and the peace of the great wilderness." The first part of the journey was comfortable enough, in a Pullman coach to Plattsburg, at the edge of the Adirondack region. There the tracks stopped, and the adventure began. Trudeau and Livingston hired a "two-horse stage-wagon, put a board between the seats, and with a mattress and a couple of pillows arranged me so that I could lie down all the way quite comfortably." Thus they traveled the rutted roads, arriving at dusk at Paul Smith's, a small and unimposing hotel. Trudeau was carried up two flights of steps by a guide ("one of the most splendid, sturdy specimens of manhood I have ever seen"), who observed as he placed Trudeau on the bed: "Why, Doctor you don't weigh no more than a dried lamb-skin!"[28]

As it turned out, Smith's was clean and cheerful. Mrs. Smith was an excellent cook, and the fresh wholesome food (including brook trout) gave Trudeau an appetite. Most important, the guides who "swarmed" around were eager to serve him. The very next morning a guide came into Trudeau's room and told him that "he had fixed the boat 'comfortable' with balsam boughs and blankets so that I could lie down in it, had put my rifle in, and if I felt up to it we could row down of the river . . . 'kind of slow' and see what we could see." Trudeau was delighted: "My hunting blood responded at once and I was soon in the boat." The weather was a "beautiful sunny June day, the sky and water were blue" and lying comfortably on his bed of boughs, the invalid-hunter spotted two deer. "I never sat up, but rested my rifle on the side of the boat and fired at the buck who, after a few jumps, fell dead at the edge of the woods." The guide loaded the buck on board, and the "triumphant" hunter was rowed back to the hotel, convinced that he would be cured.[29]

A splendid summer followed. Almost every morning Trudeau headed down to the lake, at first to be rowed about by a guide, then, as his strength returned, to row alone. Within three months he was a specimen of health. "I was sunburned, had gained fifteen pounds in weight." Before going home, he wanted a photograph, one that would evoke the oil painting of his father and his outdoor regimen. He headed into the woods dressed in hunting clothes. Rifle between his legs, Trudeau struck his pose for the photographer: an intense gaze into the distance as if watching and listening for a deer. The photograph was so prized that he inserted it years later into his autobiography, with the caption, "Dr. Trudeau, the Huntsman (1873) Three Months after Arrival at Paul Smith's."[30]

The photograph was emblematic of Trudeau's near obsession with hunting clothes. Throughout his professional career, he wore this outfit to examine patients. Even after white coats became the standard attire for physicians, Trudeau refused to discard "the knickerbockers and leather leggings of hunting days." In this garb he began a new life and earned his right to prescribe it for others.[31]

For all the gains he made that summer, Trudeau was far from cured. Soon after he returned to New York, "his old symptoms returned." Disappointed at this relapse, he decided to spend the winter in St. Paul, Minnesota, where other health seekers had apparently found a cure. But he made few gains that winter, and in the spring, "nearly as sick as the year before," he came to view the Adirondacks as "my only hope." In June 1874 he took his wife, two children, and two nurses to Paul Smith's.[32] There he met Alfred Loomis, who confirmed that Trudeau was in a "most debilitated state ... anaemic, emaciated, had daily hectic fever, constant cough and profuse purulent expectorations." Loomis advised him to remain in the Adirondacks for the winter. Trudeau hesitated, knowing the climate and having been "repeatedly warned that such a step would prove fatal." But seeing no alternative, he complied. He returned to New York periodically, but each time the symptoms reappeared, and he headed back to Paul Smith's to find relief.[33]

These regenerative experiences turned Trudeau into the keenest of advocates for the Adirondacks. The range was "surrounded by a zone of pure air" so that "diseased lungs are supplied with a specially vitalized and purified atmosphere, free from germs and impurities of any kind, and laden with the resinous exhalations of myriads of evergreens." Trudeau encouraged other invalids to follow his path. "My own personal experience and my personal observation of other phthisical invalids lead me to say that any comparison of the relative good effects of the climate of St. Paul, Minn. or of the South with that of the Adirondack region is decidedly in favor of the latter. . . . Camping out, which is the peculiar feature of this place . . . [is] an important and beneficial measure in the treatment of phthisis." The preferred arrangement was for the consumptive to arrive in June and spend four months out-of-doors, breathing the pure air and eating good food. But winter had it positive attributes as well. "Exposure in inclement weather, which this mode of life at times renders almost unavoidable, is well borne in this climate by phthisical invalids who steadily live out of doors. . . . I have seen men in camp lose their cough and gain in flesh, while it rained daily, and in the midst of occasional frosts and snowstorms." Insofar as Trudeau, Loomis, and a goodly number of eastern physicians were concerned, Go West had now become Go North.[34]

By the 1880s, then, a distinctive American system for the treatment of consumption had emerged. Whether the case in point was Colorado, California, or the Adirondacks, Americans shared a commitment to what was known as "open health resorts." These resorts constituted a spectrum of housing and camping options, ranging from boardinghouses, hotels, and private homes to ranches and camps. [35] A region and a routine, not an institution or a physician, held the key to cure. To be sure, American doctors were beginning to assume a greater importance in the daily lives of health seekers and some of the resorts were becoming more exclusive. But as yet, space, and not the doctor, counted for most.

11

The Western Narrative

THE NARRATIVES OF ILLNESS IN THE PERIOD 1860–90 WERE SHAPED BY the promotional literature of the western boosters and the testimonials of its physicians. They differed in a number of ways from those of the antebellum New England invalids. In both tone and outlook, the western narratives were far more secular and less introspective than their earlier counterparts. There were no poignant soliloquies on repentance or reaffirmations of faith. The western narratives also blurred the distinctions between the entrepreneur and health seeker. The two often moved westward in tandem in search of fortune. The New England invalids had written of vicarious undertakings, such as sea voyages, or of efforts to do good, whether for the heathen, the sailor, or the slave. The westerners, on the other hand, were attracted by the veins of minerals waiting to be chipped out of unclaimed hills as well as by the prospect of renewed health. Theirs was a physical odyssey, not a spiritual one.

George Weeks's autobiography, *California Copy*, exemplifies this new genre. The portrait that Weeks chose for his frontispiece was that of a health seeker in the guise of a civilized mountain man. Weeks stares confidently into the camera, robust, healthy, and thoroughly acclimated to outdoor living. But he had not always been so sturdy. Born in 1851 on a small subsistence farm in northern New York State, his childhood was one of poverty and abuse. His mother died when he was five (probably of consumption), and he was raised by a "stern and unloving" stepmother. In 1865, after an "unmerciful thrashing due to a false accusation," Weeks, with nine dollars to his name and the "worn and patched clothes on my smarting and aching back," ran away from home. He found a job as a mule tender on the Erie

Canal, and later through the intervention of a kindly barge captain, employment in a printing office in a nearby town. After several years he moved to New York City to become a typesetter for the *New York World* and soon had a regular paycheck, a devoted wife, and several small children.[1]

In 1875, at the age of twenty-four, Weeks began to suffer from "violent and prolonged fits of coughing," pains in his side, and profuse night sweats. He consulted Dr. Austin Flint, who warned him "never under any circumstances" to return to long hours of indoor labor. Flint also dispensed state-of-the-art medical advice: "Young man, if you care to live more than five or six months longer, you will leave this city as soon as possible and go to a warmer climate—to Florida or to California."[2]

Like generations of invalids before him, Weeks chose his destination, and the numerous testimonials of wonderful cures in California impressed him. Weeks read Charles Nordhoff's book, *California for Health, Pleasure, and Residence*; its descriptions of ranches in the San Bernadino Mountains catering to consumptives appealed to him. To finance his journey, he collected funds from family, friends, and fellow employees and, leaving his wife and children behind, he booked passage, first on a ship to Panama, then on a train across the isthmus, and finally on a steamer to San Francisco. (This roundabout route was recommended by Flint, who urged him to avoid a transcontinental train ride during the winter months.)

By the time Weeks set sail, his health had deteriorated further, and he spent most of his time on ship either in his bunk or on an "improvised couch" on the upper deck. When the steamer docked in San Francisco several months later, Weeks was still feeble and ailing. He mustered enough strength to visit a booking agency that found him lodging at a ranch—more accurately, a boardinghouse in a sparsely settled region in the San Bernadino Mountains. Weeks had to go first to Los Angeles and then take a long ride in a "dilapidated" stagecoach. Although exhausted by the final leg of the journey, the sights and smells of the orchards that lined the road convinced him he had entered "Paradise." "Mile after mile covered [and] never a minute of monotony or weariness. . . . The perfumed, life-laden air was so grateful to my weakened lungs, rasped and worn by the harsh winds of the Atlantic coast outdoors and the unsanitary atmosphere of the composing room that there was no opportunity for weariness." By the time he arrived at the ranch, Weeks was sure he would find health in California.[3]

Within a month, Weeks was strong enough to begin exploring the region. On one excursion he met a struggling rancher and beekeeper who needed an assistant to collect honey; in return for his room and board, Weeks became a "chore-man" and "commenced my outdoor life under healthful conditions." After a few months and a "steady gain in health," he heard about an abandoned vineyard, secured a claim to it, planted more vines and cultivated bees. In short order, he accumulated enough health and money to send for his family.[4]

Weeks's narrative exemplified the drama of rebirth in the West. On board the ship that took him to California, Weeks had met a Mr. Van Tassell. Apparently, Van Tassell and the other passengers were convinced that Weeks's chances of survival were so slim that they had placed bets on whether he would die during the voyage. Years later, Weeks bumped into Van Tassell in California and when Van Tassell realized that the six-foot, one-hundred-and-seventy-pound man facing him was George Weeks, a "look of astonishment, incredulity, and wonder passed over his face." "'How did you do it?' Van Tassell asked. 'I would like to know so that I may advise others.'" To which the triumphant Weeks replied: "That is easy. . . . Life in the open air, hard work, plain food, and plenty of sleep."[5]

Not only in their published writings but also in their letters back home, the health seekers boasted of their newfound virility. "The climate here is all it is described," D. M. Berry, one of the founders of Pasadena, California, wrote to his sister Helen. "I can climb mountains or hunt in chaparral all day and be well and strong at night. At Indianapolis I had to ride to the office in the street cars. My weight is a half a dozen pounds increased." Lest Helen think he was exaggerating, he assured her that his experience was not unique. "One man who came here with me in August, bleeding at the lungs . . . has become fat and strong."[6]

Just how many health seekers found a cure in the West cannot be known—the epidemiological data and mortality statistics do not exist. But the narratives of successes were so dramatic and exemplary that they effectively concealed the failures. And undoubtedly a goodly number of those who went west achieved their dreams. In the course of only a few days, Berry met several Harvard graduates who had become not only healthy but also wealthy. One lawyer from Boston was growing rich from the produce of his vineyard and fat from living out-of-doors.[7] By the 1880s the number of health seekers turned citrus growers was so large that residents of Pasadena maintained: "They came to cough and remained to spray."[8]

Dwight Heard was another spectacular success. Like that of many health seekers, his early life was marked by poverty and parental death from consumption—his father died of the disease in 1876 when Dwight was thirteen. Through the aid of a distant relative Dwight moved to Chicago, became a clerk in a hardware store, and married the owner's daughter. In 1893, he evinced the first symptoms of consumption. He took his guidance from the anecdotes of cure, went west, and purchased a ranch in Phoenix. In short order, he organized a vast irrigation project on the Salt River Valley, turned the area into a farmer's paradise, and made his fortune.[9]

* * *

The narratives promised westward-bound migrants that they would be warmly greeted by other settlers, and they were. No one refused to share a compartment on a train with a coughing consumptive and no boarding-house keeper turned him away. "Several consumptives have come here who have been totally unfit for work, and almost totally without means," the editor of the *Colorado Springs Gazette* reported in 1873. "But they are drowning men catching at straws, and are worthy of sincerest sympathy. . . . We must endeavor to bear the burden of those who are amongst us, and seek to relieve their pressing necessities."[10] This sympathetic attitude meant that well into the 1890s the most frail and least hopeful health seekers did not conceal their symptoms—not in their narratives and not in their daily encounters. As one resident observed, "They don't hesitate to inform you, that they are consumptive, and that they wish to live through a winter in order to give the climate a chance to do them some good."[11]

For all the enthusiasm, some of the narratives of illness betray a darker aspect of living with consumption. The West that many of them found was cruder than the promotional literature suggested. Brochures depicted well-designed and spacious resort hotels with airy, well-ventilated rooms, spacious porches (to ensure sunshine all day), and extensive grounds. But the reality sometimes turned out to be wooden shacks in the midst of a remote and barren plot of land, where only sagebrush and rocks dotted the landscape. The lure of the West was so potent and the health seekers so desperate that few of them investigated the accuracy of the claims in advance. But their disappointment in the accommodations they found was keen, all the more so because it was the first indication that the anecdote of cure might not be accurate.[12]

George Weeks, for example, had expected from both Charles Nordhoff's book and his conversations with the booking agent that he would be living in a handsome sanitarium in the San Bernardino Mountains. The facility turned out to be a two-story farmhouse on a barren plot. And instead of spacious, open rooms, Weeks discovered poorly ventilated "cubicles," each large enough to hold "one half-size bed, one washstand, one small bureau, one set of hooks for hanging clothes, one tallow candle and one emaciated invalid of the scarecrow style."[13]

Alfred Bacon, who had booked a room on a ranch before he left New York, was stunned when the stagecoach driver stopped before a "desolate building." Since there was no one there to greet him, Bacon "opened the door and entered the squalid room . . . [which] contained only a table, a bench, a broken stove, two bunks and a miscellaneous stack of provisions in the corner." It was not until dusk that the only other inhabitant of the ranch, a sheep herder, who was to be Bacon's sole companion during his cure, returned with his flock. Whatever else it was, this ranch was not a resort. Bacon soon learned he was responsible for all the chores, and his outdoor life consisted of herding sheep.[14]

All too often, particularly for men with few economic resources, a regimen of outdoor living consisted of working as a hired man, with tasks that were often beyond their physical capacity. Health seeking then became eking out a living under difficult conditions. "They seek some lonely bee rancher's hut in the mountains," Jennie Collier, who accompanied her consumptive brother-in-law, reported, "where they are welcome to stay if they will furnish their own bed, do their own cooking and look after themselves generally. A well man may be able to stand such a life but a sick man finds his own cooking unpalatable, a mattress on the floor not 'a downy bed of ease,' and mountain air, however delicious, not a substitute for thoughtful care and smiling faces."[15]

Other invalids lacked the hardiness to cultivate bees or care for a small grove of orange trees. "The most popular plan," Collier wrote back to Iowa from Pasadena, was "buying a small place with a cow, a horse, a chicken coop and a strawberry bed staked on it, all interspersed with a few orange or lemon trees." But as one health seeker recalled: "My hands blistered, my feet got sore, my knees knocked together, often I had to stand fifteen or twenty minutes coughing and gasping for breath, every bone in my body ached, occasionally I caved in and went home." Indeed, many partially planted vineyards and orange groves were for sale, precisely because their owners died before they could carry out their plans. As George Weeks noted, they "had waited too long before coming to this land of New Lungs."[16]

Everywhere in the West newly arrived health seekers were put off by the large number of consumptives who were closer to death than life. "Oh! What a lot of coughing suffering mortals are coming here," Berry declared. "Many too late. One man died in sight of the harbor." Weeks had imagined his companions would be active, vigorous, optimistic. Much to his disappointment, they were forlorn and enervated. Lacking the energy to exercise daily, they languished on the porch on sunny days and huddled around the single fireplace in the sitting room on rainy ones. Since the partitions between the rooms were so thin and the other boarders so sick, Weeks complained about being kept awake all night by "an almost constant chorus of coughs" and listening all day to talk of pains, coughs, and fever.[17]

Indeed western cities and towns had an army of coughing men whose demeanor and conversation contradicted the myth. "At every street corner," noted a health seeker in Los Angeles, "I met a poor fellow croaking like myself." Wherever he went, he encountered "a community [of men] with broken lungs in all stages" who spoke of nothing else but their ailments. "'Well, how do you feel today? Did you have a good night? . . . Do you cough much now?'" And the view from his window was no less distressing. "At the boarding house opposite ours, one would come on to the porch muffled in shawls, a parchment face and sunken eyes, cough, cough, cough, leaning over the hand-rail another fellow with spindle legs and shrunken form; another joins them, and still another, feebly walking to and fro, alive to save funeral expenses."[18]

Pasadena was no different. Collier wrote home about health seekers "of every possible shade of ghostliness. . . . We meet them constantly marching about the streets with a certain aimless unsteadiness which says plainer than words that hope has well nigh died out of their hearts." Her visit to the post office when mail from the East was due was most unnerving. "These poor wanderers driven from home by failing health, congregate about the doors, sit coughing upon the steps or lean against the walls with eager anxious faces, waiting, hoping for letters from home." Daily encounters with disease and death marked life in these communities. As Collier concluded, "A large proportion of the sick we meet with here never find health this side of the river of death."[19]

A physician occasionally also cast doubt on the myth, wondering whether living in primitive conditions was the ideal way to a cure. "The average ranch house," Samuel Fisk maintained in 1884, "is a miserable shanty, out on the plains, away from neighbors, where the usual diet is bacon floating in grease . . . molasses and coffee without milk." And the daily regimen often presented difficulties for invalids. "Ranch life," Fisk warned, "is necessarily somewhat rough and usually monotonous, and when it comes to herding sheep, even a vigorous man, new at the business, finds it most irksome and fatiguing."[20]

At least some among the health seekers realized that they would never experience the miracle of cure and hastened their own death. The high numbers of suicides in the towns popular among health seekers attest to the magnitude of the disappointment. In Santa Barbara, California, the suicide rate in 1893 was thirty per hundred thousand, among the highest in the world. That same year, one out of every three deaths in the town was due to tuberculosis.[21]

Why did this grimmer reality not subvert to the myth? Why were westerners so tolerant of the sick and dying? The answer, in part, rests in the number of people who had either a financial or an emotional stake in perpetuating the myth. Promoters eager to sell their land and physicians to enhance their practice had no incentive to burst the bubble. Nor would those lucky ones who had found their health in the West.[22] The only concession was to say that the chances for cure were greatest for those in the early stages of the disease and for those who gradually acclimated to outdoor living. "The sick come here too late," Dr. Charles Denison observed in 1880, "or having arrived, attempt so much more than their strength will permit, that all the good effects of the climate are counteracted." But such advice was hardly an adequate preparation for the reality that so many health seekers experienced.[23]

The change from sea voyage to western settlement, from a winter's stay in the West Indies to beginning a new life in the West, enhanced the ability of women to carry out the new health-seeking prescription. So too, the development of towns planned to accommodate families made it easier for women with consumption to migrate West. In this way, traditional medical prescriptions became somewhat less gender specific. Pasadena, California, for example, was from its inception a collective undertaking of a group of Indiana families in which husband or wife or both were consumptive. "We found," one health seeker reported in 1883, "that the majority of the inhabitants were here primarily because of poor health, either on their own part or of some member of the family." Sierra Madre was another such community. Lucy Sprague Mitchell, who would become a leading educator, joined her parents when they settled there in an effort to cure her father. She soon reported that she and her mother were the only people in town who did not have the disease.[24]

Some women did find a cure through an outdoor life and enthusiastically recommended it to others of their sex. Beatrice Harraden became a lemon grower in San Diego, a life-style, she believed, that restored her health. Together with William Edwards, a prominent physician in San Diego and himself a successful health seeker, she coauthored an advice book for consumptives that devoted a chapter to outdoor life for women. "A woman can find a great deal of satisfactory and useful work on a ranch," they wrote. "She can pick the lemons, oranges, olives, apricots, or peaches; she can sucker the trees; she can undertake the anxious task of pruning. She can superintend the curing of olives and lemons, and see after the packing and dispatching of the fruit." Other women repeated the same message. "I regard fruit culture," a woman rancher maintained, "a very healthful and paying occupation, especially for women who have children, boys in particular, growing up to assist them."[25]

The tales of women who found health through an outdoor life filtered back East and by the late 1880s influenced the prescriptions of even conservative physicians. In his widely read book *Doctor and Patient*, published in 1887, S. Weir Mitchell wrote a chapter praising "out-door and camp-life for women." He acknowledged that he had been in error thinking that this routine was suitable and appropriate only for men and wanted to "correct my error of omission." Mitchell reported a case of a "sick and very nervous woman" whom he had not been able to restore to health. "At last I said to her, 'If you were a man I think I could cure you.' I then told her how in that case I would ask a man to live." The woman agreed to undergo the "male" routine.

With an intelligent companion, she secured two well-known trusty guides, and pitched her camp by the lonely waters of a Western lake in May. . . . With two good wall-tents for sleeping and sitting rooms . . . she began to make her experiment. . . . Before August came she could walk for miles with a light gun, and could stand for hours in wait for a deer. . . . In a word, she led a man's life until the snow fell in the fall and she came back to report, a thoroughly well woman.[26]

Nevertheless, social norms still limited women's ability to go West for health. In 1880 Charles Denison calculated that of the 202 health seekers who consulted him in Colorado Springs, only 54 were women. "This," he maintained, "is due greatly to the facility with which men can leave home, take long journeys, and submit themselves to the life of 'roughing it.'" Nine years later when Samuel Fisk, a Denver physician, sampled the records of those who consulted him, he reported that only 14 of 90 were women. These findings were confirmed by casual observers. "Since coming here we have met more invalid men than women," Collier told her parents. "It is more probable that men are more disposed to seek a change of climate for health than women. When a man is no longer able to attend to business—if he can command the money—he travels. But a woman can manage her household as long as she is able to breathe, and as a rule she prefers an irrepressible kind of suicide to leaving home."[27]

Even women who did make the move West did not always adopt the medically recommended regimen. Mothers with children frequently allowed household chores to take precedence over outdoor exercise. "I know of a man who brought his wife to Denver for her health," a journalist informed readers of the *Colorado Springs Gazette*. "She needs recreation that the climate may have full opportunity to exert its influence. . . . There is no virtue in merely being here. If individuals have ever recovered from disease, it is largely because they were so situated that they could be out of doors a great deal." This sense that women were wasting a precious opportunity appeared in the narratives of health seekers. "There is no doubt whatsoever," Edwards and Harraden contended, "that it is a mistake, if not a cruelty, to bring delicate women to ranch life, unless there are ample means to pay the very large sum asked and given for household help. It is absurd to talk of the advantages of any climate from Dan to Beersheba itself, if a woman is to be weighed down by hard physical work, such as house-cleaning and washing and baking." The ideal solution for a female consumptive was to hire a strong and healthy woman to do the indoor labor while she regained her health through outdoor living.[28]

Given the responsibilities that typically kept married women at home, it was single women (some never married, others widows) who were most able to head West. The narrative of illness of Helen Hunt Jackson, the daughter of Deborah Vinal Fiske, reveals the process at work. Her mother's letters had documented how a network of female invalids supported and comforted each other within the community. Helen's letters, as well as her essays and novels, illustrate how new social and economic considerations made it easier for single women to become health seekers in the West.

Consumption, the threat of early death, and the indignities of being an orphan beholden to others shaped Helen's life. After her mother's death in 1844 and her father's increasing emotional and physical debilitation, Helen lost her home and, as she later wrote, her "birthright." Until her marriage in 1852, she was a "wanderer," living in eleven different households and boarding schools. Although she tried to meet the expectations of her relative-hosts and profess her faith, she was never able to conform to their satisfaction or comply with the constraints of the orthodox religion that structured their daily routine. As her mother had feared, she became an unwelcome guest.

During her adolescence Helen's energy was consumed by two lengthy and protracted battles: one against zealous proselytizing relatives who were determined to force her to submit to God, the other against recurring coughs and colds. Her mother's death, she recognized, "was the event which showed me only too plainly that my heart was still unreconciled. . . . I tremble sometimes when I think of the bitterness and opposition which raged in my spirit, as I saw my dear mother's form laid under the cold wet snow. But still I clung for a few months to my groundless hope. Then at last I gave it up in despair."[29]

In the fall of 1844, when Helen was fourteen, her sore throats and coughs were so persistent that the family physician persuaded her father to remove her from boarding school. But since Nathan was too frail himself to give her a home in Amherst, he sent her to Falmouth, to live with Deborah's dearest cousin, Martha Hooker. Nathan thought the change of climate and the routine of the Hooker household would benefit Helen, but the decision was disastrous. Martha's husband, Henry Hooker, a Congregational minister, was determined to have Helen profess her faith; when persuasion failed, he tried to humiliate her into submission. "The last winter that I was there a revival commenced in Uncle Hooker's society," Helen reported.

I was so opposed to it that Uncle H. felt it to be his duty to withdraw me in a measure from society, on account of my influence. This galled me, provoked me, and at the same time frightened me. I was shocked at the depth of my hatred to the cause of Christ. . . . I strove in vain to conceal all that I felt. As soon as Uncle Hooker found out what was passing in my mind, he took every means possible to increase my anxiety. He talked with me, hour after hour, all to the effect that I was the most depraved of all sinners, was in the most imminent peril etc. etc. until . . . I was fairly frightened into what I thought an actual submission of my own will and a resolution to become a Christian.

When Helen realized that it was terror and not a love of Christ that was leading her to submit, she left the Hooker household, but the ill will the battle engendered alienated Helen not only from the Hookers but also from the rest of her Vinal relatives.[30]

With no kin willing to provide her a home, in February 1847 at the age of sixteen, Helen enrolled in the Ipswich Academy, an institution headed by Eunice Caldwell, a friend of Deborah's.[31] From the start Helen complained about its isolated setting. "Nothing happens here from morning till night," she wrote to her cousin Ann. "Nobody dies, nobody gets married, nobody comes, nobody goes, nobody does anything as far as I have been able to judge, but keep themselves as much as possible out of sight and hearing of all the rest of creation."[32] Nevertheless, the academic program was stimulating, and Helen proudly wrote her father about her growing proficiency in the classical languages he had studied and loved. She longed to demonstrate to him her ability to translate Latin poetry, but during her first term at Ipswich, Nathan, in an advanced state of consumption, set out for Palestine on a final journey for health. Helen, for all her familiarity with the disease, was totally unprepared for his death. In July 1847 she received a package containing her mother's carefully bound and sorted letters, her father's diary, and a short note informing her of his death. "No words can describe the sensations of loneliness, disappointment, and discouragement which weighed down my spirit," she later wrote. "I felt that I had now no motive to *do* or even to *live*." The next year was a "painful dream." Helen, filled with remorse and raging at her loss, tried one last time to profess her faith. In this process she found some "consolation" but later believed "that it was more because I felt that such a course would please him, than anything else."[33]

After her father's death, Helen was unwilling to remain at Ipswich and asked her grandfather, David Vinal, to bring her back to Boston. There, unable to make new friends and unwilling to see old ones, she remained essentially alone, irritated by a banal daily routine. "I can sew, read, write or practice my self," she complained. "This routine can be varied by a walk . . . or *by breaking the lamp shades*."[34]

In 1849 Helen received an offer from John S. C. Abbott, the author of the best-selling guides to child rearing that her mother had so admired, to become an assistant teacher at a boarding school that he and his brother ran for young ladies in New York City. Helen accepted immediately. "Never, since my own home was closed, have I been in any situation where *home* influences in all their sacredness and strength were so binding on my heart." She conceded that although her relatives had been "very kind," there had "always been a *wall*" between her and them. "It has been *my* fault, I do not doubt," but the result was "a *separation, a want of congeniality, an utter impossibility* of sympathy which has made me sad, *how* sad you cannot know, which has often made me weep, simply because I was 'all alone.'"[35]

In New York, Helen's spirits improved, and the lively and cheerful woman that she would become as an adult began to emerge. At the Abbotts, "all was happy . . . sympathizing and congenial." But the pleasure that Helen now found in her daily life did not improve her health—her coughs persisted. In the winter of 1850 Helen's sore throat was so irritating that Dr. Horace Green was called in to examine her. Helen remembered that he was the very physician who told her father to take his final voyage for health, so she was not surprised when he informed Mr. Abbott (but not her) that her case was "precisely similar to my *father's*, except that the disease had not extended so far." Dr. Green added "that I certainly should not live long unless the disease was removed and that it was a wonder that with all the consumptive tendencies of our family, I had lived so long."[36]

Although she was twenty years old when the Abbotts' school unexpectedly closed, Helen floundered. Still viewing herself as a "ward" and an "orphan," she turned for help to Julius Palmer, the guardian her grandfather had assigned her, and he arranged for her to live with his brother, Ray Palmer, a Congregational minister in Albany, New York.[37] Although Helen was reluctant to board in another minister's home, she found there a resolution to her religious predicament and freedom from her anxieties. On the eve of her twenty-first birthday, in October 1851, she informed Julius Palmer that her life was no longer "one great hurried confused medley of mistakes, wrong doings, wishes, aspirations, vanities, absurdities, miseries." She would never be an observant Christian, but she had the inner strength to "exert as much good influence in the world as I *can*."[38]

A few months later Helen met her future husband, Edward Bissell Hunt, and in 1852, they were married. Hunt had just relinquished his post as an assistant professor in the department of engineering at West Point to become the superintendent of map engraving for the United States Coastal Survey. The courtship was intense and gay. Edward's older brother, Washington, was the governor of New York, and so there were large balls and frequent social visits. The thought of moving into her own home with her own furniture and having the companionship of a man made her happier than she had ever imagined possible.[39]

But the marriage was short-lived, marred by disappointments and unexpected tragedies. Hunt's assignment demanded that he be away from home for long periods, and Helen moved from boardinghouse to boardinghouse and from city to city. Death also stalked her. In September 1853, Helen gave birth to a son, who died soon afterward. In 1855 a second son, Warren Horsford "Rennie" Hunt, was born. The child thrived and became Helen's companion during the long separations from her husband. But then in 1863 Hunt himself died in a naval accident. Angry and despondent, Helen clung to Rennie. But two years later, in 1865, at the age of ten, he died.[40]

Bitter and evincing the symptoms considered harbingers of consumption, Helen went to live in Newport, Rhode Island. The choice was partly sentimental—the happiest year of her marriage had been spent there—and partly medical. Not only had she enjoyed better health there than at any other time in the last fifteen years, but the seaside town had recently become a popular destination for New England invalids.[41]

Shortly after her arrival, Helen met Thomas Wentworth Higginson, a well-known Unitarian minister and fiery orator who had gained a national fame as the commander of the only all-black regiment in the Union Army. Higginson was smitten with Helen. "There is a new boarder here—Mrs. (Major) Hunt, a young widow," he noted in his diary. "She seems very bright and sociable and may prove an accession." Higginson immediately invited Helen to join a social circle he had formed of literary-inclined men and women; he soon became her mentor, carefully guiding her literary efforts. With Higginson's help (he edited and revised many of the early poems and even served as an agent for her), Helen (under pen names) began to publish sentimental poetry, essays, and short stories.[42]

During the six years Helen spent in Newport, her literary success surpassed her gains in health. By 1872 she was able to publish her writing in most of the widely read magazines in the country, and her royalties more than adequately supplemented the inheritance from her grandfather. But her health was worsening, and the specter of consumption once more threatened to mar her happiness. Her sore throats and coughs became so severe that she periodically left to test the climate of the White Mountains and of Europe.

In the summer of 1872 Helen suffered from a sore throat so painful that she had difficulty eating. "You have had joy," she wrote a friend. "I have had sorrow. You are hand in hand with life. I am only waiting to go. I keep at the brave pace partly from pride I am afraid, partly from my temperament. But the heart of me is sorely tired out. I have had some little pleasure in speaking through my writings to people I do not know. Perhaps I have done a little good; but of that too, I am very tired."[43] Seeing no alternative, Helen followed the route of men and headed for California. She felt stronger there, and her symptoms disappeared. On a visit to Yosemite, she was able to hike the valleys and visit the waterfalls. She also visited the missions to observe Indian life and was captivated by its simplicity and by the ancestral customs. But no sooner did she return to Newport in the fall of 1872 than her coughs and pains returned. She found herself "irresistibly impelled" to return to the West and began to look for ways to finance a trip to Colorado.[44]

In the summer of 1873 yet another lingering sore throat turned into diphtheria, and then an attack of her "old lung trouble" further depleted her strength. Her symptoms became more ominous (she lost weight and her mass of blond curls became streaked with gray). Every time she looked in the mirror, she saw her mother's skeletal body—an incubus that she could not drive away. Frightened and despairing, she summoned enough energy to return to Amherst and visit a physician who had known her family. He advised her to head West immediately. After consulting with friends and reading the testimonials of other health seekers, she set out for Colorado Springs.[45]

It was an unusually cold and dreary November day when Helen arrived, exhausted from the five-day transcontinental journey. As she stared out at the towering mountains that rose suddenly from the long, desolate plains the only words that came to mind were "blank, bald, pitiless, gray." To Helen, the mountains were an impenetrable wall that blocked further passage to the West. Disheartened by the "sea of gray ice" that loomed above, she focused on the string of recently constructed homes and stores. The buildings were set on well-defined lots along wide streets, but the absence of shrubs and trees made them seem too small for their spacious setting. From the reports of other travelers, Helen had envisioned snowy peaks glistening in the sun, a bustling town nestled and protected by the towering mountains, but as she gazed around at the "cruel and forbidding" peaks, she had a sense of "hopeless disappointment." The town fell far short of the hyperbole of the developers and did not fit with her expectations.[46]

Nevertheless, within a remarkably short time, Helen's health began to improve, and by the summer of 1874, she was writing to friends that she planned to remain out West. "I am persuaded that it is wisest for me to stay here. I am very well indeed, and look better—some friends who came here from New York last week say than I ever did in my life." But Helen was too familiar with the capricious nature of the disease to think she had won the battle. "My throat is still weak, and . . . I am still wedded to an enemy. . . . And the dread of suffering as I suffered last summer keeps me here."[47]

Just about that time, Helen met William Sharpless Jackson. Six years her junior, he came from a poor Quaker family. He had left school young and worked first as a clerk, then as a lumber dealer and a manufacturer of railroad cars. In 1871 he was elected secretary and treasurer of the Denver and Rio Grande Railroad and went to Denver to supervise the construction and management of the spur to Colorado Springs that Palmer and Bell had promoted. When he met Helen in 1874, Jackson was the vice president of the railroad with a substantial income. With his blunt and pragmatic style, his lack of rigid convictions, and his shrewd business skills, Jackson was more reminiscent of David Vinal than any of the other men in Helen's life. On October 22, 1875, when Helen was forty-five years old, she married Jackson and Colorado Springs became her home.

Like other health seekers rejuvenated in the West, Helen became a zealous partisan of the region. "Asthmatics *must* come here. It is a sure cure for that. Bad throat and lung troubles are invariably helped if not cured. I believe half the people in this town are *one lungers*." And she, too, delighted in telling of her transformation. "Prepare to see a woman you never saw when you see me," she wrote triumphantly to one of her publishers. "I have grown so stout and strong in Colorado you will not know me."[48] Helen, once thin and delicate, now weighed 163 pounds. Small wonder she was convinced that "the destined future of Colorado . . . is to be the great sanitarium and pleasure ground of this country—the Newport of the west." For her the town was a setting for a fairy tale, a sacred shrine that lay "due east of the Great Mountains and West of the sun."[49]

Helen endowed the region with mystical powers. In her essays, the mountains "gleamed" at sunrise, "like pyramids of solid garnet, yet blue again at sunset. Sometimes in winter, they are more beautiful still—so spotlessly white, stately and solemn that if one believes there is a city of angels he must believe that these are . . . the gates thereof."[50] Colorado's canyons were the natural equivalent of Gothic cathedrals, their spires pointing toward heaven. She usually spent her Sundays in the canyons and much to the dismay of her neighbors, she would often appear just at the moment they were entering church. Dressed in hiking clothes and carrying a heavily laden picnic basket, she would climb into her carriage and head out to Cheyenne Canyon. "There are nine 'places of divine worship' in Colorado Springs," this daughter of Deborah and Nathan Fiske maintained. "The Presbyterian, the Cumberland Presbyterian, the Methodist, the South Methodist, the Episcopal, the Congregationalist, the Baptist, the Unitarian and Cheyenne Canyon. Cheyenne Canyon is three miles out of town; the members of its congregation find this no objection." These visits to the canyon became the occasion to worship nature's awesome qualities. "As I looked up from the ford to the mouth of the canyon," Helen wrote, "I was reminded of some of the grand old altar-pieces of the early churches, where lest the pictures of saints and angels and divine beings should seem too remote, too solemn and overawing, the painters set at the base, rows of human children, gay and mirthful." No wonder her version of a "holy week" was one spent hiking from Saturday to Saturday in the canyons that surrounded the town.[51]

Living in Colorado Springs also gave Helen a political mission. Beginning in 1877 and continuing until her death in 1885, she championed the rights of Native Americans. Perhaps her own losses—her sense that she, too, had lost her birthright—made her sympathetic to their predicament.

Whatever the reason, Helen carried out this secular crusade with the zeal and righteousness of the antislavery agitators of an earlier era. "I think I feel as you must have felt in the old abolition days," she wrote to Higginson. "I cannot think of anything else from night to morning and from morning to night. . . . I believe the time is drawing near for a great change in our policy toward the Indian. In some respects, it seems to me he is really worse off than the slaves; they did have in the majority of cases good houses and they were not much more arbitrarily controlled than the Indian is by the agent on a reservation."[52] Forceful, passionate, and uncompromising, Helen used her considerable literary powers to urge Carl Schurz, the secretary of the interior, and members of Congress to cede the tribes rights to ancestral lands "in such a way that they can never be dispossessed." Her most widely read and influential book, *Century of Dishonor*, is a compelling account of the callous and brutal manner in which the federal government repeatedly uprooted the tribes and reneged on its promises. Its fictional counterpart, *Ramona*, completed just a few years before her death, has often been compared to Harriet Beecher Stowe's *Uncle Tom's Cabin*. Like its predecessor, it is a tale of oppression. Set in California just before the arrival of the white settlers, it champions the cause of the Mission Indians. Helen presents them as a proud, civilized group, reduced to poverty not by their moral failings but by the inhumane treatment of the white invaders. In almost autobiographical terms, she fought to restore the status of the Native Americans, from "wards" to independent people, and to return their "birthright."[53]

Although Helen is remembered primarily for her impassioned advocacy of Native Americans, her life exemplifies the social changes and personal circumstances that led women to Go West and Live. The search for a cure for consumption was still not free of gender considerations, but a growing number of women were now able to follow a man's route to cure.

PART IV

BECOMING A PATIENT, 1882–1940

12

A Disease of the
Masses

IN 1882 ROBERT KOCH IDENTIFIED THE TUBERCLE BACILLUS, WHICH
revolutionized both the medical and the social history of the disease.
Through a novel staining method, he was able to distinguish it from other
bacteria: "Under the microscope all constituents of animal tissue . . . appear
faintly brown, with the tubercle bacilli, however, beautifully blue." This
feat accomplished, he was quickly able to prove that tuberculosis was an
infectious disease, "that it is caused by the invasion of bacilli and that it is
conditioned primarily by the growth and multiplication of bacilli." He
inoculated other animals to see whether they would "reproduce the same
morbid condition," and as he reported, they "became emaciated rapidly,
and died after four to six weeks. . . . In the organs of all these animals . . .
were found the characteristic and well-known tuberculous alterations."[1]

Koch immediately recognized the decisive implications of his findings:
on the basis of the absence or presence of the tubercle bacillus, it was now
possible to define "the boundaries of the diseases to be understood as
tuberculosis." On the one hand, it could be differentiated from other diseases such as pneumonia; on the other, it could be recognized as one common disease whether it was the lungs, intestines, or skeleton that was
infected. Koch also understood how the bacillus entered the body. Because
"the great majority of all cases of tuberculosis begin in the respiratory tract,
and the infectious material leaves its mark first in the lungs or in the
bronchial lymph nodes," it was apparent that the bacilli were spread
through the air; and there could "hardly be any doubt about the manner by
which they get into the air, considering in what excessive numbers tubercle
bacilli present in cavity-contents are expectorated by consumptives and
scattered everywhere." Koch was now confident that

in future the fight against this terrible plague of mankind will deal no longer with an undetermined something, but with a tangible parasite, whose living conditions are for the most part known and can be investigated further. . . . When the conviction that tuberculosis is an exquisite infectious disease has become firmly established among physicians, the question of an adequate campaign against tuberculosis will certainly come under discussion and it will develop by itself.[2]

Koch's discovery inspired a new scientifically derived terminology for the disease. Consumption rapidly became an arcane term, for it no longer seemed suitable to define a disease by its most dramatic symptom. The new designation, tuberculosis, linked the disease directly to its causative agent. Diagnosis now depended on the presence of the tubercle bacillus in the sputum, not the hollowness of the cough or the loss of weight. The bacillus, not the family history, held the key.

Koch's work also added to the prestige of the medical profession. Tuberculosis, to judge by levels of mortality, was the most important disease to have its causative agent isolated. Added to other discoveries—the 1874 identification by Hansen of the leprosy bacillus, the 1876 discovery by Koch and Pasteur of the anthrax bacillus, and the discovery by Neisser in 1879 of the agent of gonorrhea—this latest breakthrough inspired tremendous confidence in the new scientific method. There seemed no limit to what could be achieved. "It is within the power of man," Louis Pasteur declared, "to rid himself of every parasitic disease."[3]

And prestige bred authority. Although diagnostic capabilities far outstripped therapeutic effectiveness, physicians and their prescriptions gained new stature both in the examining room and in the community.[4] Nowhere was this more apparent than with tuberculosis. Professionals and laymen alike came to agree that medicine now had sufficient understanding of the bacillus to control its transmission and even to fashion a cure. This belief became the basis for a vigorous antituberculosis crusade made up of two distinct but overlapping camps. One group, stationed in the newly reorganized city and state departments of public health, devoted itself to preventing new cases by eradicating contagion. The other, based in a new type of facility, the sanatorium, was determined to implement a cure. But the import of this division should not be exaggerated, for it evolved slowly and lines of activity frequently crossed. Public health officials were generally comfortable in advocating confinement, and sanatorium administrators, in combating contagion. Most significantly, both camps were eager to establish their authority over persons with tuberculosis, and they imposed an unprecedented degree of regulation on the lives of Americans who had contracted the disease.

*   *   *

Two characteristics of tuberculosis helped transform the public understanding of the disease. First and foremost, tuberculosis, in contradistinction to consumption, was understood to be a contagious disease; second, it was defined as a disease of only some, not all, people, essentially the immigrant and the poor, not the middle or upper classes.

The task of spelling out the implications of contagion belonged to a cadre of physicians trained in the new biological sciences and pursuing careers in public health. As health commissioners, chief medical officers, or heads of government bacteriological laboratories, they promulgated a series of policies aimed at controlling its spread. "Science has laid before the world the cause of consumption with mathematical exactness," Dr. Lawrence Flick, a champion of the antituberculosis campaign declared, "and has given such an insight into the lives of the micro-organisms which produce it that it is possible to plan a campaign against the disease which is sure to end in victory for the human race." For Flick, as for others, the battle was nothing less than a "crusade," in which "every man, woman, and child . . . [was] to enlist in the army which is to fight this battle." Or as Dr. S. Adolphus Knopf, another leader of the movement, insisted: "It is certainly within the power of man, living in a civilized country, such as the United States, where so much intelligence, wealth, prosperity, and philanthropy prevail, to combat tuberculosis . . . most successfully."[5]

In the era before bacteriology, departments of public health had been dominated by so-called sanitarians, who located the causal elements and conveyance of disease in foul-smelling or "miasmatic" conditions. In their effort to rid the city of noxious odors and filth, they promoted massive engineering projects, including the construction of water supply and sewage systems, and initiated the more systematic collection of garbage and dead animals. To their successors, the bacteriologists, those efforts, however commendable, had been misguided. "The filth theory erroneously assumed that the infectious diseases were caused by emanations, gaseous or otherwise, from decaying matter," asserted Charles Chapin, the commissioner of public health in Providence. "Everything decaying and offensive to the sense of smell was dangerous. . . . It was boldly taught that by removing all decaying matter the infectious diseases could be stamped out."[6] The bacteriologists understood that odor, or the absence of odor, was no indicator of the danger of infection. Water that smelled clean and milk that looked pure might still be rife with virulent pathogens. The public health required scientific laboratories and coordinated epidemiological research.[7]

Public health departments set out to meet this challenge. "It is only along the line of patient investigation of each disease and practical deductions from ascertained facts," declared Chapin, "that public health work can succeed. . . . Instead of an indiscriminate attack on dirt, we must learn the nature and mode of transmission of each infection, and must discover its most vulnerable point of attack."[8] Thus, when an epidemic was caused by bacteria as in the case of cholera, typhoid, diphtheria, or tuberculosis, it was necessary first to make a microscopic identification of the specific germs attacking those stricken with the disease and then to seek out the sources of contagion and the mode of transmission. Once these were identified, public health officials would order the necessary changes and thereby contain the epidemic.

In the case of tuberculosis, public health officials understood that the route of transmission was from person to person (and not from water to person or from mosquito to person).[9] The bacilli lodging in a cavity in the lungs was coughed up in the sputum and then became airborne, coming in direct contact with another person or landing on particles of dust or other objects. The bacillus might be inhaled immediately from the air or from a dust particle containing dried but still infected sputum; it might also be transmitted directly from the sputum of an infected person, for example, through a kiss or a shared drink. All these concepts are now familiar, but it takes little imagination to grasp how astonishing and frightening they were to an earlier generation. Bacteriology gave traditional behavior unexpected meanings. Educated Americans slowly began to reckon with the fact that proximity to a person with tuberculosis could be dangerous, and common practices, like spitting, which had once seemed uncouth, could be harmful. This perception spread slowly and unevenly among the population during the next decade; but over time the implications of the findings were unmistakable and eventually bred a fear of associating with persons who had tuberculosis.[10]

The bacteriologists, recognizing almost immediately that the findings were alarming, often tried to reassure the public. In 1889 T. Mitchell Prudden, who was Edward Trudeau's teacher in the field of bacteriology, published *The Story of the Bacteria and Their Relations to Health and Disease*, in which he described for a lay audience "what bacteria do" and what precautions health-conscious citizens should adopt. He explained how the tubercle bacilli "gain access to the body" and how "if the conditions are favorable, they tend to grow, and ... form about them little masses of new tissue, which are called tubercles." The major source of transmission was the infected sputum "coughed up" from the lungs of a tubercular person, but because "the healthy body is not good soil for the tubercle bacilli," even those living with a consumptive could avoid contracting the disease. The best defense was a strong resistance, which meant that everyone should eat "good plain properly cooked food and plenty of it. . . . Get all the fresh air you can. . . . Keep clean." To be sure, the bacillus survived in dust particles and on objects, but "the individual's chances of coming into contact with the dangerous material are slight," and besides, "strong daylight or direct sunlight kill it in a few days or hours." These comforting points made,

Prudden went on to insist that persons with tuberculosis had to obey strict rules of hygiene and, above all else, to stop "promiscuous spitting."[11]

Dr. Hermann Biggs, who as pathologist and director of the bacteriological laboratory of the New York City Department of Health had established the nation's most vigorous antituberculosis program, also tried to allay the panic. "While tuberculosis is communicable," he declared in 1894, it is "communicated with far less facility than many other diseases, which are more properly called contagious." To contract it required "long exposure to infection, and intimate association with the infected individual."[12] Biggs remained staunchly convinced that although preventive measures could not totally eliminate contagion, they would help to control it. "While no one would assume," he told the Philadelphia County Medical Society in 1900, "that in a single month or in a single year all of the thousands and tens of thousands of sources of infection in a great city can be removed, yet if one-quarter or one-third can be eradicated there will be a proportionate gain, which will be increased each succeeding year." As the motto of the New York City Department of Health proclaimed: "Public Health is purchasable. Within natural limitations every community can determine its own death rate."[13]

Physicians such as Knopf, who was familiar with the plight of the consumptive poor in both Germany and the United States, reinforced this message. People could reduce the threat of contagion if they would merely "strive to be as much as possible in the open air, drink plenty of pure, clean water, keep early hours, live as regular a life as possible, avoid the saloon, and never take alcoholic beverages." Were those with tuberculosis to adhere to the same rules, the rates of the disease would be reduced further: "From living or coming in contact with a clean, conscientious, tuberculous invalid nothing whatsoever is to be feared."[14]

But none of these messages was intended to reduce the need for strict and thoroughgoing public health measures. Indeed, the newly established departments expanded their influence and budgets in response to the threat of contagion from tuberculosis. During the period 1890 to 1920, when the Progressive Era's spirit of reform dominated social policy, public health officials promoted two distinct but interrelated approaches to reduce the perils of the disease: they looked simultaneously to improve the social conditions that bred tuberculosis and to control the behavior of those with the disease. As with other Progressive Era programs, the public health movement reflected an optimism that social engineering would be able to conquer deep-rooted problems; but it also assumed that unless coercive and exclusionary measures were adopted, the physical well-being of the body politic would be endangered.

These public health campaigns built on the second critical fact about tuberculosis, that by 1900 it had become a disease of the poor, particularly of the immigrants who were crowded together in the tenement house districts. Although the death rate from tuberculosis had been declining in the general population since the 1870s, it continued to take a heavy toll among the immigrant poor. In New York City, for example, the citywide death rate from consumption in 1870 was 428 per 100,000; in 1890 it had dropped to 390. But when the 1890 mortality rate was examined district by district, critical distinctions emerged. As Dr. John Billings, the country's leading statistician and one of its most renowned librarians reported, in a "beautiful residential section" on the Upper West Side, the death rate from tuberculosis was 49 per 100,000, but in the crowded tenement sections of lower Manhattan it was 776 per 100,000. In 1900 the citywide mortality had declined still further, to 256 per 100,000, but in the poorest and most crowded districts, it hovered around 500 per 100,000.[15] In effect, the poor were the group most at risk for contracting the disease, and given the contagious nature of the disease, it might well spread from them to the entire community.[16]

Explanations as to why the immigrant population was most prone to tuberculosis, like the Progressive analyses of poverty itself, focused equally on underlying social conditions and on personal moral failings. One of the first efforts to sort out the issue was made by Knopf in his prize-winning and frequently reprinted essay *Tuberculosis as a Disease of the Masses and How to Combat It*. He identified those susceptible as the innocent victims of poverty or those who through personal vice had only themselves to blame for their misery and illness. Thus, his roster included the "temporarily or permanently enfeebled," as a result of "alcoholism ... [and] other intemperate habits," or "through privation or disease." Having contracted tuberculosis, they then, through "ignorance or carelessness," spread "their infectious sputum everywhere without any regard to the danger." In turn, their neighbors, some because of intemperance and others because of privation, lacked the necessary resistance to fight off the bacilli.[17]

The vision of the poor as victims not only of low wages but of a deadly disease prompted some Progressives, particularly the cohort of settlement-house workers, to advance a broad reform agenda. Defining the city as their laboratory, they set out to investigate social conditions the way that physicians investigated bacilli; and they intended to use the data they accumulated on the causes of poverty and disease to marshal legislative support for remedial programs. They became convinced that tuberculosis flourished when families were crowded together in "dark interior rooms" and had the poorest sanitary arrangements, when they had "the least nutritious diet and often spent time in the saloons and the beer halls." Thus, to combat both poverty and disease, they sought to remodel tenement housing, eliminate sweatshops, reduce the hours of labor, abolish child labor, establish municipal bathhouses, sterilize milk, purify water, and construct playgrounds and parks ("the lungs of a great city"). In effect, the grand Progressive program would improve the quality of life and thereby eradicate tuberculosis.[18]

A number of physicians shared this commitment. As Knopf declared, reform could best be realized through "the combined action of a wise government, well-trained physicians, and an intelligent people."[19] Dr. Edward von Adelung, a health officer in Oakland, California, deemed tuberculosis "a ministering angel in disguise, for it tends ultimately to force better drainage, better dwellings, better modes of living, more fresh air, sunshine, cleanliness, rest and recreation."[20]

Nowhere did physicians and settlement-house workers cooperate more closely than in reform of tenement houses, as witness the New York State Tenement House Commission Report of 1900. For fifty years would-be reformers had pronounced tenement houses "prolific sources of moral degradation and physical suffering" and proposed the design of model houses that would eliminate foul odors even as it reduced the propensity to immorality. The 1900 report followed in this tradition but imbued the campaign with a new power and specificity. Tenement-house living was correlated not only with crime, prostitution, and alcoholism, but also with tuberculosis—which threatened the wider community and intensified the need for change.[21]

The 1900 report included maps of the city districts with special markings to show the correlations between tenement houses and tuberculosis. Superimposed on "poverty maps"—which marked the buildings in which families had applied for charity—were "disease maps" with black dots indicating buildings with a high number of cases of tuberculosis. "It was appalling," the commission reported, "to note the extent of this disease; nearly every tenement house had one dot on it, and many had three or four, and there were some houses that contained as many as twelve. . . . The connection between this disease and the character of the tenement houses in which the poor people live is of the very closest."[22]

Public health officials readily explained the correlation. Biggs of the New York City Department of Health, and Dr. Arthur Guerard, a bacteriologist in the department, emphasized the absence of light and air from the tenements. Since the tubercle bacillus "is readily destroyed by sunlight, or even diffused daylight," Biggs declared, "the danger of infection is largely diminished by thorough ventilation." In bright and roomier quarters families "will be less exposed to infection, because of less overcrowding, more sunlight, more air, and better ventilation in their dwellings."[23] Enacting tenement reform legislation, Guerard insisted, would eradicate the problem. "Tuberculosis, though an evil much to be dreaded, is not an inevitable decree of fate, not an unavoidable dispensation of Providence, but, like many other ills . . . the remedy for it exists to a great extent in ourselves."[24]

Knopf was even more enthusiastic about the potential benefits of housing reform, nimbly moving between social and moral arguments. "Think of the difference between the old tenement, which we desire to abolish, and the new one we desire to erect," he declared. The old tenement was "a bee-hive of humanity living in filth and dirt, well-nigh without light and air . . . disease breeding in every room; a hot-bed of tuberculosis and other conta-gious diseases from which are spread the foci of infection throughout the city among old and young, poor and rich alike." The new tenement was "a well-regulated city within a city, its citizens living in airy, sunny rooms . . . which make the longing for the rum shop less, and create a love for temper-ance and purity; a home where infectious diseases can be controlled and from which the most bitter foe of mankind, 'the great white plague'—con-sumption—can be ultimately and lastingly banished."[25]

But even as they made the case for reform, city and state health officials advocated a second and very different kind of strategy, one that looked not to social conditions but to individual behavior. Persons with tuberculosis had to learn to follow rules of hygiene, and if they did not comply voluntar-ily, public health commissioners would have to impose penalties. Thus, the campaign moved along a spectrum from persuasion to outright compul-sion, with each measure justified by an appeal to the welfare of the commu-nity.

In the 1890s public health officials mounted an educational program to teach everyone the new lessons of hygiene. "At least one-half of the existing sickness and mortality from tuberculosis could be prevented within the next two decades," calculated Johns Hopkins medical school professor William Welch, if only the public had a "clear understanding of the modes of con-veyance of the disease."[26] Targeting the immigrant community, the New York City Department of Health in 1894 published a pamphlet "Informa-tion for Consumptives and Those Living with Them," translated it into various languages (including German, Italian, and Yiddish), and over the next decade asked settlement-house workers and charity organization workers to distribute it. The pamphlet carefully explained the rudiments of contagion. ("Consumption is a disease which can be taken from others and is not simply caused by colds. . . . It is usually caused by germs which enter the body with the air breathed.") It then set forth general measures for pre-vention. ("It is not dangerous for other persons to live with a consumptive if the matter coughed up by the consumptive is at once destroyed.")[27] As part of this campaign, public school teachers had students memorize rules of sound health habits (avoid spitting, cough only into handkerchiefs), and settlement-house club leaders taught members a list of dos and don'ts (open the windows, let in sunlight, prepare nutritious meals, discourage alcohol consumption). In 1901 the department reported that each year since it was printed, the inspectors had distributed between twenty thousand and fifty thousand of the circulars in the tenement-house districts.[28] By 1912 the number of languages in which the circular appeared had also increased—it was now also available in Bohemian, Finnish, Polish, Slovak, Ruthenian, Swedish, Armenian, Spanish, and Chinese.[29]

However important these general educational efforts, they could not substitute for the direct instruction and supervision of persons with tuber-culosis. Before such an agenda could be accomplished officials had to know precisely who the infected were. A partial list could be compiled from the rosters of dispensaries and hospitals, but that would identify only those suf-ficiently motivated to seek treatment, the ones who might already be atten-tive to the rules of hygiene. The more difficult task was to locate those too isolated or frightened to go to a hospital, the ones who were probably unable to read a circular or too dissolute to remain on the list of a charity organization. They were likely to be least mindful of hygiene and most threatening to the public health.[30]

To meet this challenge, a number of departments of health, none more energetically than that of New York City, advocated registration laws requiring physicians and other health providers to supply them with the names and addresses of all persons diagnosed with tuberculosis.[31] By 1904 fifty-nine cities reported having similar ordinances.[32] Once these depart-ments had the names of those with tuberculosis in hand, they dispatched a sanitary inspector to the home to initiate a program of education and supervision.

It was a large order, but departments believed each element indispens-able. The inspectors initially were to give "verbal instruction . . . about the danger of infection and the care of the sputum."[33] The inspector would explain how important it was for tuberculars to sleep alone, use their own utensils, expectorate into sputum cups, and cough into napkins (that would be burned), and they would also teach the proper regimen of diet and rest. They would periodically examine the other family members to see if they were developing the disease, and if they were, they would be sent for treat-ment. In the event that the family moved, the inspectors arranged for the premises to be thoroughly disinfected before the next occupant moved in.[34] Should the family prove uncooperative, the inspectors were to initiate for-mal procedures to take away the children and institutionalize the sick.

Public health officials enthusiastically and aggressively justified every intervention. Biggs was the first to do so, in the mid-1890s, as he set out the New York City policies; but variations of his justifications for intrusive new laws were echoed by other public health officials as they promulgated similar policies. A tuberculosis registry, they all argued, was essential to the reduction of contagion. "The cry has been raised again and again," Biggs observed,

that for humanity's sake pulmonary consumption must not be pronounced a communicable disease, and the friends of patients often
declare that they prefer to expose themselves to the chance of infection
rather than have their dear ones banished, or treated as if they were
plague-stricken; but this is all the sheerest nonsense.

The stakes were so high as to justify the most exceptional intrusion of state
authority into the life of the individual.[35] "The government of the United
States is democratic," Biggs insisted, "but the sanitary measures adopted
are sometimes autocratic, and the functions performed by sanitary authorities paternal in character. We are prepared, when necessary, to introduce
and enforce, and the people are ready to accept, measures which might
seem radical and arbitrary, if they were not plainly designed for the public
good, and evidently beneficent in their effects." Or as Charles Chapin put
it: "Our business, daily and hourly, leads us to the depletion of men's pock-
ets and the restriction of their liberty. We cannot expect the thanks of those
who feel themselves aggrieved."[36] Guarding the public health might
encroach on individual liberties, but the common weal required it.
    Departments of health moved step-by-step to realize this mandate. First
they registered the tubercular. In New York, for example, the department
added tuberculosis to the official list of communicable diseases in 1893;
physicians were "requested to notify" it within ten days of the name and
address of their patients diagnosed as tubercular. The case would be registered and come under the "direct surveillance" of the department's corps of
inspectors, unless the physician agreed "to provide the instruction necessary
to prevent the spread of contagion." Four years later the department made
registration of tuberculosis compulsory. It was listed as an "infectious and
communicable disease . . . dangerous to the public health," and it became
the "duty" of all physicians to inform the department of every case.[37]
    Although the New York register was not a public document, private and
public organizations often gained access to it. In 1894 one New York industrial insurance company, which also underwrote life insurance policies for
workingmen, wanted to match the names on the registry with those of their
policyholders so as to screen applicants and deny benefits. The company's
contracts contained a clause allowing them to void a policy should the
holder die of tuberculosis. On the death certificates, physicians often mis-
stated the cause of death, listing it as pneumonia or chronic bronchitis, in
order to protect the policy and thereby provide the family with money for a
funeral and perhaps to pay their own fees. The Department acceded to the
company's request, believing that the effort would contribute to controlling
the spread of the disease. It reasoned that workingmen with tuberculosis
tried to remain on the job as long as possible, not only to earn the weekly
wage but to keep the insurance benefit; if, however, they knew that the

insurance policy would be voided, some might resign sooner and thus reduce the likelihood of transmission.[38]

To be sure, many private physicians, medical societies, and charity organization workers opposed mandatory registration. Physicians wanted to curtail the authority of public health officials. Their motives were undoubtedly mixed: some feared losing their patients; others were concerned about violating the confidentiality of the physician-patient relationship. Whatever the reason, they protested what they called "bacteriological edicts," which they found "offensively dictatorial and defiantly compulsory." To give the department "official control" of people with tuberculosis, they maintained, was "unduly magnifying the importance of its bacteriological department" while intruding on their professional prerogatives.[39]

Medical societies and social workers also complained that registration imposed too heavy a burden on the tubercular poor. In 1894 the College of Physicians of Philadelphia passed a resolution protesting the New York policy. To treat consumptives "as the subjects of contagious disease would be adding hardship to the lives of these unfortunates, stamping them as the outcasts of society. In view of the chronic nature of the malady it could not lead to any measures of real value not otherwise obtainable." In this spirit, Edward Devine, the president of the Charity Organization Society, the largest private relief organization in New York City, urged the department to use its authority sparingly. "Registration of all cases, whether in tenements or palaces, whether in the city or country," should not "be followed by any unnecessary interference . . . [or] any other invasion of privacy or personal hardship."[40]

But these sentiments did not deter public health officials who remained convinced that protection of the public health trumped all other considerations. By 1908 eighty-four cities required both registration of the tubercular and disinfection of lodgings, procedures that led to discrimination in housing and employment. Landlords refused to rent to the tubercular. Insurance companies invalidated their policies and employers refused to hire them. Many municipalities and states passed laws specifically prohibiting persons with tuberculosis from working in dairies and bakeries, others barred them as teachers in public schools.[41]

Biggs remained convinced that registration and supervision were in the best interest of the community, and he was warmly supported in this position by Robert Koch himself. "Public opinion is now ripe for such action," Koch wrote Biggs in 1901. "I hope to secure the inclusion in this country of the compulsory reporting of such cases of pulmonary tuberculosis as are in a communicable state although I am finding strong opposition to such a step. To meet this opposition I wish to cite the example of the free American people who have of their own free will accepted the limitations of their own liberties in the interest of public health."[42] Biggs also garnered support from some ordinary physicians. "The health authorities are granted the right to separate cases of smallpox and certain other infectious diseases from their families and friends," Dr. De Lancey Rochester told his New York colleagues. "The same right should be accorded them with regard to the greatest destroyer of them all—tuberculosis." Dr. Charles Ingraham, writing in the *Journal of the American Medical Association* in 1896, asked: "How far can the Government carry legal measures designed to control tuberculosis, and not infringe upon the natural rights of American citizenship?" His answer: "It is estimated by competent authorities that 450 persons die every 24 hours in the United States from tuberculosis. A disease which is responsible for a human fatality so large and so continuous should be classed with dangerous contagious affections, as one requiring the strictest hygienic management designed to minimize the infection arising from each individual case."[43] Thus, over the first decade of the twentieth century the campaign to educate the public gained momentum,[44] and as its message spread throughout the country, so did the fear of associating with persons who had contracted tuberculosis. The more the department of health officials stressed the danger, the more they bred a fear not only of the disease but of associating with those who had it. By 1903 this fear had earned its own sobriquet: *phthisiophobia.*[45]

Nowhere was this apprehension more apparent than in the efforts of some public health officials to exercise their police power and ban the interstate travel of persons with tuberculosis. From their perspective, those who undertook a voyage for personal health were actually spreading the disease and endangering the public health. Anyone with the disease, but particularly those with careless habits and limited budgets, ought not to be riding for days in closed railroad cars (their route marked by a trail of dried but infected sputum on the seat cushions), then moving from boardinghouse to boardinghouse, coughing at communal dining tables, and spitting on the streets.

The fiercest battle to restrict the interstate travel of persons with tuberculosis took place, not surprisingly, in California.[46] In 1900 its State Board of Health proposed regulations to ban their entry, convinced that the entire southern region was becoming the "tubercular sanitarium for the whole country." As one of the proponents of the measure, Dr. George Kober, declared: "Why should this glorious State be stocked with consumptives and their offspring? Instead of this State producing a people with mental and bodily vigor . . . we shall have a race weak in mind and body, and deeply tainted with a predisposition to consumption." [47]

Opponents successfully fought the measure, for reasons of practicality as well as equity. For one, the border was so long and the modes of transportation so varied that no screening system could work. "All passenger trains would have to be delayed several hours till all the passengers could be examined," remarked Norman Bridge, a physician who had found his cure in California. "The general appearance of the travellers could not be relied upon to tell who are dangerous consumptives, for some mortally sick ones look in the face very well, and nine-tenths of all tuberculous patients could easily hoodwink any inspector."[48] For another, a residue of compassion for the tubercular remained. Dr. F. M. Pottenger, president of the California Anti-Tuberculosis League, pleaded: "What one of us has not a friend or dear one who is afflicted with this disease?" The tubercular "are not criminals. It is no fault of theirs that they are afflicted, but it is the fault of society collectively for not teaching the manner of preventing tuberculosis. . . . The society which would add unnecessary stigma to them is culpable and inhumane."[49] Even a number of public health officers found the measure foolish. Dr. Edward von Adelung urged his California colleagues to reject the quarantine "because it is eminently unnecessary"—education was sufficient. So, too, the Tuberculosis Committee of the state's Medical Society found that exclusion "is impractical, unconstitutional, inhumane, it is unscientific and entirely unnecessary."[50]

Although a ban on interstate travel was beyond the pale, and no state enacted such legislation, the fear and hostility that underlay the movement persisted and found other means of expression. If the state could not discriminate among newcomers, private parties could. Thus, boardinghouse and hotel owners turned away the sick, particularly those without substantial resources or family and friends. Town fathers readily reimbursed the railroads for giving the homeless tubercular a lunch basket and ticket back home. Western physicians did their part to restrict the flow. "When will our professional brethren in the East learn," declared Dr. George Kress, "that to send advanced cases to the West with no financial means to enable them to supply themselves with that food and environment that really forms a most important part of climatic treatment, is not only a sin of omission, but one of commission."[51] And many eastern charitable societies urged both social workers and physicians to remember, as Lillian Brandt of the New York Charity Organization Society put it, that "for a consumptive in any stage of the disease to go to a health resort with the idea of supporting himself while he gets well is folly, if not madness. . . . There is no climate which will avail to cure consumption if the other elements in the treatment are privation, worry, and homesickness. . . . It is useless . . . to go to the most favorable climate unless one has the means to meet a year's expenses including a reserve for emergencies."[52]

Public health officials had recourse to one final weapon in their campaign to control contagion: the power to confine anyone found "liable to jeopardize the health of others." Increasingly, during the first two decades of the twentieth century, they obtained authority to "employ summary measures" to commit such a person to a special facility until "he shall no longer be a menace to the public health." The primary goal was to confine the poor who had tuberculosis. The nightmare case was an infected tramp, but the legislation extended to include anyone not meeting the standards set by the public health authorities.[53]

Support for this measure among city and state officials and members of the medical profession increased, particularly as it became more evident that the departments would exercise their authority almost exclusively against the vagrant, the poor, and the immigrant. Most city councils and state legislatures considered the commitment of the tubercular "a valid exercise of the police power of the state."[54] In 1896 Dr. Charles Ingraham urged the American Medical Association to promote a network of state hospitals in which indigent consumptives who were careless in their hygienic habits could be "*sentenced* by health officials for a greater or less term, according to the seriousness and persistence of their offense." Without such compulsion, "we can not hope to gain any apparent control over the disease, for the majority of such indigent in their ignorance and carelessness scatter sufficient infection to perpetuate tuberculosis, though all other sources were perfectly eliminated." In 1909 William Welch, in a major address to the National Association for the Study and Prevention of Tuberculosis, urged compulsory confinement of the most recalcitrant. "In dealing with patients who are a serious menace to the community," he declared, "who cannot or will not be taught to take proper safeguards against the infection of their fellow-men, I think that the health authorities should be empowered to place them in proper institutions." At that same meeting Dr. John Billings, Jr., of New York City's Department of Health, urged his colleagues to press for compulsory commitment laws in every state. In this way, "the consumptive tramp, roaming from one dispensary to another, moving from one lodging house to another can now be removed to our institutions and kept under supervision."[55]

To implement this program, the New York City Department of Health in 1903 dedicated one pavilion of its contagious disease hospital, Riverside, to the recalcitrant tubercular. The roster of its potential inmates, as public health officials enumerated them, was lengthy. Generally, the "public nuisance" headed the list, which also included the tubercular who had been discharged from hospitals because they were "undesirable patients" or had "violated the regulations of the institutions." Typically they were the "homeless, friendless, dependent, dissolute, dissipate, and vicious consumptives . . . which are likely to be most dangerous to the community." Also on the list were "consumptives living in lodging houses or . . . inmates of public institutions" who would not voluntarily enter the hospitals to which they had been sent. They were joined by patients living at home who were "sources of danger to their family" and lived in "unfavorable . . . sanitary conditions." Finally, there were those already in hospitals but who were demanding discharge against medical advice.[56]

Riverside Hospital was soon holding all of these types of people.[57] Charity workers dispatched the tramps, and nurses and inspectors, the dissolute parent.[58] For example, Mary Jones, a tuberculosis nurse, recommended to the New York Department of Health that John Standish, a dying consumptive, be removed from his five-room flat, where he lived with his wife and five children. As Nurse Jones informed her supervisor: "I have been visiting this case of tuberculosis for 6 weeks, paid 8 visits, but have been unable to secure observance of those precautions necessary to prevent infection of others. [I] therefore recommend removal by force if necessary to Riverside Hospital."[59]

So too, physicians at public hospitals were happy to transfer patients they found bellicose or obstreperous, requesting the police to send an ambulance to transport the "fractious and intractable" patients. In this way, Riverside became as much a dumping ground for the recalcitrant as a public health facility. As with other new custodial institutions, its inmates were the discards of other caretaker facilities. Although, as we shall see, the numbers confined against their will were not large, having tuberculosis had become grounds for a loss of liberty.

13

Confining for Cure

THE NEW UNDERSTANDING OF TUBERCULOSIS IN THE BACTERIOLOGICAL era bred not only a fear of contagion but also a heady optimism about the prospects for cure. Now that the bacillus was identified and its characteristics known, physicians would be able to make an early diagnosis and to devise effective remedies. To be sure, there were neither chemotherapeutic agents to kill the bacillus (as streptomycin eventually would) nor vaccines to protect against it. Koch's own experiments with tuberculin were judged unsuccessful after an initial wave of enthusiasm. Rather, the principles of bacteriology more generally and the epidemiology of tuberculosis more specifically established new paths for therapy, and these led directly to the sanatorium. A generation of physicians, social reformers, and philanthropists were convinced that confining the tubercular in these facilities would promote not only societal well-being by isolating those with the disease but also individual well-being by implementing a therapeutic regimen. The sanatorium satisfied both the drive to coerce and cure. Inside it, fear met hope.

It was a fear and hope that paid almost no attention to considerations of gender. The overriding concern of public health officials was to control the spread of contagion—it did not matter whether the carrier was a man or a woman. As for cure, physicians recommended the same course of treatment regardless of gender. Almost all sanatoriums admitted, and imposed the same routine and discipline, on both sexes.

The first institutional treatment of consumption took place in Germany in the middle of the nineteenth century. In contradistinction to American prescriptions to travel for health, the German approach, as practiced by Drs. Hermann Brehmer and Peter Dettweiler, emphasized the importance of medical supervision in what they referred to as "closed institutions." In 1859 Brehmer opened a facility specifically for the treatment of lung diseases at Gorbersdorf in the Prussian province of Silesia. He was attracted to this particular town because it apparently had very few reported cases of consumption. Brehmer attributed this phenomenon to the "diminished atmospheric pressure" at high elevations that "demands an increase of heart action and a subsequent increase of metabolism."[1] He also reasoned that an environment that rendered inhabitants less prone to a disease would help those afflicted with it.

Brehmer's institution, really more a spa than a hospital, laid out on extensive and well-manicured grounds, served only the well-to-do. They followed a prescribed regimen of rich food and moderate exercise; their three daily meals were supplemented by snacks as well as by milk, wines, and cognac. Brehmer decreed that physical activity "must be in accordance with the strength of the patient and the condition of the disease at the time," and it was his responsibility to prescribe the precise amount of activity for each resident. One rule applied to everyone: to avoid physical and mental fatigue and not strain the heart or lungs by violent or prolonged exercise. Some of the residents were limited to "lung gymnastics," that is, deep breathing, while others took daily walks, at first on level promenades and then later along carefully graded mountain paths. Brehmer even placed benches at close intervals along the paths so that his patients could rest as needed.[2]

In 1876 one of Brehmer's physician-patients, Peter Dettweiler, modified and popularized the Brehmer regimen at a private facility he established at Falkenstein, near Frankfurt. Dettweiler faithfully followed Brehmer's dietetic rules but revised his method of open-air treatment. Unlike his mentor, Dettweiler was convinced that the typical consumptive is "a physical and usually a nervous weakling and needs much more rest than one ordinarily takes." Accordingly, his routine, what he called "permanent or continuous fresh air treatment," required residents to sit outside for most of the day in reclining chairs (known as cure chairs) on protected verandas. In this way, they breathed in "pure air" while sheltered from the rain, wind, and snow. Dettweiler made no special claims for the climate of Falkenstein. Aside from the quality of the air, the town was indistinguishable from others in southern Germany. But Dettweiler, even more than Brehmer, underscored the importance of medical supervision. To effect a cure, physicians had to monitor their patients' regimen closely.[3]

Dr. Paul Kretzschmar, a patient and disciple of Dettweiler, introduced these conclusions to American colleagues in a very incisive way. He linked the advantages of the closed institution directly to Koch's discoveries in bacteriology and to the wretched condition of the new immigrants. In several seminal papers delivered in 1888 and 1889, he presented the principles of the Brehmer-Dettweiler regimen in these terms, sparked a debate on the merits of closed versus open institutions, and laid the groundwork for the American sanatorium.

Soon after completing his own cure at Falkenstein, Kretzschmar moved to New York, establishing his practice in a poor German neighborhood in Brooklyn. His experience in Falkenstein, his readings in bacteriology, and his recognition of the plight of German immigrants were all factors in his advocacy of closed institutions modeled on the Dettweiler system.[4] Aware that American physicians were wedded to considerations of climate and travel for health, Kretzschmar first argued that open health resorts, in which the sick lived without medical supervision and followed a physically demanding life out-of-doors, violated Koch's findings in two ways. First, it disregarded the possibility of contagion. Second, and far more important, it ignored what had recently been learned about the relationship between disease and a lowered "resistance."[5] To combat (or for that matter to prevent) tuberculosis required increasing the "vitality and the resisting power of the cells in the body." As Kretzschmar insisted: "It should be our endeavor so to combine *all* remedial forces at our command as to strengthen and invigorate the great complex of cells—the general organism—and thereby to enable the diseased organ to resist the destructive invasion of the tubercular bacillus." [6]

In keeping with the idea of enhancing resistance, Kretzschmar advised those with tuberculosis not to "select resorts where the well find rest and recreation or outdoor sports." Rowing, hiking, hunting, and climbing were activities for the healthy. To live outdoors like an Indian was to overtax an already "enfeebled organism." The effective treatment of tuberculosis required entering an institution and following a medically supervised regimen designed to increase the "remedial agents." Persons with tuberculosis had to follow their own special routine, not mimic that of the healthy. Indeed, in his account, the tubercular had to be protected from the healthy, not the other way around. They "suffer in a much higher degree from living among well people than the latter do by the presence of the former."[7]

The critical figure in this regimen was the physician. He was both "remedial agent and scientific researcher," and his knowledge of how the bacilli thrived and spread set the treatment regimen. "The greatest importance in obtaining favorable results," Kretzschmar told his American colleagues,

> is the treatment of phthisical [tubercular] patients within institutions where they are constantly under the personal supervision of an attending physician. . . . The smallest details of the patient's life are controlled by the supervising physician and nothing of any importance is left to his or her

judgment. The daily exercise in the open air, the use of lung-gymnastics, the administration of stimulants, even the changing of garments, are matters not left to the judgment of the patients.

The physician "should have the widest possible control over *everything* that might influence the condition of the patient either favorably or otherwise, and *such* a supervision cannot be maintained outside of a well-regulated sanatorium."[8] The physician who achieved this authority would produce large numbers of cures. "Under appropriate treatment," concluded Kretzschmar, "if the disease has not made too much progress and if the treatment is continued for a sufficient length of time, *more than one-half of all cases of bacillary phthisis should be cured, and will remain so if the patient will live accordingly afterward.*"[9]

The new design transformed the relationship between the physician and the sick. In the sanatorium, invalids became patients, that is, entirely passive, with all decision-making relegated to the physician. Consumptives— whether on shipboard in the 1830s or out West in the 1860s—had been on their own, choosing their own destinations and setting their own routines. Of course they visited doctors and got their advice, but ultimately they exercised a large measure of personal freedom. Patients, by contrast, led lives that were far more circumscribed. Confined to the sanatorium, they were obliged to follow the directives of the physician, to respect his judgment in all matters, and to take his prescriptions as orders.

This revolution was clearly perceived by contemporaries. The stark comparison between invalid and patient is not merely a reflection of a post-1960s sensibility to patient rights; rather, it was well appreciated at the time and served as the basis for opposition by American physicians to European practices. Samuel Fisk, president of the Colorado State Medical Society and a physician who had found a cure in the West, opposed Kretzschmar's arguments by citing his own and his patients' case histories.[10] He distinguished carefully between diagnosis and treatment, allowing that bacteriology had led to major advances in identifying the disease, but "the introduction of the germ theory and the demonstration of the bacillus has not aided us much" in terms of therapy. For all Koch's discoveries and Kretzschmar's claims, "the best accepted plan of treatment is the climatic."[11]

Fisk objected most strongly to the doctor-patient relationship advocated by the Germans. Not that he denigrated the role of the doctor. "A climate, like any other therapeutic measure," he contended, "has to be used discreetly to obtain the best that can be gained from it, and this can be attained ... from consulting those who have had experience in it." A knowledgeable physician offered important advice "to the regulation of

diet, exercise, clothing . . . the ventilation of the rooms, the regulation of
the hours of sleep—in fact, the regulating of the invalid's life."[12] But Fisk
rejected the notion that proper supervision required setting up an institution and anointing the physician as its head. He bridled at the idea of confining the tubercular to facilities "run on a system with almost clock-like
precision." Anyone afflicted with the disease was entitled to be "his own
master, to live, always subject to direction, of course, but without surveillance, in a boarding house, hotel, or at his own home. . . . The majority of
patients will use due care, if the importance of the subject be presented to
them."[13]

In his arguments, Fisk sounded thoroughly American and especially
western. "I think that it should never be lost sight of," he insisted, "that a
phthisical invalid is a human being, usually of mature years, who values his
independence, who chafes under discipline of any sort, and who hates and
detests being schooled again, or being huddled with other invalids like a
flock of sheep." Framing the issue in personal terms, Fisk told his colleagues: "I have been a consumptive invalid myself, and many of you have
also been in the same condition yourselves and I appeal to you, if you do
not feel with me, that as a consumptive you would rather live as a man,
under the plan pursued in Colorado, than be caged with a crowd of hollow
coughing consumptives in any sanatorium, even though it might have covered walks and a winter garden, suitably warmed and ventilated." Sanatoriums did not fit with the American ethos.[14]

Nevertheless, for all the efforts to link the open institution to American
values, it was the German system of closed institutions, or sanatoriums, that
triumphed. By 1900, 34 sanatoriums with 4,485 beds had been opened in
the United States. Twenty-five years later, there were 536 sanatoriums with
673,338 beds.[15] Why did the sanatorium movement spread so rapidly?
Why did the European closed institutions replace the American open
resorts? The answer rests, in part, on social considerations. There is no
overestimating the fear of contagion among both the public at large and
public health officers, or the appeal of the new system of cure. But there is
also a biographical component to the story, the extraordinary influence of
one particular, really charismatic, figure—Edward Livingston Trudeau.
Trudeau established the first American sanatorium at Saranac Lake in the
Adirondacks, and the choices he made about location, admissions, and regimen set the model for the American sanatorium.

The transforming year in Trudeau's life was 1882, and for reasons that went
beyond Koch's discoveries. That year the tubercular Trudeau was so frail
that active exercise left him short of breath. He had been living in and
around Saranac since 1876, following an outdoor routine and occasionally
treating others who arrived in search of a cure. He continued to hunt from

a seat in a rowboat, a method that required "only slight exertion and kept me out of doors all day." However limited his progress, he was convinced that he owed his life to this exercise, to the purity of the air in the Adirondacks, and to a wholesome diet. These features, and surely not the "inclement and trying" climate of Saranac, enabled him to survive and divide his time between "medicine and hunting."[16]

The first of the 1882 incidents so critical to Trudeau was his coming upon an article in the *English Practitioner* describing the Brehmer-Dettweiler regimen. He was intrigued by their design, mostly because the emphasis on pure air, rest, modest exercise, and a rich diet almost exactly mirrored his own routine. Moreover, the atmospheric conditions in Gorbersdorf and Falkenstein resembled those in Saranac Lake. In fact, the Brehmer-Dettweiler cure so validated Trudeau's own experience that he was eager, as he later wrote, to make "a test of this new method in treating some of my tuberculosis patients."[17]

That same year Trudeau read about Koch's work and, unlike many of his American counterparts, was immediately excited by its implications. "I became strongly convinced of the soundness of his deductions and the far-reaching importance of his discovery," Trudeau recalled, "and intensely anxious to test his experimental results." He was so fascinated by Koch's ability to stain and identify the tubercle microorganism that he wanted to learn the technique and replicate the experiments. ("Every step," he said of Koch's research, "was proved over and over again before the next step was taken, and the ingenuity of the new methods of staining, separating and growing the germs read like a fairy-tale to me.") He himself owned a microscope but had little idea how to use it. "I knew nothing of bacteriology," he confessed, and "had never heard the name [of Koch] before. I lived in a remote region which made access to books, scientific apparatus, or other physicians impossible."[18]

Neither his illness nor his ignorance deterred Trudeau. He first shared his enthusiasm for Koch's methods with his mentor, Alfred Loomis, but Loomis was skeptical—he simply "didn't believe much in 'germs.'" Trudeau then obtained a letter of introduction to Dr. T. Mitchell Prudden of the Columbia College of Physicians and Surgeons. Prudden had worked in Koch's laboratory, and Trudeau went down to New York to see if he would teach him Koch's methods of staining. Prudden was courteous, gave Trudeau a specimen of the bacilli, and had his laboratory assistant show him "where the stains were and . . . some simple directions for each step to be taken." Even so, Trudeau found it difficult to replicate the experiment. During the first three days, I "stained my fingers, my clothes, even my shoes" but had no success with his specimen, staining "too much or too little, so that the germ remained invisible under the microscope." Eventually, he mastered the technique and was ready to "study some of my doubtful cases by this test."[19] He returned to the Adirondacks and set up a laboratory with rudimentary equipment so that he could conduct his own peculiar experiment to "determine how far extremes of environment favor or arrest the progress of germ infection."[20]

Trudeau, as he reported in abundant detail to the 1887 meeting of the American Climatological Association, collected fifteen rabbits and divided them into three cohorts. He inoculated two of the three cohorts with tuberculosis, and then placed all three "under conditions best adapted to answer in the results." Group 1 was inoculated, "confined in a small box . . . in a dark cellar . . . deprived of light, fresh air, and exercise," and fed limited rations. Four of these five rabbits died within three months; the fifth was killed a month later and at the autopsy, its right lung "was found solidified and shrivelled." Group 2 was not inoculated, but the rabbits were placed in a small box in a freshly dug hole in the middle of a field and fed small amounts of food once a day through a trapdoor in their box. Four months later, none had developed the disease but they "were emaciated . . . their coats . . . rough." Group 3 was inoculated and "at once turned loose on a small island" near to Trudeau's camp. For the next four months, from June to September, they lived "in the midst of conditions well adapted to stimulate their vital powers to the highest point attainable." Not only was food naturally available but Trudeau added "an abundant supply of vegetables." One rabbit died a month after the inoculation, but the others "remained apparently in perfect health, and so active had they become that two of them could only be captured with the aid of a gun." Later, on autopsy, their "organs were healthy and . . . the points of inoculation could not be made out."[21]

The design of Trudeau's experiment and his interpretation of its results highlight his ability to amalgamate disparate theories into support for his own favored outcome. The rabbits of Group 1 living in dark cellars—read tenements—died quickly. The rabbits of Group 3 who roamed freely in the wilderness and enjoyed abundant food all thrived. The experiment not only demonstrated to Trudeau that damp cellars, inadequate food, and the absence of sunlight exacerbated tuberculosis but that wholesome food, pure air, hours of sunshine, and freedom of movement effected a cure. Two additional observations, one drawn from wildlife and the other from purported experience of Native Americans, confirmed his findings for him. "Animals and game birds, which, in their wild state, are never known to die of tuberculosis," noted Trudeau, "rapidly succumb to the malady when placed in confinement." By the same token, "North American Indians, among whom phthisis is practically unknown while living a savage life, are decimated by consumption when placed under the trying restrictions of a more civilized mode of existence." The conclusion was thus unassailable: "All measures which tend to increase the vitality of the body cells have been found to be

precisely those which are most effectual in combating tuberculosis . . .
hygiene, climate, and feeding—in other words, a favorable environment—
have alone given results which have stood the test of time."[22]

Those who read Trudeau's findings were impressed by them. To Kretzschmar, they revealed both the devastating effects that resulted "when both
bacillary infection and unhygienic surroundings are made to co-exist in
tuberculosis," and the value of fresh air and out-of-door life "for all living
creatures." So, too, none other than the renowned Johns Hopkins professor
of medicine William Osler asserted that "a patient confined to the house
particularly in the close overheated, stuffy dwellings of the poor . . . is in a
position analogous to that of the rabbit confined to a hutch in the cellar;
whereas a patient living in the fresh air and sunshine for the greater part of
the day has chances comparable to those of the rabbit running wild." Even
Loomis, who had been so skeptical of germ theory, praised Trudeau. "It
seems to me," he commented at the American Climatological Association
meeting after Trudeau concluded, "that this is one of the most valuable and
carefully prepared papers that we have had before this society. . . . This line
of study is going to help us to explain our clinical facts."[23]

Armed with these findings, Trudeau decided to open an institution for the
treatment of tuberculosis at Saranac Lake. His Adirondack Cottage Sanatorium, like his laboratory investigations, began as an experiment. But his
results seemed so impressive that within ten years, the facility had set the
standard for treating tuberculosis. In light of the commitment of American
physicians to the open resort system and the anecdotes of cure that it had
spawned, Trudeau's achievement was all the more remarkable.

In establishing the institution, Trudeau intended to duplicate the German method. Rejecting the western model, he insisted that "it is not so
much *where* the consumptive lives as *how* he lives that is of the most importance, and that the pulmonary invalid cannot be left safely to his own
devices as to his mode of life in any climate."[24] But in accepting the
Brehmer-Dettweiler methods, Trudeau encountered a problem that they
had not confronted—how to attract patients. In Germany spa going was an
entrenched habit of the well-to-do. But who would come to Saranac?
Loomis, for example, had long been encouraging his patients to go to the
Adirondacks for a cure, but without much success. In 1882 one hotel for fifteen to twenty guests was "adequate to take care for all the visitors at
Saranac Lake."[25]

Trudeau took an altogether novel approach to solving this problem. He
would serve the poor, constructing a "few cottages at Saranac Lake" at
modest cost. Those with the least resources and options would become his
subjects; in return for subsidized rent and free medical consultations, they
would test the routine of open-air treatment.[26] Loomis, as usual, proved

essential to the project, agreeing to examine his worthy but poor tubercular patients without charge and to send to Trudeau those unwilling or unable to seek a cure in the West. (Selecting this population made the experiment acceptable in two ways—absent Trudeau, these patients would not be receiving any treatment, and other physicians would not find his efforts competitive.) Loomis himself remained wary of the therapeutic value of the experiment but readily conceded: "We need such institutions certainly for those patients who are not able to take care of themselves. . . . When we look at the manner in which consumptives die in our general hospitals, and the unpleasant life that they lead while they are dying, it seems to me that we are stimulated to help them—if we cannot cure them, to help them to a more comfortable way of dying."[27]

Although Trudeau had not anticipated it, limiting admission to the worthy poor gave his project a powerful philanthropic appeal. To his amazement, he proved to be a highly successful fund-raiser. He first approached the men and women who had personal experience with tuberculosis and had spent their summers at Saranac Lake. Thus, one afternoon, when he and Anson Phelps Stokes, a wealthy merchant and banker, were sailing, Trudeau outlined his plan. "I expressed the wish that some of the poor invalids shut up in cities might have the opportunity for recovery which the climate offered and which had done so much for me." Stokes immediately pledged $500. Several weeks later, Mrs. Stokes held an "open-air fair at her camp," which turned into an annual fund-raising event.[28]

With the first subscriptions in hand, Trudeau gained entrée to the benevolent wealthy of New York, and in their living rooms over tea, he described his project and asked for their assistance. Often he met with skepticism. "Most people couldn't understand just what I wanted to do, because, they always argued, consumption couldn't be cured; an aggregation of such invalids would be so depressing that no one would stay in such a place, and besides, the region was so inaccessible—forty-two miles from a railroad—and the climate so rough that my plan seemed to them entirely visionary." But frequently the wealthy, inspired by his enthusiasm or by the sight of this frail physician wanting to use his remaining strength to help the poor, gave him funds. Trudeau, a pragmatic man, tailored his appeal to suit his potential donors. He told some of them that he wanted to test the Dettweiler methods at a "little hospital for consumptives in the Adirondacks." To others he emphasized the humanitarian aspects of the undertaking. The "little hospital" became a "little institution at Saranac Lake" where the poor "could come for less than cost and remain as long as necessary."[29]

Trudeau even modified the design of the facility to attract donors. "I knew," he said later, "it would be easier to get some of my patients to give a little cottage which would be their own individual gift, rather than a corresponding sum of money towards the erection of larger buildings." But none of this bothered him, for, as he frankly conceded, "I had no knowledge whatever of what sort of buildings to plan for such a sanitarium, nor was such information to be found in books then."[30]

Despite or because of this flexibility, the enterprise thrived. After one year of "begging" as he called it, Trudeau had collected $5,000, a sum that was more than enough to conduct his experiment.[31] By 1900, fifteen years after it opened, the Adirondack Cottage Sanatorium had twenty-two buildings, clusters of small cottages, a large administration building, a library, a chapel, and an infirmary. It had become a "little village" for the poor with tuberculosis.[32]

However varied Trudeau's message, it was the prospect of curing tuberculosis that most deeply animated him. He took considerable hope from the new science of bacteriology. In his sanatorium a well-equipped laboratory was an "indispensable requisite" for "the study of the disease and the diagnosis of obscure cases." Trudeau and his staff conducted a variety of experiments at Saranac, for only in this way "can we reach satisfactory conclusions as to the real value of the specific methods of treatment . . . or make any progress in the development of such methods." Trudeau was convinced that "it is to these methods that we must look in future for much-needed light upon many of the unsolved problems relating to etiology, prophylaxis and disinfection."[33]

The design and the routine of the institution also reflected Trudeau's belief that tuberculosis was treatable, although the character of his interventions appears to have had less to do with science than tradition and anecdote. "The principal aim of the modern sanitarium treatment of tuberculosis," he declared in 1897, "is to improve the patient's nutrition and increase his resistance to the disease, by placing him under the most favorable environment obtainable. The main elements of such an environment are an invigorating climate, an open-air life, rest, coupled with the careful regulation of the daily habits and an abundant supply of nutritious food." Trudeau was convinced that this regimen would cure the disease, certainly in its first appearance. "Early phthisis is therefore a disease which should be treated, and which yields under intelligent management a fair proportion of cures." Indeed, Trudeau was eager to limit admissions to patients in "the earlier stage of the disease, or with a fair chance of more or less complete restoration to health."[34]

The regimen at Saranac faithfully followed the Brehmer-Dettweiler method. Like them, Trudeau instructed patients to "gradually accustom themselves to leading an outdoor life, that is, to remaining eight to ten hours in the open air each day. This should be done gradually. . . . Little by little the open air sitting and walks are to be increased until the entire day is spent out of doors in all kinds of weather." He also supplied a rich diet—

patients received three full meals a day and a glass of milk every four hours. And in this same spirit, Trudeau wanted the physician to monitor the daily regimen. "Patients," his rule book announced, "will be informed by the physician how much exercise their case requires."[35]

Trudeau was all the more prepared to empower the physician because most of his first patients were uneducated and foreign-born. Charity was critical to the sanatorium's admission policy. The facility accepted the person whose "pecuniary circumstances . . . make it impossible for him to pay the usual prices asked at the hotels and boarding houses of the region."[36] But charity, as is often the case, imposed a rigid code of behavior. The rules, reminiscent of those in city almshouses and hospitals, not only set the time for waking, eating, and retiring and explicitly prohibited drinking and smoking, but also duly noted: "Patients are requested that, as the sanitarium is run not for profit but only for their own benefit, they should individually do all in their power to keep the place looking neat and protect the furniture and other property from injury." Anyone whose behavior was "obnoxious to others" or who "violates the rules of the establishment" would be discharged—apparently disobedience trumped cure.[37]

Trudeau taught hygienic procedures to prevent the spread of the disease (now in the sanatorium and, he hoped, eventually back in the tenement house). The facility itself was designed to avoid the spread of infection from patient to patient. The cottages were well ventilated; partitions separated the individual sleeping spaces from the common sitting room, which, in turn, was in "direct communication with the veranda on which the outdoor plan of treatment is carried out." Accordingly, each patient had "so large an air space as to make it difficult, when rigid precautions as to the care of the expectoration are enforced, for the buildings to become contaminated."[38] The staff also gave patients extensive and repeated instructions about the proper disposal of expectoration. Trudeau placed spittoons throughout the facility and was prepared to penalize "indiscriminate spitting" by dismissal. "The presence of the consumptive," he always maintained, "entails little or no risk where the expectorated matter is properly cared for." In fact, he boasted in 1903, almost twenty years after the sanatorium opened, that "none of our employees or servants has been known to develop consumption."[39]

To confirm the success of his experiment, Trudeau collected data on the discharge status of former patients. In 1903 the staff located 1,066 of the 1,500 patients who had been treated by Trudeau and learned that one-third of them described themselves as "well." Although the overall percentage was not impressive, Trudeau observed that of the "well" group, fully two-thirds had been incipient cases. Thus, his conclusions supported his hypothesis that those who received "an early diagnosis" and went immediately to a sanatorium for treatment could expect to be cured.[40]

* * *

The American sanatorium in its development looked to the Adirondack Cottage Sanatorium and Edward Livingston Trudeau for guidance. Almost every physician and organization about to construct a sanatorium paid a visit to Saranac Lake to meet Trudeau and tour his facility, and usually they came away convinced that a well-run facility could cure the disease. Like Trudeau, they believed that persons with tuberculosis were victims trapped by circumstances beyond their control; a sanatorium stay would liberate and restore them to a productive life.

This vision of rescue shaped the charitable impulses of philanthropists even as it energized the public health crusaders. To Jacob Schiff, a leading figure in Jewish charities, the sanatorium promised to "restore the health of the countless numbers of men and women who, afflicted with consumption in its early stage, often perish, but could be saved, if adequate provision existed for their proper treatment."[41] In this same spirit, Lillian Brandt of New York's Charity Organization Society urged voluntary organizations to administer such facilities. "More than a hundred thousand deaths," she maintained, "are caused by consumption each year in the United States. . . . There is imperative need for free sanatoriums for early cases and of sanatoriums for persons who are able to pay five or six dollars a week."[42] What Trudeau did for the poor in Saranac, the argument went, ethnic, religious, and social groups should do for their own.

Because the sanatorium was so quintessentially a charity movement, social criteria were as important as medical criteria in setting admissions policy. In large cities the charitable bureaus directed potential applicants to organizations on the basis of ethnicity or religious affiliation, for the sanatorium, like the voluntary, not-for-profit hospital, considered each bed as a gift reserved for the most worthy recipient. Indeed, with applicants outnumbering beds well into the 1920s, the organizations screened the pool all the more rigorously. The United Hebrew Charities, for example, sponsored and funded sanatoriums in Denver as well as New York; its social workers met together with its physicians to determine which applicants should be accepted and where they should be sent. If recommended to the National Jewish Hospital, a second screening occurred, this time by the hospital's own physicians and representatives in New York. The National Jewish Hospital also insisted that patients had to come with two sets of warm clothing, including rubber boots, and with a guarantee from their home charity society that it would pay for the return ticket.[43]

All the while sanatorium officials expected gratitude as well as complaince from the patients. Stony Wold Sanatorium, another Adirondacks facility, was opened by a Trudeau admirer to treat working girls in the initial stage of tuberculosis; its admission committee, aptly called the "appreciation committee," tried to make certain that all those accepted would think of themselves as "guests."[44] Other facilities tried to screen out those who were friendless, single, or homeless, or who had a criminal record or a mental or physical disability. Some facilities were so determined to admit only cooperative patients that they insisted that patients pay, or more likely, get someone to pay, a portion of the cost of the stay.

Some of the eagerness to institutionalize the poor stemmed from a belief that they could not be trusted to follow medical prescriptions without supervision. "On account of home conditions and great poverty it is next to impossible to maintain discipline with such patients in their homes," Dr. Lawrence Flick declared. "They often will not sit out in the open air because they have no convenient place to sit in. . . . They will not take the diet. Even when supplied with milk, they will divide it up with other members of the family rather than use it for their own recovery." Apparently, they lacked the resources and the discipline to cure themselves on their own.[45]

These facilities varied in a number of ways, in terms not only of admissions policies but also of prescribed routine. Directors, boards of trustees, and staff introduced their own policies, reflecting personal history, preferences, or ethnic and religious values. Moreover, since many of the physicians in charge of the sanatoriums had tuberculosis themselves (they stayed on either because they were too frail to practice elsewhere or because they thought that the stigma of the disease would not allow them to build up a practice), they often tried to introduce whatever regimen they believed had worked for them. Hence, everyone subscribed to the general tenets of open-air treatment, rich diet, and moderate exercise, but there were many interpretations of what these principles meant in practice. As to what constituted the right rich diet, in 1908 Irving Fisher, a professor of political economy at Yale who had cured at Saranac Lake, compared the diets in ninety-five American and European sanatoriums. To his dismay, he found that "there is still no fixed theory in regard to nutrition in tuberculosis. . . . Diet in most consumptive sanatoriums is unsystematic and extremely varying. . . . There is disagreement as to the extent to which the appetite of the consumptive can be trusted or should be forced, and as to the number of calories . . . fat, and carbohydrate which he should consume." Some sanatoriums insisted on 5,500 calories a day; others supplied only 2,500 to 3,000. Some directors who had been cured on a vegetarian diet made their sanatoriums vegetarian; others thinking that cells needed more proteins and fats fed their residents a dozen eggs a day and a quart of milk. As Fisher sadly concluded, it all "centered on opinion."[46]

Variations were as prevalent in prescriptions for physical activity. Almost everyone opposed vigorous exercise and demanded that newcomers have total rest for the first few weeks. The common understanding, at one with Trudeau, was that in people with tuberculosis "the organs and tissues have now an extra burden to bear. Exercise which in health would help to build up the normal body and increase resistance to disease, in this illness, when injudiciously carried out, leads to much harm, weakening the resisting powers and hastening the progress of the disease." Beyond this tenet, however, there was little consensus.[47] Some superintendents liked to keep patients in cure chairs all day; others, like Dr. Alexius M. Forster of Colorado Springs, believed that "graduated systematic exercise improves the discipline in the institution."[48] Still others tried to define a middle way. "Neither rest nor exercise should be prescribed to the exclusion of the other," Dr. F. M. Pottenger, who ran a sanatorium in Los Angeles, maintained. "Both must be employed." And still others had their patients follow a graduated program, from rest to exercise to manual labor, which they then called "productive exercise." In this spirit, the medical staff of the Loomis Sanatorium (named in honor of Alfred Loomis) in Liberty, New York, explained that manual labor was "the form of exercise" they relied on; it included "forestry work, road-building, gardening, mowing lawns etc." The directors unabashedly argued that this policy did "add interest and zest to the patient's sanatorium routine, and thus is conducive to better discipline." It also reduced expenses—surely a welcome by-product, even as it made superintendents defensive. "I do not think," insisted Dr. Forster, "that it is the object of those of us who are interested in the development of graduated exercise to make workhouses of our sanatoria. It is primarily our object to recognize that we have the moral and mental welfare of our patients to look after, as well as the physical." Others were less certain that the distinction between workhouse and sanatorium would be maintained. "If charity tuberculous patients are to work while they are being treated," Dr. Pottenger cautioned, "the work should be carefully measured and suited to the patient and his condition."[49] But there were few ways to make certain that such admonitions were heeded.

It was the city, county, and state sanatoriums that were most prone to confusing cure with discipline and confinement with coercion. Public facilities were even more likely than charitable facilities to lose sight of their therapeutic mission.

As was true of many other tax-funded institutions, the public sanatoriums were places of last resort, serving the rejects of the not-for-profit system, those too marginal even to apply to them or those considered a serious danger to the public health.[50] Even so, there was a considerable variation in quality among them. The more desirable were the state sanatoriums, particularly those located in rural regions; the less desirable were the municipal sanatoriums, especially those proximate to the tenement districts. After surveying 221 facilities in 1926, Godias J. Drolet reported to the New York Tuberculosis and Health Association: "It is to the country, in a sanatorium, that a patient wants to go, where undoubtedly he has a better chance for recovery, rather than in the old hospital." Drolet found that county sanatoriums had 97 percent of their beds filled while hospitals located in the cities reported 82 percent occupancy.[51] The very worst were the wards or facilities holding prisoners or mental patients with tuberculosis.[52]

Some public institutions tried insofar as they could to emaulate not-for-profit facilities and take the patients who, based on past history, appeared to be most compliant and likely to be cured. A number of state sanatoriums, for example, levied a small weekly charge, not so much to balance their books as to keep out the riffraff. These facilities also gave preference to new cases over the chronic. One Boston physician, Dr. Joseph Pratt, complained that the Massachusetts State Sanatorium rejected patients "with a good fighting chance for recovery," either because they could not afford the fee or because "the disease is too far advanced."[53] For its part, the New York State Sanatorium required payment either from the patient or from his town's department of charities, in this way hoping to take in the worthy poor and keep out the dissolute. To the degree that such strategies succeeded in skimming off the most respectable and treatable among the poor, city and county facilities were left to serve what were presumed to be the most chronic and least worthy patients—and it was not an assignment they relished.

Not surprisingly, city and county sanatoriums defined their responsibilities as narrowly as possible. Smaller municipalities gave one ward in the almshouse to the tubercular; larger ones reserved a building. Neither setting usually provided more than a shelter for the dying. Cities like New York, confronting thousands of cases of tuberculosis among its immigrant population, were compelled to establish more elaborate systems, but here, too, the design looked more to custody than cure.

Hermann Biggs, New York's energetic and ambitious public health officer, devoted some twenty years to organizing a system of care for the poor tubercular, but his efforts took him in a very different direction than that taken by Trudeau. First, he tried in 1893 to reserve a ward in each municipal hospital for the tubercular. But the numbers of patients always exceeded the number of available beds, and so inevitably patients with tuberculosis were scattered throughout the hospital.[54] Next, to handle the surplus from the municipal hospitals, Biggs took over a recently vacated building on Blackwell's Island (in New York's East River) that had housed the insane. The Tuberculosis Infirmary of Metropolitan Hospital, as it was called, was in actuality an almshouse for those with tuberculosis.[55] Admitting anyone with the disease, it was soon seriously overcrowded, particularly in winter, when hundreds of beds lined the corridors. Within a month of arrival, one-third of the patients had died and half of the remainder had left.[56]

In 1906 Biggs was finally able to raise sufficient funds to open Otisville—

his version of a real sanatorium in the Catskills—for the city's poorest residents.[57] Eschewing rich diets and long periods of rest, the regimen at Otisville was designed to be spartan and austere, as befit the social class of its patients. Convinced that the "rest cure" had no place in a facility for the poor, Biggs substituted what he called a "work cure." "The treatment by long-continued rest (which in my judgment has been carried to too great a length)," he maintained, "often returns the patient with arrested disease but physically unprepared for any lucrative manual occupation." In Trudeau's type of sanatorium, "a working tuberculous person has been converted into a fairly healthy loafer." Accordingly, at Otisville the rest cure lasted one week, followed by "measured walks." These were "personally supervised by the Captain of the Walking Squad, a kind of patient trusty who kept his charges moving. The measured walks gave way to the "work cure"; at the end of three weeks patients were assigned to daily tasks that increased in rigor as the stay progressed.[58]

Convinced that six months was too long a period to confine the poor, Biggs set a three-month limit for Otisville. The few who remained longer were the most diligent workers, those who provided "exceptional service." But Biggs's problem was not an excessive number of patients who wished to stay on but the speed with which most of them left. Many were gone after thirty days—most against medical advice.[59]

Supplementing his almshouse and would-be sanatorium was Biggs's Riverside Hospital, which, as we have noted, was intended to confine, involuntarily, the tubercular whose "dissipated and vicious habits" endangered the health of the community.[60] But in planning as in execution, Biggs could never decide just what kind of facility Riverside was, hospital or prison. It was regularly short of basic supplies, including sputum cups, which meant that patients neither practiced nor learned basic hygienic measures. Discipline was supposed to be strict, but patient-inmates spent their days playing cards and wandering about the corridors.[61] Serious infractions were to be punished with solitary confinement. But as Robert J. Wilson, the superintendent of hospitals, noted in 1914: "There are neither police officers to govern nor cells or quiet rooms in which to confine these recalcitrant ones. The only weapons in the hands of the hospital authorities are those of argument or persuasion."[62] In the end, Riverside was too prisonlike to be a hospital and too hospitallike to be a prison.

The failure in New York was typical of the outcomes in other cities. A 1912 committee appointed by the National Association for the Study and Prevention of Tuberculosis investigated twenty-five municipally funded facilities in five major cities and reported that they held friendless immigrants and vagrants. As in almshouses, the population fluctuated with the weather, so that in winter "the patients go to them for shelter," and in warmer weather they leave. These facilities had not even attempted to provide the rudiments of treatment (few had porches or a regimen of rest) or of education (the committee noted everywhere "defective methods of disposal of sputum, [and] insufficient instruction of patients in the methods of prevention"). Patients who were strong enough to be out of bed were assigned chores, which they often refused to perform. The only disciplinary authority that officials had was to discharge patients for "bad behavior," but since they were carrying a contagious disease, such punishments, at least from a public health perspective, were not sound policy. Nor was the commonly practiced policy of granting "leaves of absence," for that meant that the patients would "mingle for days among their relatives, friends, etc.," spreading the disease wherever they went. The municipal sanatoriums, concluded the committee, were indistinguishable from almshouses or workhouses. They served as a "place of last resort to the narrow group of cases, in the extreme stages of physical and economic helplessness."[63]

The many variations that characterized the sanatorium system of care were altogether familiar not only to municipal officials and physicians but also to persons with tuberculosis. For patients, this diversity put a premium on manipulating the system—learning how to avoid the health inspector or how to gain admission to the best facility. Many patients recorded how they fared in this process, giving us our third and final set of narratives of illness: living and dying with tuberculosis in an era of contagion.

14

In the Shadow of the Sanatorium

THE NEW UNDERSTANDING OF TUBERCULOSIS THAT INFORMED THE PUB-
lic health and sanatorium movements transformed the lives of both men
and women with tuberculosis. Defined as contagious by public health officials, they incorporated these negative judgments into their own self-iden-
tity. They referred to themselves as "tbs" or "lungers," the diseased organ
representing their personas. They were "a special species," morally as well
physically disabled.

In the bacteriological era patients did not have to break their physician's
code about a diseased lung to learn that they had tuberculosis. Physicians
were now less likely to be evasive in their diagnosis.[1] In part, the change
reflected the power of the new diagnostic technologies. Instead of having to
judge the meaning of a rattle as heard directly or as amplified by a stethoscope, they now were able to see into the lungs via an X ray (Deborah's
Vinal Fiske's fantasy realized) or, by using a microscope, to identify the
tubercle bacillus in the sputum. But the change also reflected both the
physicians' fear that an uninformed patient would spread infection and
their hope that a patient diagnosed early would be susceptible to cure.

Although many patients presented themselves to the physician with
marked symptoms of the disease—dramatic weight loss, blood-streaked
sputum, and persistent cough and fatigue—the news that they had tuberculosis and the prescription to leave the community and perhaps enter a
sanatorium often came as a surprise. Many did not follow the advice and
continued to work for as long as possible or remained in bed at home.[2]
Those who did comply were nonetheless stunned by their sudden exile. In
their letters, they invoked the term "banishment." In 1898, Irving Fisher, a
professor of political economy at Yale, explained his departure to Saranac
Lake by announcing: "I have been banished by my doctor."[3] Edwin Davis

French, a well-known engraver, sent the same message back from Saranac in 1897: he had undergone an "unexpected banishment to this corner of the wilderness."[4] To make matters worse, the banishment was of indeterminate duration—lasting six months, a year, perhaps a lifetime.

Contracting tuberculosis was so stigmatizing that beginning in the 1890s and persisting through the 1930s those who were diagnosed with the disease often failed to inform family or friends. In 1909 James Williams, a newspaper reporter in Washington, D.C., told his parents in as casual a tone as he could muster that he had suddenly decided to spend the winter in Arizona for "a complete rest." Williams related his plans in so light-hearted a manner that his father believed the trip was "a mere lark."[5] John Ward Stimson referred to his "misfortunes of health" or vaguely to a "disease which threatens," in order to explain why he was "practically handicapped for several months."[6] In 1912, when Edwin Alderman, the president of the University of Virginia, learned his diagnosis, he quickly arranged for a leave of absence, and he and his wife went to Saranac Lake. Alderman instructed his secretary to tell people that he had been working too hard and was taking a vacation in the woods.[7] Even those more ready to be candid hesitated to be completely honest. "The truth is," Fisher wrote a friend, "I have a threatening of tuberculosis."[8]

Patients confirmed for one another the wisdom of hiding the disease. Anne Ellis repeated the tale of an indiscreet young woman who discovered that "people were afraid of her, and she felt like an outcast, a leper. Added to this the doctor would not permit her relatives, not even her fiancé, to enter her room, and when she left [to go West] they had to make their farewells through an open window." Better to lie than suffer such isolation and humiliation.[9]

Families and confidants were as secretive as the sick themselves. They told friends that their spouses or siblings were taking a much needed "rest" or "vacation," and they cited other physical ailments to account for sudden departures. When Robert Ferguson, a former Rough Rider with Teddy Roosevelt, learned he had tuberculosis in 1908, he and his wife immediately set out for Saranac Lake, leaving his mother-in-law to inform friends that "Bob is resting up for a slight operation for piles."[10] The mother of Charlie Moses told family and friends that Charlie was in college in upstate New York when in fact he was trying to cure his tuberculosis. The result was that "no one ever knew that I had tuberculosis," a disease, he maintained, "you were supposed to conceal."[11]

Although the stigma was pervasive, the experience of those diagnosed with tuberculosis varied by time, social class, and place of residence. In the 1880s or early 1890s, they did not suffer as much discrimination as their counterparts did in the first decades of the twentieth century, as phthisiophobia became more widespread. The well-to-do were better able than the poor to shield themselves from its impact; and immigrants living in large cities were more likely to encounter significant discrimination than rural residents. Thus, in 1893, when New York City made registration of the tubercular compulsory, the rich as well as the poor did everything possible to avoid having their names entered on health department lists or having their homes visited by inspectors.[12] Private patients, eager to be spared the embarrassment, coaxed their doctors to bend the rules, something that was often easily accomplished.[13] Immigrants who used public dispensaries had their own strategies to prevent losing a job, insurance, or lodging. Some gave a false name or wrong address at the dispensary, or they moved without notifying the department, or they brazenly told the inspector that they were not the person she was looking for. Indeed, under even the best of circumstances, it was difficult for public health inspectors to keep track of the poor tubercular.[14] Immigrants often Americanized their names and altered the spellings. How was a health department clerk to know whether the woman that the dispensary listed as Ethel Kahn on Delancey Street was not really Yetta Cohan who lived on Rivington Street, or the Etta Cohen on Orchard Street? And of course, if Ethel Kahn left town, there was no possibility of follow-up, for health departments did not cross-list names.[15]

Persons with the disease who went West after 1890, particularly to less densely populated areas, had no way of predicting the local response. In Colorado and California some residents who themselves had found a cure there empathized with health seekers; others who worried more about the prospects of contagion were downright hostile. To be sure, money and respectability could smooth the way, as the experience of the Cutting family demonstrated. "Where to go?" mused Justine Cutting in 1910, as the family searched for a town in which her brother, Bronson, could seek a cure and they could live comfortably. "The world was open to us," she observed. "For the cure to be successful, it must not be some dreary place which would be like a prison in which one would count the days and weeks and months—years perhaps. There must be some pleasure and interest, some charm to make up for the disappointment of an interrupted career." Gradually, "by process of elimination" they "hit on New Mexico," finding it ideal both from a "medical standpoint" and a "psychological" one.[16]

They were not disappointed. The Cuttings built a comfortable and airy home and carried on an active social life, dining regularly with the governor of the state and the editor of the local paper. After a year Justine was satisfied that Bronson was "living a most normal and sensible life." Eight years later Bronson felt strong enough to purchase the *Santa Fe New Mexican*, and in 1928, to become a United States senator.

In the 1890s and into the first decade of the twentieth century, those with ample resources found a welcome in Colorado Springs. They socialized with the healthy and were often invited to tea and dinner. Philip

Washburn, who resigned his pulpit at the Episcopal church in Northampton, Massachusetts, in 1893 after he contracted the disease, found that tuberculosis was no barrier to his continued employment as a minister or to his enjoying a full social life in the Colorado town. "The social demands of this place are tremendous," he told his mother shortly after his arrival in the fall of 1893. "There are teas all the time and calls are numerable." Any limits on activities, he found, were self-imposed. "Invalids have to be careful or they are worn out by social attentions before they know it."[17] Washburn bicycled daily, and he occasionally joined a football game. "I was making calls," he told his mother, "when I saw ball playing going on. . . . I knew some of the young men and soon I was with them. . . . I did not . . . do anything violent but I had an hour's splendid exercise in the sunlight, and showed the youngsters that age and theology have not robbed the boat of all cunning."[18] (He would be pleased that the athletic field of Colorado College is named Washburn Field.)

Communities like Colorado Springs tried to maintain a tolerant attitude toward the tubercular. "We do not regard the tuberculous invalid with any of the aversion and morbid fear so frequently shown in many places," one resident informed the readers of the *Journal of the Outdoor Life*. "We know that after years of contact with them, our permanent population has not suffered to any appreciable extent." In fact, she reminded her readers, most of the homes in the town had been built with tuberculosis occupants in mind. "Many private residences are equipped with several porches in which the entire family sleep in preference to their bed-rooms . . . the great number of new houses and cottages contain some provision for the sleeping porch." Sleeping out, like camping out, was part of the western ethos; it was an activity common to both the sick and the healthy.[19]

For those with limited personal resources, however, discrimination even in the more tolerant West increasingly became a fact of life. In the prebacteriological era, health seekers had lived more or less freely on vacant plots of land; in 1905 the tents of homeless consumptives in Colorado Springs were still scattered along the banks of the river and filled its only park. But over the next several years, as Dr. Ernest Sweet of the U.S. Public Health Service observed, popular attitudes changed and residents viewed the tubercular as "becoming more parasitic . . . [and] potentially, if not actually, harmful."[20] After spending one week in El Paso in 1908, Will Ross commented: "If a tuberculosis patient came to town with enough money to support himself, he was welcomed; indeed, they were glad to have him. If he arrived broke and didn't quickly get a job, he was given short shrift. A ticket to the next town was the usual procedure, and his exit was supervised by the police."[21]

Given the fluctuations in attitude, "passing" was the best way to avoid discrimination. Thomas Galbreath reported having no difficulty finding a boardinghouse when the landlady thought he was healthy. But when another boarder complained about Galbreath's cough, he was asked to leave. He had better luck in a second boardinghouse where "everyone coughed." None of them, he was amused to note, admitted to tuberculosis: by their accounts, these were "dyspeptics, rheumatics, nervous wrecks, heart patients, kidney patients, ear patients"—anything but tuberculosis.[22]

Thus, exchanges between landlady and prospective boarders took on the character of a ritual. After two days of having the boardinghouse keepers shut their doors in his face, Will Ross devised a new strategy. When the landlady asked "the inevitable question," he answered: "Well, not in the way you are thinking of. I'm down here for my health, but I'm troubled with stomach trouble and have to rest for a while." Satisfied by his answer, "the deal was closed." Several days later, he overheard a man requesting a room for himself and his wife. When the landlady asked where the wife was, the man answered, back in the hotel with "a little stomach trouble." The next day the wife arrived on a stretcher and never left her room.[23]

These stories worked only if the symptoms were not pronounced. Those who coughed uncontrollably had trouble finding a place to live unless some good samaritan intervened. When Anne Ellis arrived on a stretcher in Albuquerque, New Mexico, she was told that no boardinghouse or hotel admitted people on stretchers. The brakeman on the train, a complete stranger but a Mason like her son, brought Anne and her daughter to the boardinghouse of a friend and smuggled her "past his landlady, [and] gave her his room for the night." But the next morning, Anne recalled, "we could not hide with my rasping cough, my labored breathing," and the landlady informed her that "it was against the law . . . to take in anyone suffering with T.B."[24] Sydney Haley, who had frequent hemorrhages and very little money, reported similar incidents when he traveled in Texas in 1908. Although he was finally able to persuade a family to board him, he was nevertheless ostracized. "I was granted the precious privilege of . . . having my food passed out to me on a tray at the kitchen door," he reported, "so that I could carry it off to my cell and eat it in solitary grandeur. I soon discovered that my landlady had a special knife, fork, and plate, and a special tray covered with a special napkin . . . in a special corner of the kitchen . . . all for my most especial benefit—to keep the deadly contagion from spreading." In 1904 Henry Sewall, a Denver physician with tuberculosis, summed up the experience of almost all his fellow patients when he wrote: "TB is a good respectable disease if you have money, but without it, it is a mean low-down business."[25]

A few did manage to penetrate hostile communities, but even they remained very much on the margins. Mae Goodwin was able, with help, to rent a cot and mattress and the right to pitch her tent in the backyard of one boarding house and to sit "by the fireplace during the day."[26] Never-

theless, she took care not to linger in public places so as to avoid confronta-
tions with the healthy, and, let it be said, others among the sick. "I get tired
of seeing such careless consumptives as there are here," she told her
mother. "Most everyone looks well but you can hear them coughing all
over town on a morning early. I guess it is partly the Drs. fault that they are
not careful about spitting."[27] Eventually, Mae staked a claim on a plot of
land on the outskirts of Santa Fe, where she raised and sold produce and
chickens. Out of sight, she lived her final years.

The poorest individuals generally faced the harshest reality, although
some among them became adept at negotiating the system. There were
those immigrants who learned about the cures to be had in Colorado even
before they learned English. They carried letters of introduction to relief
societies from charity workers, physicians, or clergymen, testifying to their
good character and asking for help in taking up residence in the town or
gaining admission to the local sanatorium.[28] Thus, Hyman Goren, a thirty-
six-year-old tailor from Boston, arrived in Denver in 1904 with a crumpled
letter from a Boston physician in his pocket. "To whom it may concern,"
wrote Dr. M. Ziselman. "This is to certify that Mr. Hyman Goren of
Boston is the victim of General Pulmonary Tuberculosis and has been
under my care for several months and I sincerely recommend him to Denver Colorado as there is no cure for him in the Eastern States."[29]

Barney Goldberg, a twenty-four-year-old immigrant from Austria, used
a similar letter to persuade a fully booked Denver sanatorium to let him
take his meals there until he could be admitted. "The man is absolutely
destitute," one board member testified. "His friends have collected several
times donations to support him. He is an intelligent and deserving man."
The strategy worked—Goldberg became a day patient and soon thereafter
received his bed.[30]

Not all the migrants were so lucky. A substantial number, homeless and
lacking any resources, ended up in tent colonies outside the town limits.
Located at least a mile beyond the last bus stop, these places carried such
sobriquets as "Bugsville" or "Lungers Camp."[31] The tent colony outside
Tucson stretched as far the eye could see along the barren desert floor.
("When a sick person needed a place to live," recalled Dick Hall, who
arrived in Tucson with his tubercular mother in 1909, "he somehow got a
tent set up in this area.")[32] On first appearance, their sheer size made them
appear to be established institutions, but in reality the sites were unplanned
and neglected. Sewage was primitive, the water supply unprotected.

Hester Shigley's own demeaning experience in a tent colony provided
the material of a short story. Her protagonist, "one of those pathetic 'health
seekers,' who throng the West and the Southwest, looking for a miracle to
overcome that slow death which preys upon them," went to a hotel and
"was about to be shown to her room, when, noticing a suspicious little

cough the clerk said, 'Beg pardon, Madam, but are you sick?' Having
learned by experience that 'sick,' so used, was meant to apply only to those
who were victims of tuberculosis she gave a quiet affirmative. 'Then,' said
the clerk, 'We can't give you a room. It's against our rules to take lungers.'"
The health seeker tried other hotels but was greeted repeatedly with the
words, "'I never take sick people!' until she felt that, as the leper of old, she
ought to cover her face and cry, 'unclean, unclean!'"[33]

The worst was yet to come. With no boardinghouse keeper willing to
take her and no other alternative, the fictional Hester accepted the offer of
a sympathetic stranger and went to Granite Glen, the tent colony outside
of town. Although she was grateful for a place to live, she felt "deserted by
God and man." At Granite Glen, the sick nursed each other to the best of
their limited ability, sharing their tales of "want and desperation." Suicide
was frequent. One young man in the last stage of the disease, "having no
friends, and feeling himself utterly without hope . . . ended that life that
seemed so useless a thing to himself and the world."[34]

Not only in fiction was suicide a route out. "Sometimes life was too
much to bear," noted Dick Hall, "and a victim would end it." But the tent
he left vacant did not stay empty for long. "He was soon replaced, however,
by others who hoped for a cure in the dry air and bright sunshine of Arizona. It was a desperate and sometimes a heroic gamble, which many lost
and few won." As Hall concluded, the colonies were "truly a place of lost
souls and lingering death."[35]

Given this increasing hostility, it is not surprising that many people with
tuberculosis, both rich and poor, took up residence in the shadow of a sanatorium. It was a choice that physicians endorsed, hoping it would promote
compliance. "Such a patient," Dr. Frederick Knight advised, "should go to
a community of such patients, where a hygienic mode of life is the rule.
Here he can have his own house and family if he likes, but the general tone
of the place will make him follow the directions of the physician, and he
will have plenty of company in outdoor life." The preferred retreat for
many wealthier patients and their physicians was Saranac Lake, New York.
Those with fewer resources went to towns with state sanatoriums, such as
Rutland, Massachusetts. In both locations, patients gained access to physicians skilled in treating tuberculosis and enjoyed the tolerance of residents
in these one-industry towns.[36]

The arrival of the sanatorium transformed small farming communities
like Saranac Lake and Rutland. Some residents, particularly in Rutland,
were wary of the prospect of having a tuberculosis facility located in their
midst. But they soon profited from its presence, finding jobs working in the
sanatorium itself, or in running boardinghouses for the sick. Farmers also
benefited as they enlarged their herds and flocks to supply the large quan-

tity of eggs and milk the sick required. This prosperity may not have eradicated stigma, but it certainly made townspeople more empathetic to the patients.

Physical evidence of the change in these towns was marked. "Cure cottages," for example, began to dot the landscape; their most prominent architectural feature was a large porch. "We passed a few houses, houses such as are seen only in Saranac," recalled Marshall McClintock. "Houses with porches on every side, at every corner, porches tacked precariously on all sides, jutting out from second and third floor rooms. The porches were screened and glassed and on all of them were men and women lying in long reclining chairs. Men and women lying silent and unmoving. . . . On some porches we could see white iron beds and in the beds lay patients, looking quietly out the windows, looking at nothing."[37] Those on the porches confirmed the impression. "I do nothing all day but lie here staring at the mountains," Elizabeth Mooney wrote to her family. "I wish they would rearrange them a bit."[38]

The well-to-do rented houses in the exclusive neighborhood and associated only with their own kind; the poor, particularly in such a setting, were considered not only ill-mannered but also contagious. Boardinghouses often served a single ethnic or religious group—there were Jewish boardinghouses, Italian boardinghouses, and so on. Yes, everyone lived with or off of tuberculosis, but that commonality did not obliterate other distinctions.[39]

For both the public and the medical profession, the place that appeared to exemplify the peculiar characteristics of the sanatorium town was Saranac Lake. "You have tuberculosis," Dr. Lamson, a physician, straightforwardly informed Helene McClintock; he immediately ordered her to "go to Saranac at once. . . . [It] is the best place to cure." Helene protested that several friends had been unhappy there, complaining that there were "nothing but sick people all around you. I couldn't stand it." But Dr. Lamson replied firmly and authoritatively: "You don't know the place. . . . It is wonderful. It is beautiful. It is not depressing at all. It is the best place to be because everything there is arranged to care for people with tuberculosis."[40] With similar enthusiasm, John Lathrop's physician advised him to "find a house or boarding house for the winter. . . . Sleep on an open porch every night; sit on it all day long or at least nine hours in each twenty-four."[41] In effect, Saranac served as a sanatorium without walls. Not surprisingly, its population soared, going from four hundred residents in 1880 to four thousand in 1910 to six thousand in 1920.

For over half a century, Saranac attracted a contingent of very wealthy persons with tuberculosis. (A number of them went on to become owners of the "great camps" of the Adirondacks, where the lore of the region and of the magic of an outdoor life was passed from generation to generation.) Congregating in neighborhoods with strict zoning laws and the most stringent regulations on the disposal of waste, these wealthy cure seekers created a community of their own. Members of the group paid each other formal visits, with all due attention to the silver laid out and the food and drink served. On some occasions guests were expected to dress for dinner (black tie), and it was not uncommon in this circle to have butlers on hand.[42] Invitations to high tea, a daily ritual in Saranac, were in demand, and the rule was that all who were strong enough to visit did so. The conviviality of the guests made them forget for at least a few hours why they had been banished there.

The well-to-do carried on what one literary critic in another context has called "serious gossip," which enables strangers to "share experience by sharing stories" and gain a "sense of solidarity."[43] Knowing who else was in Saranac made the disease more tolerable and less disrespectable. In this spirit, Charles M. Palmer gleefully informed Robert Ferguson, who had left Saranac Lake for New Mexico, about some newcomers. "The best man among them is Alvin Untermeyer, son of the late Samuel, whose wife . . . is quite ill." Other notables included Mrs. Adolph Ludenberg, who was "fitting in nicely, and beginning to see things in a proper way," and "a number of nice Boston people." Medical progress was not always welcome, especially if the patient was a good host. "Mrs. Louis Agassiz Shaw of Boston . . . has been the season's social star," Palmer told Ferguson. "She is very young, very rich, and . . . has entertained us all very much. . . . Mr. Shaw is only slightly ill and I am afraid they won't come back next winter."[44]

Given the climate of Saranac, the medical emphasis on outdoor living, and the rewards of an active social life, the wealthy made a fetish of being impervious to the cold and ignoring the extremes of the weather. No one canceled a tea or dinner party because of a winter storm. By 1915 this attitude had become so much a part of town life that Saranac Lake became known, in the words of a local physician, as a town with an "outdoor conscience." "We all like the zero weather better than thirty to forty above," Edwin French insisted. And he went on to assure one friend that "I have not forgone my walk a single morning on account of the cold."[45] In this same spirit, proficiency in winter sports was esteemed, particularly those sports requiring expensive clothing and equipment. Ice-skating rinks and toboggan runs were built and kept well maintained. The weekly races and skating exhibitions were well attended. A distinctive, unisex winter outfit became the uniform of the well-to-do who took their cure at Saranac—a coonskin coat that reached from right below the nose to the ankles.

The mix of high living and an outdoor ethos culminated in a spectacular annual February winter carnival, the costs of which were borne by the wealthy. A welcome diversion, the carnival was also the occasion for the sick to show family visiting from Boston and New York how well they were doing. Moreover, in Saranac, as elsewhere, carnival overrode social distinctions. Townspeople mixed with the residents of the cure cottages, and there were even some patients from the sanatorium. Everyone marveled at the carnival's centerpiece, an ice palace that the town residents constructed from the design of a local architect.

The highlights included a parade through town. Some of the elaborate floats depicted storybook tales that celebrated a hero who conquered all against considerable odds; others glorified hunting and fishing, and still others conveyed a didactic message about the value of hygiene and prevention. The finale was an illuminated procession across the ice with an elaborate fireworks display. It all served to make taking the cure in Saranac almost respectable.[46]

But carnival, of course, was the exceptional moment. What most impressed visitors to Saranac was its eerie quiet. "The silence of the town was uncanny," McClintock reported. "We thought the president had died and put the village in mourning. Our room faced the main street, but even with the window open not a sound came to us. We sat expectantly, waiting for noise, for sound of life. Silence, quiet." The town took its routine from the cure. "After the big midday dinner," continued McClintock, "came the rest period, from two to four, universal throughout the town. For two hours, absolute silence and rest. Sleep, if possible. Dogs were kept inside. Children were kept quiet by hook or crook. No deliveries were made. No talking, not even whispering. No reading. No writing. Rest. Rest and quiet."[47]

For Saranac's less wealthy health seekers the "cottage system" developed. Those who were on the waiting list of the sanatorium often stayed at one of these cottages, hoping to be admitted sooner if they were on the spot when a vacancy opened up.[48] Almost all the cottages were small, essentially slightly enlarged family dwellings and not mini-institutions with their own medical and nursing staffs. Boarders were expected to engage their own physician. Proprietresses often recommended a particular physician, but in Saranac, unlike other sanatorium towns, physicians did not have a commercial interest in the boardinghouses.[49]

While some attempted to reserve a cottage before their arrival, the majority just showed up—without a reservation and without a referring physician. Their numbers were considerable, for example, fifteen hundred in 1920.[50] To handle the press for rooms, a representative of the local antituberculosis society met each train and escorted those without a reservation to the Riverside Inn, which the society had purchased to provide temporary housing for new arrivals. Once at the inn physicians interviewed and examined them, sending those without any resources but with some prospect for recovery (if there was a vacant bed) to Raybrook, the New York State Sanatorium, just a few miles out of town. To those who had the money for room and board they gave a map that identified each official boardinghouse; the representative circled the three to six that had vacancies "at rates within their means and where conditions are best suited to their particular needs." Some took their cure in the cottages; others hoped it was only temporary, until a bed came available in the sanatorium.[51]

It was not unusual for the proprietress herself to have been a patient, like her boarders living in the shadow of the sanatorium. There were Saranac cottages to fit almost all social and medical criteria. There was one for Jews who wanted kosher food, others for Greeks and Cubans in which house-keepers spoke the native languages. There were cottages that catered to cir-cus performers or fraternal orders. Cottages were also classified by medical needs. Some were designated "up cottages," for patients who were ambula-tory, others were designated "nursing cottages," for those following a regi-men of bed rest.[52] So, too, lodge brothers in Saranac kept in close contact with their counterparts elsewhere and provided special hospitality when a member came to town. Thus, when Louis Andrews arrived in Saranac on May 3, 1902, he found a delegation of Odd Fellows waiting for him at the station. "I was carried to a private boarding house which they had secured for me previous to my arrival," he noted. The lodge had arranged for him to occupy one of the less expensive rooms, on the third floor, but when the proprietress saw how sick he was, "she voluntarily took me to a room on the second floor." Such a welcome was unimaginable outside a sanatorium town.[53]

The homogeneity of the boardinghouses alleviated some of the pain of separation from family and friends. In that sense, the lodging system was reminiscent of the invalid communities on St. Croix, if somewhat more artificial. "I was in a house with sixteen girls," Isabel Smith recalled, "all of whom were in the same pickle that I was. I was no longer alone, isolated with an infectious disease, but one of a crowd with which I could associate freely. What if I *did* have to lie in bed—so did everyone else. What if I *was* far from home—so was every other patient, not only in this house but in the whole town. I was no longer an individual singled out by a cruel fate, but a rookie in an army of the undefeated." Nonetheless, living in a con-fined space with the same group of sick people and doing nothing all day but stare out at the same scene could be suffocating. As one patient recalled: "A year's proximity to 'lungers' had taught me that where any number, from three to one hundred, are herded together, there is sure to be more or less discussion of symptoms that is bound to 'get on the nerves' of any one who believes that a sufferer can conquer his ills only by resolutely turning away from the contemplation of them and centering his thought on some object outside." He finally chose "solitary confinement," that is, a pri-vate porch.[54]

* * *

Saranac had its clear divides. Sanatorium patients were generally of a lower social class than those residing in the town. Not only were there the rich who set themselves off from others, but ordinary townspeople marked themselves off from the patients. As eager as they were to provide services and make their living from those taking the cure, they did not want to be mistaken for them. Thus, in the town's own terms, there were the "pioneers," as the original settlers were called, and there were those who came for a cure. The pioneers cultivated a manner of dress and social mores that bespoke prowess and robustness. They boasted of their hunting and fishing skills and hired themselves out as guides. It was not difficult to know who was who in the town: the rich taking a cure wore their coonskins, the locals, their pontiacs, and the rest, an assortment of sweaters and coats.

But one critical element connected everyone in Saranac, and that was the personal style and attributes of Trudeau himself. From 1885 until his death in 1916, Trudeau was the uniting force of the town, loved and respected by pioneers and patients alike. When his daughter died (of tuberculosis) in March 1893, the town mourned with him. "I have just come from the funeral of Miss Trudeau," Philip Washburn wrote to his mother. "Her death has been looked upon with grief by the whole community. There was no school this morning and the shops were closed. The service was at 2:00 and the church was crowded with a reverent and sorrowful congregation. The church was filled with flowers."[55]

Trudeau never attended the fancy balls and parties (even when the proceeds went to the sanatorium). Ascetic by temperment and because of his own illness, he spent what energy he had on his patients. In turn, his own health was a great concern to them. Trudeau had the rare ability to make each patient feel special. In letters to him they conveyed the admiration he inspired. "I have never thanked you for your great kindness to me, which I have indeed appreciated," wrote Bayard Cutting, Jr., who like his brother Bronson also had tuberculosis. "To tell the truth, it made me feel very guilty to have you devote so much of your strength and energy to me at a time when you were in bad health yourself, and needed all the rest you could get. I suppose you hear the same thing from everybody but you must allow me to tell you what a great privilege I consider it to know you and to have been under your care."[56] Alexis Stein, another of his patients, told him: "You have been indeed as a rock in a dreary land to [my wife and me]." Knowing that this might be his last letter, Stein continued: "I do hope physically that you are having some comfort and that the 'tb's' are leaving you alone. As you used to say to me it is remarkably easy to be philosophical about the boil on the other fellow's nose. But oh, it must be magnificent when you have to lay by, to be able to look back on a good work accomplished and to know you have some right in the ranks of those 'whose path is as a shining light.' And that you can do. How few can."[57]

Trudeau's skills brought fewer therapeutic victories than he would have liked. He himself was rarely free of symptoms, and his own ambivalence about repeatedly having to take the cure was acute. "I am sorry to say I am in the grip of the enemy again," he wrote to one of his benefactors in 1908.

> Life is . . . principally made up of bed, my room, my invalid chair, my lit-tle porch and last but not least, that dreadful spit cup and the other acces-sories I know so well. I don't think however I can ever get *used* to illness and I have looked at the outside porch and that chair everyday this winter and been thankful I didn't have to live that kind of a life. But Fate has decreed I am to go back to it so I am trying to be cheerful about it and read novels and enjoy the fresh air.[58]

Many of his patients, including Bayard Cutting and Alexis Stein, fared no better, although they did not fault him. Occasionally, but only occasion-ally, did someone take Trudeau's poor health as evidence of the deficiency of his purported therapy. "People arrive here nearly everyday who *insist* on seeing me," Trudeau once noted. "One woman . . . had come all the way from New Orleans. . . . So I had her admitted—she wanted to be examined. I told her I was sick and could not examine her. 'Well what is the matter with you?' I said if you really want to know, Pulmonary Tuberculosis. And then she put her hands up in despair. 'And you who have such a reputation, why don't you cure yourself?'"[59]

More often, Trudeau's standing as physician and human being drew a large number of people, both the ordinary and the celebrated, to Saranac. The town never did become "a refreshing place," as Philip Washburn noted after he left it for Colorado Springs. The climate was dismal and there was no escaping a "consciousness of invalidism," which made the place appear "more desolate than ever." For all the efforts at carnival and dinner parties, Washburn complained about a "crude barrack-like air about everything . . . where the library was the nearest approach to civilization."[60] Nevertheless, Saranac continued to attract many of the tubercular, mostly because Trudeau gave patients a good measure of hope, and the town gave them a good measure of protection.

Rutland, Massachusetts, the site of the Massachusetts State Sanatorium, had little of the fame of Saranac and almost none of its amenities.[61] But it, too, attracted a cadre of persons with tuberculosis—those still lower down on the social scale, in effect, the worthy poor. They were drawn to Rutland not by a charismatic physician but by the sanatorium itself. Some of them lived there while awaiting admission to the facility; others stayed on even if they were denied admission because their case was too advanced. And still others treated it as an aftercare center and remained post-discharge. The town was organized to serve all three groups, with a mixture of efficiency, commercialism, and tolerance. But if Saranac represented first class, Rutland was steerage.[62]

Whatever quaintness had originally characterized Rutland gave way to a busy and profitable service industry for the tubercular. "In every yard, field, and piazza in the town," a visitor reported, "there were tbs wrapped in blankets sitting on reclining chairs often in front of tents that provided some protection from the wind, rain, and snow." They needed lodgings as well, so "the gossip at the store . . . had it that widow so-and-so who had never made a dollar except in blueberry picking time, was gathering in six or seven each week and suffered no inconvenience from having the windows in one room open all night." Soon all were expanding their homes, adding a porch along the front, purchasing extra blankets and reclining chairs, and enlarging the chicken coop or the herd.[63]

Within a short time the widows and farmers had to compete with a growing number of former patients eager to make a living running boardinghouses. Having been patients themselves, they were able to provide not only room and board and empathy, but also instructions, acquired first-hand, on how to cure. "Ex-patients," as one Boston physician explained, "had an advantage over the residents of the town. They had learned the rudiments of the treatment." Better than the others, they stood ready to impose a "regimen that is very exacting."[64]

The most famous boardinghouse in Rutland was run by John Huntress, who opened it in 1899, shortly after his discharge from the facility. "We all felt an interest in each other, much like a large family," Huntress insisted, "making one happy to be alive." On his tenth anniversary, he noted: "There are many patients scattered over the country who got their first lesson here. It was a pleasure to see the progress they would make; it certainly gave one courage to keep up the fight."[65]

Two other groups in Rutland soon went into the boardinghouse business—the physicians themselves and the charitable societies. It was not unusual for one doctor to own several homes, sometimes affixing the label of "private sanatorium" to them, and running a for-profit venture. The physician hired the housekeeper, set out the regimen, and himself provided all medical services, the fees for which were included in the weekly rent. Of course, they were well situated to keep their rooms filled through self-referral, taking the number and types of patients that they wanted. Thus, David Butler, first a patient then a doctor at the sanatorium, over time purchased eight houses in town, each able to accommodate eight to twenty-one patients. Some had private rooms; others were run on the "ward system." Butler combined them all into the Rutland Cottage Sanatoriums, which had a total of one hundred beds and eighty-five acres of land, more than enough for the cows, chickens, and vegetable gardens that provided the patients' food.[66]

There were few amenities in Rutland. No wealthy group underwrote the cost of winter carnivals; instead of sledding and figure skating, the lodgers shoveled snow. Not surprisingly, the lore of the town is minimal, contained in a few typed transcripts of reminiscences, a handful of press clippings, and a small stack of sanatorium reports. But if the magic was minimal, the degree of comfort was considerable. Better Rutland than a municipal sanatorium, an almshouse, or an airless tenement.

15

The Sanatorium Narrative

THE IMAGES IN THOMAS MANN'S *THE MAGIC MOUNTAIN* HAVE DOMI-nated popular understanding of the meaning of a sanatorium stay. The most enduring impressions are of pampered patients wrapped in blankets sitting out-of-doors, eating hearty meals accompanied by good wines and brandy, removing their thermometers from beautifully lined boxes to check their temperatures three times daily, and engaging in lengthy discussions as ethereal as the alpine setting in which they reside. Yes, physicians were often authoritarian and unapproachable, and patients had their feuds, grievances, and passions; right beneath the surface calm ran a fevered sexuality. But Mann's sanatorium is scarily seductive. Time moves to a different rhythm. Every aspect of daily life takes on startling intensity. The mundane considerations of the everyday world below recede. Put down the book and one intuitively understands why Mann fled the Davos sanatorium where his wife was recuperating, afraid that otherwise he would succumb to its bewitching allurements.

In *The Magic Mountain*, as with any great work of the imagination, fact mingles with fiction in a way that at once illuminates and obscures reality. To enter into the world of the American sanatorium, to read the narratives of illness it inspired, whether in autobiographies (*The Plague and I*) or weekly patient newspapers (*The Fluoroscope*) is to be reminded repeatedly of the many nuances of sanatorium life that Mann captured.[1] But it is also to learn how fundamentally different was the experience of many Americans. It is more than a matter of American sanatoriums being exercises in charity and not spas for the wealthy, with patients coming more often from the poor and working classes than from comfortable bourgeois backgrounds. Rather, it is the utter incongruity of invoking a term like magic, when profound unhappiness, disappointment, and despair were the dominant emotions. To see the sanatorium from the inside, from the perspective of the patient, is to see it in the first instance as an incarcerative institution, a superb example of Erving Goffman's "total institution."[2] And then to go on, to read deeper in the patient narratives, is to see it as a waiting room for death: the possibility of escape (through cure) is ever present, but the dread of failure is pervasive.[3]

Patient memoirs and writings on the sanatorium are far more constricted in angle of vision than were the nineteenth-century narratives of illness. The earlier genre was a *life* history, which told the reader about childhood and family, ambitions and achievements (whether in finding salvation or wealth). The sanatorium literature, by contrast, was essentially an encounter with disease, with staff, and with other patients. In effect, the sanatorium so encompassed the life of the sick and so isolated them from all other experiences that it turned being a patient into what the sociologist Talcott Parsons has called a career. And the narrators find their plot line in the career: how they entered it, how they managed it, and for the fortunate ones, which included most of those who published their accounts, how they left it.

The sanatorium narratives generally describe conditions in the 1920s and 1930s, by which time the facilities had become larger and the routine more rigid.[4] Although many of the physicians and nurses were former patients, the sanatorium rules and regulations promoted a distance between staff and residents. Hence, these narratives do not contain poignant passages relating empathetic exchanges with physicians. The doctors emerge as aloof and uncaring figures, very different than the images of Trudeau; apparently in the process of curing their lungs they had lost their hearts. To be sure, the narratives are in one sense success stories, for the patient-authors recovered at the sanatorium. But they tell an angry and bitter tale, depicting the regimen of cure in terms of humiliation and denigration. One had to give up a personal identity and become an inmate. It was like making a pact with the devil, sacrificing dignity in return for health.

None of this is to imply that there were no contented patients in the sanatorium. Indeed, if the narrators are to be believed, they too were compliant patients, albeit hiding their frustrations. Moreover, oral histories collected in the 1980s from patients who were at the sanatoriums in the 1920s and 1930s contain fond memories. As Charlie Moses reported to historians Ruth and Neil Cowan, the eleven months he spent at Raybrook, the New York State Sanatorium, were "the happiest . . . of my life. . . . It was a place which opened my eyes to the world." As Moses recalled the experience, he saw "things which I never would have seen, things which I never would have done if I had been in the city. . . . When they told me that my eleven months were finished and it was time for me to go home, I was very unhappy. I was going back to reality."[5]

Nevertheless, the predominant tone of the narratives of illness that emerge from the sanatorium is one of unrelenting hostility. The narrators make no effort to put themselves in the place of the staff. There are no sympathetic soliloquies in which they imagine what it was like for physicians and nurses who were grappling with their own disappointments to deal with very sick and very frustrated young men and women. The accounts are one-sided—not a balanced portrait of the sanatorium but a compelling account of what it meant to be a patient.

The stories often open at the moment of diagnosis: the doctor has pronounced the disease to be tuberculosis, and the narrators offer a lengthy, defensive, and apologetic explanation of how and why they contracted it. It was not their fault, they insist. They were victims of circumstances beyond their control, unwittingly exposed to the disease. They were not guilty of dissipation or immoral behavior. "For years," explained Anne Ellis, "I had driven myself, never realizing . . . that I was working beyond my strength. I was a widow and the breadwinner for myself and children . . . and I had bent over a sewing machine or cook stove, never relaxing." Hard work and, out of necessity, overwork mixed with bad luck were the sources of her illness.[6]

Betty MacDonald offered a similar defense. Divorced and raising two children, she lived with her mother to save money. No one in the family had tuberculosis, and just two years earlier, she had qualified for a life insurance policy. A diligent employee, MacDonald was a secretary in a government agency; the problem was that she had been forced to work in an unventilated room at a desk next to a man with the unmistakable symptoms of the disease. When she suggested to her supervisor that her coworker might have tuberculosis, he merely responded: "Who don't?" To prove he was the source of her illness as well as to get the money to cover the cost of a sanatorium stay, MacDonald sued the government, and although she never received compensation, the employee in question turned out to have the disease. MacDonald was an innocent victim—her negligent supervisor and coworker were at fault.[7]

In this same style, Will Ross told his readers that he bore no culpability for his illness. He kept regular hours and did not overwork. Born in 1888 into a stable family in Appleton, Wisconsin, he insisted: "I never lived in squalor, I never went hungry, I didn't grow up in the crowded streets of a big city." Nor did he have an inherited predisposition to the disease; his forebears had been "sturdy. They were rugged, long-lived people who never heard of the forty-hour week and . . . lived uneventful lives." But why the illness then? Or as his mother kept asking: "Where did you get it, son?"

as though it were a sexually transmitted disease. Ross frankly did not know—he was as puzzled as anyone else—but he was certainly not to blame.[8]

The narrators insisted on their lack of culpability, not only because they wished to dissociate themselves from the charge of dissipation, but also because the next step in their career as patients, the introduction to the sanitorium, made them feel the more guilty. They experienced initiation as punishment; every procedure reinforced the sense that they were criminals. Entering the sanatorium was like entering prison.

MacDonald was quickly admitted to the Washington State Sanatorium, Firland, which she called the "Pines." Indeed, because she had two small children, MacDonald was quickly moved up on the list. At first elated by the news—the reputation of the place was for delivering cures and she believed that her stay would be brief—her euphoria faded quickly. She went for her preadmission physical examination to a clinic, which was housed, she reported, in the same building as "the police station, city jail, emergency hospital and venereal disease clinic." The clinic itself was a "depressing place," with unfriendly and unsympathetic nurses including one who "shouted questions at me and I shouted replies, which was very embarrassing owing to the nature of some of the questions." The clinic required not only a chest X ray but also a Wassermann test; the association between syphilis and tuberculosis made the visit all the more painful.[9]

By the time the examination was over, MacDonald viewed her forthcoming stay in a sanatorium in much darker terms. As she packed her bags, she mused about what lay ahead, almost convinced that a diagnosed tubercular faced an ordeal worse than that confronting a convicted criminal. "Being sent to an institution," she observed, "be it penal, mental, or tubercular is no game of Parcheesi and not knowing when, or if you'll get out doesn't make it any easier. At least the criminal knows what his sentence is."[10]

For many the only analogy to entering the sanatorium and undergoing the intake process was imprisonment. "Memories fall thick and fast upon me as I attempt this reconstruction of my sojourn at River Pines," wrote Frank Burgess, "but of those outstanding, the one really depressing is of the moment when I arrived at the door of my 'prison.' I saw it swing open on great hinges like the mouth of some devouring monster.... Above that engulfing portal I seemed to read from the infernal gates: 'Leave hope behind, all ye who enter here.'"[11] Or as Iva Marie Lowry, a former nurse, bitterly contended: "If a criminal thinks he is the only social outcast, let him take heart. There are some of us without blemish or without breaking a law of society that are still as much of an outcast as he who robbed or murdered. One enters a jail; the other enters a sanitarium. Each comes out 'branded for life!'"[12]

H. Leivick, a widely read Jewish poet and playwright (best known for his often produced play *The Golem*), had a similar reaction to his stay in a sanatorium. Leivick was born in Russia and became active on behalf of the Jewish socialist Bund. In 1906 he was arrested for illegal revolutionary activity and sentenced to life and hard labor in Siberia. In 1913 Leivick escaped and went to the United States. He eventually became a patient in a Denver sanatorium, which led him to compose the poem "Sanatorium."

> *Gate, open;*
> *doorsill, creep near.*
> *Room, I'm here;*
> *back to the cell.*
>
> *Fire in my flesh,*
> *snow on my skull.*
> *My shoulder heaves*
> *a sack of grief.*
>
> *Good-bye. Good-bye.*
> *Hand. Eye.*
> *Burning Lip*
> *charred by good-bye.*
>
> *Parted from whom?*
> *From whom fled?*
> *Let the riddle slip*
> *unsaid.*
>
> *The circling plain*
> *is fire and flame;*
> *fiery snow*
> *on the hills.*
>
> *Look—this open door*
> *and gate. Guess.*
> *Hospital? Prison?*
> *some monkish place?*
>
> *Colorado! I throw*
> *my sack of despair*
> *on your fiery floor*
> *of snow.*[13]

This sense of being a pariah was reinforced by the location of the facilities—beyond the town limits, far enough away to discourage visits and exchanges. Although the rural settings were often attractive, the isolation and the absence of people moving about the grounds gave the facilities an air of gloom, exuding disease and suggestive of death. "We entered the Pines by a long, poplar-lined drive," MacDonald recalled. "On either side were great vine-covered Tudor buildings, rolling lawns, greenhouses and magnificent gardens. It might have been any small endowed college except that there were no laughing groups strolling under the trees. In fact, the only sign of life anywhere at all was a single nurse who flitted between two buildings like a white paper in the wind." Maybe it would have been wiser, MacDonald thought, to buy a one-way ticket.[14]

The encounter with the intake nurse and the numerous rituals of admission convinced even the most acquiescent narrators that they had entered a prison. For many the epiphany was the moment they were handed the thick institution rule book and told, then and there, to sign a form saying that they had read it and promised to abide by it. This was standard practice in practically every sanatorium—the Adirondack Cottage Sanatorium as well as the tuberculosis workhouse on Blackwell's Island—and the signing often took place even before the newcomer was examined by a physician or assigned a room.[15] Almost all of the narratives comment on this traumatic event. To the staff the signing ceremony may have symbolized a contract with a compliant patient, but to the narrators it was an unmistakable, and indelible, mark of the abjectness of their condition.

Upon admission to the Adirondack Cottage Sanatorium, Marshall McClintock related how he was given a "rule book, which I was supposed to read and sign. It had my number on it—8027. I felt worse than ever. Like a prisoner. And the book was full of rules, lots of rules. Everyone must be out of doors . . . between nine and twelve-thirty and between two and five. Everyone was expected to go to bed in the afternoon. . . . Everyone must be in his cottage at nine o'clock and lights must be out at ten. . . . The rules seemed endless and my heart sank."[16]

The experience of Sadie Seagrave at a midwestern state sanatorium was identical. Here intake was in groups; all new admissions were expected to arrive between three and four-thirty in the afternoon (between rest hour and supper), so that they did not disrupt the routine. Once assembled, they were escorted to the office of the head nurse

> where we were asked to sign our names to the book of a thousand rules (more or less). We were not given time to read them but before the place for signature was a statement to the effect that the foregoing rules had been read. I suppose this gives the management a right to say that igno-

rance of the law excuses no one. I'm wondering what would be said to a person who couldn't read, even if he had time. . . . By the time the nurse was through with us, we were through with her. She showed us our lockers and beds, and said supper would be ready in twenty minutes. We put a few things away, and then sat by our beds until the bell rang.[17]

If the rule book signing was the first ritual, the second—one that the narrators found equally demeaning—was the way many sanatoriums washed and scrubbed the newcomers. To the staff, it was an appropriate procedure for new arrivals at a hospital; to the patients, it was evidence that they were unclean. At public sanatoriums it was standard procedure to read the patients the rules, then send them for a haircut, a bath, and a set of clean clothes. The fact that MacDonald had bathed and visited a beauty parlor right before going to the sanatorium did not exempt her from the ritual. She explained to the nurse "that I had had a bath not three hours before but she didn't even look up. She said, 'Makes no difference, rule of the Sanatorium is that all incoming patients must have a bath. Get undressed.'" As the nurse washed her newly permed hair with green soap, more rules were recited: "Patients must not read. Patients must not write. Patients must not talk. Patients must not laugh." The nurse next rummaged through her suitcase, examining disdainfully even the pictures painted by her children—"I had brought [them] to remind me of home." By the time she was put in a wheelchair and taken to her ward, MacDonald was no longer a neophyte. In the course of a few hours, she had become an inmate.[18]

The rationales given by physicians to explain their emphasis on rules only made the patients more apprehensive. No one, of course, ever hinted that the edicts were to serve the convenience of the staff or were a medical ritual to remind them that they were now in a facility that valued cleanliness. Rather, they were presented as therapeutic—the patient who followed them would be cured and those who violated them would not. Thus when Everett Morris, the senior physician at Cook County Tuberculosis Hospital, Chicago's municipal tuberculosis facility, delivered the "ABC Talk" to groups of newcomers (given year after year from a printed script), he conceded that having to follow so many rigorous rules might seem onerous. "We may appear to some," he declared, "as being too drastic, too severe with *our discipline*. But to the man, to the woman who is really in earnest our rules are not objectionable. The very first thing one stricken with consumption must realize is—it's a man's, a woman's job to get well. . . . It's a matter of business." To make certain that his audience did not think that they were being singled out because they were in a public facility, Morris quoted Dr. Charles Minor, superintendent at a private facility in South Carolina: "It does not matter so much about what the patient has in his lungs—it's what he has in his head." Putting his own gloss on the dictum, Morris added: "That is very true. Your getting well depends very largely on yourself. Tuberculosis is intensely personal and must be treated as such by the patient. . . . It takes a lot of determination, a lot of grit and a good stiff backbone, not a wishbone, to beat the game."[19]

The message to the patients was clear enough: it was up to them to manage their cure, essentially by following the rules and thinking positive. It was not simply a matter of resting and eating the right diet—they had to have the will to be cured! "Complete rest doesn't mean lying here in bed reading a newspaper," the admitting physician informed Will Ross. "A little of that will be all right after you get to feeling stronger, but right now I want you to lie as nearly motionless as you can manage. Don't even think if you can avoid it. Once you have gotten yourself thoroughly disciplined to rest the way I want you to, you will be well started on the road to a cure."[20]

The mottoes decorating the sanatorium walls reiterated the message: "Everything that is not rest is exercise. If you have nothing to do, don't do it here." And the instructions in the rule books were even more explicit. "Getting well depends on the patient. Rest, fresh air, good food, and later, regulated and supervised exercise all help. But if the patient doesn't have the will power, honesty, and character to obey the rules, nothing will save him." Staff bluntly informed patients who seemed especially strong willed or energetic that for them recovery might prove impossible. "Taking the cure is going to be difficult for you," the admitting physician warned MacDonald. "You have red hair—lots of energy, you're quick, active, impatient. All bad for tuberculosis. Discipline will be hard for you. The cure of tuberculosis is all discipline."[21]

From the staff's perspective, the rhetoric of willpower and discipline served a variety of purposes. It helped to make patients comply with the rules and thereby simplified their job. It also shifted the onus of responsibility for delivering a cure: a failure reflected on the inadequacy of the patient, not the potency of the therapeutic regimen or the staff's skills.

But from the patients' perspective, the rhetoric increased their own sense of guilt; it also bred defiance. "One knows what to expect," Sadie Seagrave wrote back from the sanatorium. "So far I have not felt any particular inclination to break any rules, except talking in rest hour occasionally, but perhaps I'll feel more unruly when I feel better physically. I have not felt any of the restrictions a special hardship but there seem to be a number of 'bugs' (slang for a tuberculous person) whose chief aim is to see how many infractions of the rules they can get away with, even to their own detriment."[22]

Whatever the friction, staff kept emphasizing the need for obedience and willpower. They saw it as the best way to keep up patients' morale, even when—and the rest of this sentence was more often unspoken than articulated—even when they witnessed fellow patients dying around them.

It was the presence of death that ultimately gave the sanatorium its character, stamping it in ways that distinguished it not only from prisons but also from general hospitals. In general hospitals, patients entered and left on a relatively frequent basis. Length of stay was measured in days or weeks, but not usually months. Given the heterogeneity of diagnosis, patients rarely came to know each other as intimately as sanatorium residents did. Rarely did they reach the point of identification that made another's death a foreshadowing of their own. In the sanatoriums, especially in not-for-profit facilities, patients stayed on long enough to forge bonds, to create a distinctive subculture, and to read their own fate in the progress of the symptoms of others.

An elaborate patient subculture developed within the sanatorium. At its core was an extensive communications network—with its own language, mores, and rituals—that kept patients (even those in the infirmary) in touch with all aspects of life in the institution. A group of "up patients," those convalescing, passed messages and gossip to others, arranged clandestine meetings, and even threw parties with bootleg alcohol. The close ties between patients were based not only on the shared disease but also on the shared sense of their own unworthiness, the stigma imposed on them by outsiders and to a degree by the rule book–minded staff. "We were like one family," Katharine Sturgis recalled of her stay in the Eagleville Sanatorium near Philadelphia, "very close to each other because of the suffering and the attitude of the public that we were lepers." Or as MacDonald observed: "We had everything in common, and we were firmly cemented together by our ungratefulness, stupidity, uncooperativeness, unworthiness, poverty, tuberculosis and longing for discharge."[23]

Even those who initially tried to keep their distance from other patients changed with the passing of time, as memories of home, family, and friends, faded. "During my first few months," Malcolm Logan recalled, "I tried as far as possible to hold myself aloof from my surroundings. I was wholly intent on becoming cured and leaving as soon as I could. It was impossible, however, to maintain this detached attitude, for the ties binding me to the life I had left were gradually loosened. At first I had many letters and visits from my friends . . . [but] their forgetfulness . . . forced me to thrust reluctant roots into this alien soil."[24] MacDonald spoke for all sanatorium patients in observing:

At first when my visitors told me of happenings in the outside world I was vitally interested and relived each incident vividly with the telling. Then gradually, insidiously, like night mist rising from the swamps, my invalidism obscured the real world from me and when my family told me tales of happenings at home, I found them interesting but without strength, like talk about people long dead. The only real things were connected with the sanatorium. The only real people, the other patients, the doctors, the nurses.[25]

The isolation that followed was acute. The sanatorium did little to try to alleviate it, however: visiting was discouraged, as befit an institution serving a population that was both contagious and on the brink of despondency or rebellion. MacDonald was told upon arrival that her two children were permitted to visit only once a month for ten minutes. Moreover, if they, or any other visitors, arrived before official visiting hours began (Thursdays and Sundays between two and four in the afternoon) or stayed too late, or were noisy, her "visiting privileges would be removed for an indefinite length of time."[26]

The newsletters put out by the sanatoriums give intimations of the impact, both positive and negative, of this subculture on the patients' lives. The publications were under the direct supervision of the administration and were intended to be an "inspiration" to the patients. Modeled on the *Journal of the Outdoor Life* published at the Adirondack Cottage Sanatorium, they were "to impart useful medical and hygienic information, to cheer and encourage patients . . . to create opportunities for the development of literary skill . . . [and] useful employment along the lines of occupational therapy." The superintendent or staff physician typically wrote the lead article, reiterating the links between compliance, cheerfulness, and cure. Contests were held to choose the title of the magazine and among the winners were "Grit-Grin," "The Optimist," "Pep," "Pluck," "Spunk," Smilin' Thru'," "Sunbeams," and the Hebrew "Hatikvah" (Hope).[27]

But inevitably, whether through oversight or indifference, another reality crept into the poetry, short stories, and gossip columns that the patients contributed, giving a more textured picture of sanatorium life. Thus, in the closed world of the patients, privacy and even private ownership practically disappeared. Clothing, radios, and love letters became communal property. "We leave to your own discretion the way to welcome newcomers to the Pisko Building," wrote two long-term patients at the Denver National Jewish Hospital. "Some choose to ignore them altogether. Others look them over carefully, the very first thing, to estimate and compare the hip and bust measurements with their own. At any rate, you should take a subtle peek into the new girl's locker to see if there is anything of interest in the line of clothes. If she can be used to your advantage, then take her off in a corner somewhere and welcome her to the Pisko building." In turn, they counseled new arrivals that "that no girl is supposed to buy anything . . . if anyone else has something she could use just as well."[28]

There was no point in trying to keep correspondence confidential, for gossip was the lingua franca of the facilities. "Up patients" had learned to decipher the most illegible return addresses and to open and then reglue the paste on any envelope. "If you can't add anything to a choice bit of gossip," new patients at the National Jewish Hospital learned, "then keep your mouth shut. There is nothing duller or more uninteresting than a story that has been repeated over and over with no alterations. Use your imagination and add color and drama to the gossip." Their counterparts at the Colorado Springs Cragmor Sanatorium were told: "*Talk much; listen little.* Being reticent in a sanatorium will inevitably class you with the servants."[29]

The best gossip—and the most daring, exhilarating, and desperate subversion of the sanatorium rules—involved sexual relationships between patients. The sanatoriums' term for it was "cousining," evoking both the illicit character of the liaison and the depth of the intimacy that characterized all patient relationships. Even before newcomers had acclimated to the facility, they were asked whether they were ready to cousin. McClintock reported that at his first dinner a patient struck up a conversation, asking where he was from, about his family, and then: "His eyes sparkled and he smiled as he began to talk about cousining. 'Well, if you have a wife in town you won't be so interested in cousining, will you?' 'No, not particularly.' 'Oh that's what they all say when they first come here, but in a few weeks they are at it strong. You'll see. There's plenty of it, married or not.'"[30]

Cousining was, of course, prohibited by the rules; it disrupted institutional routines, and a resulting pregnancy was dangerous to the health of the woman, to say nothing of the implications for the offspring. Women were offered sterilization, although one cannot be certain how many of them underwent the procedure. Staff also took careful note if male and female patients were spending too much time together and tried to discourage intimacy. But the force of the ban only made the liaisons more exciting. "Rules prohibiting affairs of the heart are strictly enforced," reported one patient, Arnold Lamden, "and offenders who succumb to the lures of Cupid are severely punished." Nevertheless, "love does exist, and the more it is discouraged, the more it flourishes."[31]

There were almost as many reasons as there were patients to explain the sexual intensity within the sanatorium. Boredom and loneliness provoked by prolonged isolation was one element. Or, to turn the point around, relationships inside cushioned losses on the outside. The nightmare story, told as fiction in a sanatorium newsletter but so often true to life, was of Dave, with a girlfriend "built strongly and beautifully," who for a time visited regularly. But Dave stayed on in the sanatorium, unable to shake his fever or stop hemorrhaging, and one day the news arrived: "The girl married someone very suddenly. Dave left the hospital to go East. On the train he died." The writer's ambivalence over how to end the tale said it all: "It was only a coincidence that when the girl went, he went. The one cord was snapped, so what was there to it now?"[32]

Moreover, forming a sexual relationship was one of the few ways patients could assert their individuality in a situation where they were forced to spend their every hour with people not of their own choosing. No matter if the romance soured. "In this world," wrote Bill Haking after his sanatorium experience, "each selects his companions . . . and if an acquaintanceship terminated disastrously . . . that is the individual's misfortune and a product of his own lack of intelligence in selection." Or as another patient, Joseph Walsh, declared: "We hear the argument that . . . love and tuberculosis should not mix. Be that as it may. . . . To love, even unrequitedly, is better than to have never loved at all. Love is God's gift to mankind—a gift which recognizes not an obstacle worthy of perpetual opposition."[33]

Moreover, cousining was a way to cope with one's own physical disabilities. For some, it was an assertion of physical integrity over the impairments of the disease. "The vision of a broken body," Lamden insisted, "and a pair of germ-ridden lungs is not strong enough to thwart love." For others, it was coming to grips with their own limitations. "It is very difficult for a normal person," Haking insisted, "to adjust himself to the sedate and unstimulating life that his tuberculous mate must lead. One-time patients are best suited to each other."[34] And cousining for women patients might also keep alive the prospect of someday having a family.[35]

Cousining also relieved the boredom of spending day after day in bed or in a cure chair, cut off from everything that made life interesting. Only by remembering the awful monotony and dreariness of sanatorium life can the excitement over cousining be fully appreciated. Imagine the dreariness, as MacDonald captured it, of "lying in bed at The Pines day after day, week after week, month after month, engaged in pursuits such as listening to the split, splat, splat of the rain hitting the gutter outside my window." She lost track of the days of the week: "I only knew them as . . . bath day, fluoroscope day, visiting day, supply day or store day."[36] No wonder, then, as Lamden remarked: "The paths of love in the sanatoria are not strewn with roses. But happiness without pain and fear is not happiness enough. The pains of love are as welcome as its pleasures." Or as Haking noted in more therapeutic terms: "Love gives one . . . a new lease on life. . . . The will to recover is an important factor of recovery. In the instances where love is successful, I sincerely believe that love is beneficial rather than detrimental to one's recovery."[37]

The weekly movies became the occasion not only to watch a fantasy but also to play it out. The event was naturally the highlight of the week— "looked forward to eagerly," remembered one patient, for it helps "to make the time pass more pleasantly." Women reported primping for hours before the movies, putting on makeup and curling their hair; the men shaved for the occasion. If the sanatorium allowed it, street clothes were worn, and if not, then clean pajamas and robes. "The most amusing situation was the first movie," one patient reported. "Being one of this strange, intimate audience—garbed in robes and slippers . . . and chatting hectically against time—created more of an impression than the picture itself." [38] Indeed, the only rival to the movies was the occasional dance for patients almost fully recuperated. The event was so good for morale that bed patients were sometimes allowed in as well.[39]

All of this became grist for the gossip columnists in the patient newsletter. They were both seers and matchmakers, with each entry in the "All of Us" or "Private Lives" column an item to be savored. It mattered little that the sounds of coughs competed with the peals of laughter; ever so much could happen from the time the lights were turned off for the movie until the staff herded everyone back to the sex-segregated wards. The tidbits sound puerile, what one expects from adolescents at summer camp, but they reveal not only how infantilizing a sanatorium stay was but also how desperate residents were to bring some diversion and pleasure into their lives.

> Did anybody notice Matty Valenza showing up at the movies with a red smear over his lips? He said it was the strawberries handed out at Sunday's supper. . . . Vinnie "shortpants" Gonzales . . . says Helen (Avila) only laughs at his ardent protestations at Sunday night movies—We have to smile a bit also at these hit-and-run romantic scenes on Sundays. They should be captioned "Love Between the Second and Third Bus.". . . It must be a charming little domestic scene indeed: Kitty McLaughlin mending Tony Ottarski's socks. . . . And what are these ominous things we hear about that already legendary romantic idyll involving Carol Lichtenberg and Johnny Testa?[40]

* * *

However much the sanatorium resembled other institutions, it had one unique feature—the omnipresence of the shadow of death. Apart from it, nothing can be understood about sanatorium life, whether it was staff enforcing rules or patients seeking sexual pleasure. Staff tried to brush it off with aphorisms about being strong and determined. But in countless ways, some personal, others collective, the sanatorium experience was at its core an encounter with mortality.

The initiation often occurred on the trip to the sanatorium. Will Ross remembered being met at the depot by a convalescent patient, Paul, whose job it was to bring the outgoing mail and departing patients to the train and return with the incoming mail and new arrivals. "The sanatorium was about a mile out of the city," Ross reported. "As we walked along the station platform, we passed a truck on which rested an undertaker's shipping case. Paul patted the box familiarly. 'There goes one of our customers,' he said with a chuckle." And just in case Ross missed the point, Paul took the back road to the facility in order to pass a cemetery. "'I wanted you to get a good look at this,' he remarked. 'I like to bring new patients this way and scare 'em a little.'"[41]

Each sanatorium had a counterpart to Paul. In the Pines, MacDonald's guide was a highly depressed chronic patient, Charlie Johnson, nicknamed "Laughing Boy." The only time Charlie laughed was when he broke the news to an initiate. "'You're new here, ain't you?' Charlie greeted MacDonald. 'Well, I been here five years and I seen 'em come and I seen 'em go. Some go out on their feet but most of 'em go out in a box. How bad are you?' I said that I didn't know but that I only expected to stay a year. 'Ha, ha!' he laughed mirthlessly. 'A year. That's what they all say when they first come. . . . The only one who ever got out in a year was a woman who had cancer of the lungs. They let her out in three months—feet first.' Then Charlie laughed some more."[42]

Even seemingly formal and routine questions took on a very different meaning. One patient recalled that he was shaken when the admitting nurse asked him to pay for his room a week in advance, "secured from me my home address and the name of a person to be notified in case of my death," and then asked him "to deposit the price of a ticket home." Each one of these requests could only mean that she expected him to die at the institution.[43]

Occasionally, the official sanatorium literature hinted at the grim prospect of therapeutic failure, but it was framed as positively as possible. "On entering the sanatorium," John William Parker recalled, "I was handed one of the official rule books given to all entering patients. On the inside of the back cover was printed in black type for emphasis a poem to the effect that I (or anyone else having tuberculosis) was in an awful fix but it was up to me to be brave and put up as good a fight and live as long as I could. Even if I didn't live very long . . . I would have the satisfaction of dying in the knowledge that I had put up a good fight." The message unnerved Parker, who had come to the sanatorium confident of a cure. "The effect of this masterpiece of pessimism was the same as that of a bucket full of water on a camp-fire. I immediately lost a good large chunk of my fighting spirit and was about to give up the battle."[44]

Usually the facility was so insistent on maintaining a positive attitude and rewarding the residents who did that its rules actually prohibited crying in public. It took new arrivals a while to obey the injunction. As one character in a play produced at a sanatorium commented about a new patient: "She has been crying her eyes out since she came." And then added in a flippant tone: "You know how it is the first few days at the 'san.'" Only when alone in bed could patients release pent-up emotions. Anne Ellis, for example, was determined to be a model patient, to observe all the rules and get well, to be cheerful all day long. But at night she did give in to her fear and frustration. In the sanatorium, she maintained, "I learned the meaning of many things: fortitude, patience, unselfishness, joy, sacrifice. I learned that it isn't sporting to whine; that in order to keep up your neighbor's courage as well as your own you must take everything lightly." But she also learned something else: "I know, too, that in the darkness of night you lay aside the garment of well-being and give up to the deepest anguish, smothering sobs under the pillow. The uppermost thought in your mind is that others must not hear you."[45] This was the secret that everyone shared, and she put in into verse:

Since I laugh all the day I am called an inspiration to others.
But in the darkness of night, when I cough and hear my neighbors coughing,
(Even the engines in the railroad yards cough),
I am lonely and afraid and cannot inspire myself.[46]

Although sanatorium officials did not usually allow patient newspapers to become too morose, the darker side of the experience occasionally crept through.[47] The *Killgloom Gazette*, a small, short-lived publication at the state sanatorium in New Mexico, printed a poem that was more graphic than most. Entitled "The Undertaker's Refrain," it read:

So who'll be the next, who'll be the next,
As this bright new year rolls round,
To be laid out in a gorgeous shroud
In his casket underground?

Chorus

In Fairview on the hill
There's a tiny lot we'll save,
We feel it will
Just fill the bill
While you will fill the grave.[48]

Each time someone died, the tension between the staff and patients mounted. Some patients decided to leave the facility AMA (against medical advice), others decided that there was no point in following the sanatorium rules. Living on the edge, they might just as well do as they pleased—why die without ever having lived?

None of the emotional expressions was unique to sanatorium patients—those who died of consumption at home or in the West undoubtedly experienced them. But the sanatorium was a hothouse, and its isolated and charged atmosphere intensified every feeling, even as it provided a ready object, be it staff or fellow patient, upon which to discharge it. The sensations were that much sharper, and the responses that much angrier, because the sanatorium had appeared to strike a bargain—do as we say and be cured—and not kept its end. When death, not cure, was forthcoming, patients were left confused and angry. One encounter reported by McClintock captures the dynamic. He was given the room of a patient who had just died. "Did he go home?" another patient asked. McClintock explained that the dead patient had been scheduled to go home that very week but unexpectedly "threw a hemorrhage." He and his fellow patient then shared their surprise. McClintock observed that "he cured better than anyone in the whole place." "I know it," the other patient agreed. "And some of these guys that chase around and get drunk, play the women, sneak out late at night—they get along all right. It makes you wonder."[49]

Deny as staff might, there was no shielding the patients from the omnipresence of death, even in those facilities that served the incipient and not the chronic case. For Sadie Seagrave, knowledge came her very first night as a patient. "I'm here, and how can I ever stand this exile," she confided to her fiancé back home. "The rain drips, drips, drips and they say little Nat died last night. The girls on the porch where I have been put say they are going to stay awake tonight to hear the wagon come to take him away. Somebody on the porch is coughing and choking, and I want to get away from all this gloom. I won't stay. I *won't*." But Sadie did stay, hoping her fate would be a cure.[50]

It was the patient subculture, not the administrative personnel, that forced the confrontation. Sometimes it was cruel, as with people like Paul and Charlie; sometimes it was tinged with black humor. Indeed, the oddity would have been the absence of black humor in this outpost of death. So patients called the lidded sputum cups their "music boxes," which when opened played "Nearer My God to Thee." They joked about the sound of the undertaker's voice and the hoofbeats of his horses, with frequent references to leaving "feet first" or to the "Pine Box Special," the evening train that took the coffins back to the city. At one sanatorium party night prizes were given out for tables with the most original decorations. First prize went to the table that put tombstones at everyone's place filled out with the date of their birth and the date of their death. The old-timers talked about these things with a "breezy, lighthearted, and nonchalant attitude," at once taunting and measuring the newcomers—those who flinched or recoiled were likely to be picked on again.

There were patients who publicly at least clung to the official version that those who followed the rules would be cured. Their articles in the patient newsletters promoted obedience and good cheer. "Because the fight is primarily the patient's," wrote Eleanor Remy in the *Journal of the Outdoor Life*,

> we belittle the physician's part, and hence his advice. Because others break rules and recover, we reason that we can do likewise and overlook the fact that had these 'others' obeyed orders they would the sooner have won their victory. . . . The best antidote to this mental poison, which has killed more patients than most wars, is a habit, which should be acquired at the early stages of the fight, of obedience to and co-operation with a competent, sympathetic doctor. . . . To become a 'cure,' patients must cast off their old life of action and thought in order to acquire passivity, new modes of thought and new self-control.[51]

Other patients tried to find something positive about the sanatorium experience, even when the outcome was the death of a fellow patient. They would talk about an eerie beauty, or how those barely able to walk would bring flowers, or sit and talk with the dying. But more numerous were those patients who fiercely and angrily rejected this view—self-styled "realists" who distained both "ward rats," and "pollyannas." The ward rat was the patient who tattled, reporting infractions to the staff. As one ditty put it:

> *I'm a very model patient which nobody seems to know. . . .*
> *If I see folks do aught that's wrong I always tell the nurse. . . .*
> *In spite of this I'm not well liked,*
> *One patient called me "rat."*[52]

It was the pollyannas whom the realists found most irritating. Lamden, when appointed editor of the National Jewish Hospital *Fluoroscope*, informed his fellow patients that he would forthwith reject articles in which "the authors with the zeal of converts and the enthusiasm of martyrs, tell of their metamorphosis from utter despair and resignation to a life of hope faith and joy." That he was never allowed to carry out his order only increased his dislike for the rhetoric of the pollyannas.[53]

The realists in every sanatorium rebuked anyone who would "extol suffering." To a patient like Arno Eldi, articles along the lines of "I am Glad I Had Tuberculosis" or "Tuberculosis—A Blessing in Disguise" were an outright fraud. Did these authors genuinely "consider spending two or three years in an atmosphere reeking with the smell of the sick room—and human pity an enjoyable experience? Do spasms of coughing and feverish tossings and aches and pleural pains constitute the only means to a successful and useful life?" In his terms, tuberculosis and a sanatorium stay were a terrible curse. "I am robbed of all the physical pleasure I loved. I can't play tennis, nor skate, nor swim, nor even walk at a manly pace. . . . Tuberculosis robbed me of my youth, and with it of my faith and my independence. It made me lose the world and gain nothing, except perhaps a callousness that leaves me indifferent in [the] face of death, a cynicism that shattered the finest ideals I ever cherished." The disease was an "evil to be denounced . . . not to be flattered and coaxed." In the end, "the fight against tuberculosis vexes with as much bitterness and disappointment, with as many sacrifices and tragedies. The false prophets will have to raise their voices in their cries of 'Hosanna and Hallelujah' in order to drown out the pathos in our lives and the pain from our hearts."[54]

But it was the rare patient who stayed in either one of these roles for long. The oscillations in mood between hope and despair were frequent. "It was an extreme optimism," McClintock observed, "just as the pessimism was extreme when it occasionally held sway. On one day in every twenty-five a lunger laid plans for committing suicide. But before he could get far enough towards carrying out the plans the old optimism and cheerfulness returned."[55]

As with any confined population, sanatorium patients had harsh words for what they took to be the callous and inattentive attitude of the staff. In one sanatorium play, scenes 2 to 7 were identical, repeating the identical encounter between physician and patient:

DR. (very breezily): Good morning.
PATIENT: Good morning, Doctor. Do you know that I have lost 5 lbs.?
DR.: (greatly surprised) You have? This will take looking into. Good morning.
PATIENT: But, but. (Doctor is gone. Scenes 3, 4, 5, 6 & 7, Ad infinitum.)
FINIS.[56]

It may well be that these patients were especially discontented because they had expected more sympathy. Probably aware that a disproportionate number of doctors and nurses at the sanatoriums had themselves contracted tuberculosis, they anticipated the empathy of fellow sufferers. But however well intentioned a nurse was, it was almost impossible to keep dispensing this kind of nurture over time to a highly demanding population. Some of the more perceptive patients understood the problem, even if knowledge did not bring forgiveness. "The staff at The Pines had but one motivating factor—to get the patients well," conceded Betty MacDonald. But "this motivating factor, like policeman's nightstick was twirled over our heads twenty-four hours a day." Once it may have been different. "In the beginning the staff at The Pines had undoubtedly been more sympathetic, more understanding, more interested in each patient as an individual, but years and years of working with people who clutched their tuberculosis to the like a beloved old shawl and dared the doctors and nurses to get it away

from them . . . had finally worn off any little facets of sympathy and tender-
ness and left the system smooth, efficient and immutable." In effect, she
concluded, staff told patients: "'We are going to make you well and the
shortest distance between two points is a straight line. . . . Here is the line,
either follow it or get out.'"[57]

A recurring tension between staff and patients turned acute on the issue
of discharge. Patients were bitter about the seeming indeterminacy of their
stay and the refusal of the staff to discuss it with them. Staff had every reason to avoid such discussions—telling those who were not making progress
of their likely fate was too painful, and those who were on the mend might
be tempted to leave too soon or stop adhering to the regimen.

For the patients, however, the silence was unbearable. In an effort to
make the inexplicable seem rational, they devised a series of benchmarks to
gauge their prospects for discharge. "The only way we could tell whether
we were getting well or dying was by the privileges we were granted," Mac-
Donald observed.

> If we were progressing satisfactorily at the end of one month we were
> given the bathroom privilege and fifteen minutes a day reading-and-writ-
> ing time. At the end of two months, if we continued to progress our read-
> ing-and-writing time was increased to half an hour, we were allowed to
> read books and were given ten minutes a day occupational therapy time.
> At the end of three months we were given a chest examination, along
> with the other tests, and if all was still well we were given three hours'
> time up, one hour occupational therapy time and could go to the
> movies.[58]

Even patients who had passed all benchmarks did not know when they
would go home. As MacDonald reported: "A discharge was supposed to be
a complete and wonderful surprise." But since all discharges at the Pines
occurred on Mondays after rest hour, anxiety mounted as the day wore on.
All, from the sickest to the healthiest, were "jumpy with anticipation and
lay in their beds during rest hours, stiff and prickly with hope. . . . When
weeks, even months had gone by without a single discharge, we'd relax or
rather droop and make morbid plans for our third Christmas, our fourth
summer at The Pines." But then, let one patient be released, and the tension mounted all over again.[59]

No wonder, then, that patients so frequently left the sanatoriums against
medical advice—more frequently the municipal and state facilities than the
not-for-profit sanatoriums. Superintendents everywhere tried to stem the
flow, without great success. They had neither the resources nor the inclination, regardless of what public health departments said, to enforce compulsory confinement. So they cajoled the patients, holding out the prospect of
cure. "All must admit," conceded the director of the Pennsylvania State

Sanatorium, "that out of every ten patients who leave Mont Alto at least eight are making a mistake, a fatal mistake, going home too soon, wasting the time they did spend and wasting the state's money. This is the reason Mont Alto cannot point to more cures; the patients won't stick."[60]

These sentiments notwithstanding, anywhere from 10 to 30 percent of sanatorium patients left within a month of arrival.[61] If health and resources permitted, they remained outside, perhaps holding a job, perhaps bedridden at home. But if they suffered a relapse or the support system crumbled, they were soon seeking admission again, if not to the first facility (which might prohibit readmissions) then to another one. But this time, however, they arrived hardened to the experience. They were not fooled by the driver who rode by the cemetery or flustered by the patient who asked if they cousined.

EPILOGUE

THE GREAT TWENTIETH-CENTURY INNOVATION IN THE TREATMENT OF tuberculosis, rivaling Koch's identification of the tubercle bacillus, was Selman Waksman's discovery of streptomycin. The breakthrough came not from a sanatorium laboratory, as Edward Trudeau had anticipated, but from the Department of Soil Microbiology at the New Jersey Agricultural Experiment Station of Rutgers University. Waksman had spent many years analyzing soil-inhabiting microorganisms; these microorganisms live together, constantly interacting, and some of them prevent the growth of bacteria and fungi through their production of chemical substances (which would later be labeled antibiotics). One species of microorganism, the actinomycetes, was particularly active, and the Waksman team was studying them, hoping to find substances that would kill bacteria that infected humans (which was not particularly difficult) but would do so without excessive toxicity (the test most of them failed).[1]

As is so often the case in science, chance favored the prepared mind. The actinomycete that would yield streptomycin was found in 1943 on a swab taken from the throat of a sick chicken brought to the station by a New Jersey farmer who had noted its difficulty in breathing and wanted to prevent the infection from spreading to the rest of his flock. The lab team identified a soil microorganism (that the chicken had picked up by pecking in the dirt) in the swab sample, investigated its properties, and learned that it was active against an especially wide variety of bacteria but did not appear to be highly toxic to animals. When Dr. William Feldman of the Mayo Clinic visited the Waksman lab in November 1943, interested in antimicrobial activities of the agents it was purifying, Waksman told him about streptomycin and soon sent him a batch to test in guinea pigs infected with tuberculosis. Within a few months Feldman was reporting successes.[2] In July 1944 he began clinical trials in humans, and by June 1946, the Waksman-Feldman collaboration had established the "first effective chemotherapeutic remedy for tuberculosis."[3] Waksman was justifiably proud of the achievement. As he wrote on the twentieth anniversary of the discovery of streptomycin: "Thus, a disease that less than two decades ago was still regarded as the greatest threat to the health and life of man, a threat that hung over the heads of the people like the sword of Damocles, has been reduced to the tenth position or even farther back, among the killers of human beings."[4]

However stunning the accomplishment, two important qualifications are in order. For one, the disease had been on the wane in the United States, even among immigrant groups, though not among blacks, before streptomycin.[5] In 1930, the death rate from tuberculosis was down to 70 per 100,000; in 1945, to 40 per 100,000. In 1954, ten years after the introduction of the new drug, it was 10 per 100,000.[6] Second, streptomycin was more toxic than had first been appreciated and not effective against all strains of the bacillus. However, two additional chemotherapeutic agents, para-aminosalicylic acid (PAS) and isoniazid (INH) were soon developed, and later, an additional agent, rifampin, was added. With these drugs at hand, the history of tuberculosis in developed countries seemed at an end.[7]

The first to celebrate the arrival of the new therapies were the sanatorium patients. The drug went to the acute patients; the more chronic had to wait their turn. Thus, Isabel Smith, who had lived in Saranac Lake since 1928, initially in a boardinghouse and then as patient #9049 at the Trudeau sanatorium, remarked how she "watched with envy the remarkable improvement they produced in certain selected patients—and wished desperately that I had not been crossed off the list."[8] Her turn finally came. In 1949, over a period of four months, she was given gradually increased dosages of streptomycin and PAS, and the results were beyond her most optimistic expectation. "I breathed not only more easily but less often, and so far as my wheeze and cough were concerned—well, things were becoming mighty quiet around here." In April 1949 a guinea pig was injected with her "germs." Two months later, her physician "hurried into my room with a smile on his face *that I will never forget.* 'Isa you're *negative*' he cried. 'Your guinea pig is hale and hearty!'" Smith was overjoyed: "Always before, for twenty-one long years, since 1928—my germs had remained hale and hearty and it had been my poor guinea pig who had died."[9]

Smith's experience was shared by many others. *Time* magazine reported the sudden and miraculous transformations that occurred in 1952 when patients at the Sea View Hospital in New York's Staten Island began a course of the new "wonder" drugs. "All 44 patients with fever had a temperature drop to normal within two weeks, most of them within a week, some in a single day. Patients who had picked apathetically at their food became ravenous; they called for third and fourth helpings of cereal. . . . Weight gains were amazing. . . . Those who had been bedridden for years were now 'dancing on the wards.'"[10]

As cures mounted, the sanatoriums began to close. In November 1954, as *Life* magazine reported, the last patient left the Trudeau sanatorium, leaving "only the recumbent figure of Edward Trudeau . . . resting beneath his blanket of bronze on which winter now had spread a softer shroud."[11] Some of the facilities, like the White Haven Sanatorium founded by Lawrence Flick, simply ran down. A few, like the National Jewish Hospital, went on to specialize in research and treatment of other forms of lung disease. Others, such as the Trudeau sanatorium and the Loomis sanatorium, were bought by entrepreneurs and turned into conference centers. Still others were converted into caretaker facilities for the mentally disabled or the elderly.[12] Perhaps the most symbolic passing of an era took place in Davos, Switzerland, the onetime home of Mann's magic mountain. "The treatment of tuberculosis has entered on a different phase today," Thomas Mann observed in 1953, for "most of the Swiss sanatoria have become sports hotels."[13] The only remnant of their past were the number of rooms with balconies and porches.

Progress was so remarkable that some observers confidently predicted that tuberculosis would never again threaten the population. "This disease will hardly ever disappear completely," E. R. N. Grigg informed the readers of the *American Review of Tuberculosis* in 1958, "but it is expected to cease to be a public health problem, and before the end of this century it may become so rare in the United States as to constitute a medical curiosity."[14]

Over the 1960s and 1970s, it did seem as if Grigg had been right, that tuberculosis would be remembered only for the public health policies and individual habits that lingered. Public school and hospital employees were still required to have chest X rays and ordinances prohibiting spitting remained on the books, but these measures seemed more a token of inertia than reasonable methods to prevent contagion. So, too, one found families that insisted on sleeping with windows open, although they could not remember why they did so. I met one couple at a summer barbecue who happened to remark that they slept on their balcony almost all year round; when I asked why, their only answer was that their grandmother always insisted on it. Not surprisingly, family research soon turned up the fact, always kept secret, that their grandfather had been in a sanatorium. And in this same spirit, the cure chairs at Saranac Lake became valued as furniture antiques, now sold as "Adirondack recliners."

These survivals aside, by the 1980s tuberculosis had become, medically speaking, altogether uninteresting—not that the disease had entirely disappeared from this country.* It still cropped up among nursing home residents and newly arrived immigrants. But when it did, a drug regimen of isoniazid and rifampin seemed to take care of the problem. Within two weeks the sputum of infected patients would be negative for the bacillus; and provided that the regimen was followed for six months to a year, the disease would be cured.

None of this, of course, held true in underdeveloped countries, which is where I most frequently and poignantly encountered it.[15] In the course of medical human rights missions to low-caste Indian communities and refugee camps along the Thai-Cambodian border, I found the disease to be endemic and the drugs not consistently available. Refugees from Cambodia, for example, displayed the most dreaded symptoms of untreated tuberculosis. In 1989, at a hospital unit at Khao-I-Dang, a refugee camp at the Thai-Cambodian border, a nurse introduced me to a young man who had just arrived. He was emaciated not only from the deprivations incurred on a long journey but also from the final stages of tuberculosis. As I looked at his frail body (he weighed just thirty kilograms) and saw his sallow sunken cheeks and hollow chest, I suddenly realized just how Deborah and Harriet must have appeared to their contemporaries. The link to the past was all the stronger when I noticed in the corner of the ward two young children watching over their mother, who was dying of tuberculosis. In these settings the disease was still claiming those in the prime of life, and leaving orphans in its wake.

By 1989, however, we had all come to understand that the sanguine predictions about the eradication of tuberculosis, indeed the end of the era of deadly infectious diseases, were wrong, as was the belief that death was the fate only of the elderly and not the young. First it was human immunodeficiency virus (HIV) disease that made us humble, and then it was the return of tuberculosis, all the more frightful because it so often appeared in a multidrug-resistant form.

No warning signs prepared us for HIV, and so the responses both in the gay community and in the medical profession were slow and hesitant in the first years of the outbreak. No one was prepared to grapple with a deadly disease that was striking down the young—not the doctors who

---

*The exception that proved the rule occurred one morning when I was on rounds at the Columbia-Presbyterian Medical Center. We saw an elderly patient who had spent time in a sanatorium in the 1930s and had undergone a number of pneumothorax procedures. His chest X ray revealed the scars left by the earlier treatment. The sight was so unusual that students and residents from nearby wards were called over to look at it. The senior attending explained the assumptions about "resting the lung." The juniors could not hide their astonishment, or smug sense of superiority.

attended them, not the friends who found themselves going from one funeral to another.[16] To put these events in context, it was helpful to turn to history. Suddenly, events around the plague in fifteen-century Florence had a compelling relevance, as did the early-twentieth-century experience with tuberculosis and syphilis.[17] Historians and ethicists combed the past to locate the origins of the medical duty to treat and the right to intervene in individual lives in the name of public health, as well as an understanding of how a society coped with the death of the young.[18]

In each instance, the story recounted here has a contribution to make to contemporary events. As I surveyed the record, doctors and nurses had not shied away from treating patients with tuberculosis, even though a number of them contracted it while doing so. It turned out that the sanatorium was a place where these health care professionals first came as patients and then stayed on as staff.[19] To my surprise, this shift in roles did not soften the experience of confinement for other patients—Hollywood aside, doctors do not necessarily undergo transformations after they become patients. Nevertheless, the professional record set a standard for medicine in confronting HIV disease.

By the same token, the ways by which nineteenth-century communities made certain that the dying did not go through their agonies alone took on a new meaning. Not that we could ever re-create the religious impulses that underlay this response or structure our own communities around the values of earlier ones. Rather, the historical experience alerts us to the possibilities of shared grief, and here, too, sets a standard that might be approached, even if it could not be matched.

As public health policies were being formulated for HIV disease, the precedents set around tuberculosis at first served as negative reference points. The compulsory character of reporting, the right to insist on X rays, indeed, the idea of establishing a single-disease hospital for treatment were all rejected.[20] A rights model, not a public health model, prevailed, not least of all because the first HIV patients were middle class, educated, and perhaps most important, politically organized in advance of the disease.[21] They stood in marked contrast to the great majority of tuberculosis patients of the early twentieth century who were poor, uneducated, and politically unorganized.

None of this, however, prepared us for the resurgence of tuberculosis. There were warning signs, but almost all of them were missed. In retrospect, it is obvious that HIV disease, by compromising the host immune system, would leave the patient susceptible to tuberculosis. Moreover, epidemiologists did not flag the fact that as early as 1979 New York City rates for tuberculosis were beginning to climb; that year 1,530 new cases were reported, a 17 percent increase over the year before and a reversal of a

century-long pattern of decline. Then, between 1980 and 1991, the number of cases in New York City climbed from 1,514 to 3,673, an increase of
145 percent. Even more worrisome was the fact that 19 percent of the
microorganisms were resistant to the two most effective and least toxic
drugs, rifampin and isoniazid.[22] This resistance resulted from the fact that
many of the patients had begun a course of therapy but failed to complete
it, thereby fostering the emergence of drug-resistant strains.

It was not until 1991 that public health officials sounded the alarm,
acknowledging that the disease was back with a new force and deadliness.
In keeping with tradition, tuberculosis was a disease of those without social
privilege, in this case, African Americans, the homeless, and those with
HIV disease.[23] Not surprisingly, panic and precedent led to calls to re-create the sanatorium and reinvigorate the power of health departments to
confine patients with tuberculosis, especially those who had demonstrated
noncompliance. Newspapers and magazines dug through their files and
found pictures of rows upon rows of patients sitting outdoors in their cure
chairs. It all seemed benign, perhaps even therapeutic.

But the historical reality ought not to be glossed over. Before we rush to
resuscitate the sanatoriums and empower departments of health, let us not
forget that the stigma society attached to the disease and those who had
contracted it affected almost every aspect of life inside and outside the facility. To the medical profession and the sanatorium founders, the facilities
were a gift to the tubercular. To many patients, however, they were more
like prisons than hospitals, in which the prescience of death, not the
promise of cure, was pervasive. Department of health officials were earnest
in their efforts to secure the public good, but again, persons with tuberculosis found the policies too intrusive and often manipulated the system for
their own ends.

Perhaps the most important contribution that this history can make to
public policy is not to offer a series of recommendations but to emphasize
the importance of angle of vision. The stories told here demonstrate what
disease meant to invalids, health seekers, and patients, not only in terms of
physiological changes and social impact, but also ultimately, in personal
terms. As we formulate plans to combat tuberculosis as well as HIV and
other dreaded diseases, indeed, as we design a national health policy or
think about rationing schemes, we should remember that we are in a profound way affecting individual life chances and life choices. This is finally
why it is so important to write the history of disease from the perspective of
the patient.

APPENDIX

Because archives rarely classify their manuscripts by disease categories, identifying the letters and diaries of persons with consumption or tuberculosis was a complicated and time-consuming task. Occasionally, archivists would remember that a family collection told a particularly poignant story of the disease, but other strategies were required for locating manuscript collections as well. Biographical dictionaries provided me with clues. Sometimes they listed the disease that caused the subject's death; other times they would note a series of early deaths of family members. Several infants might die shortly after birth, or the mother and/or father might die before the rest of the children were grown. Given my interest in identifying persons with the disease, the mingling of childbirth, infant death, maternal and paternal invalidism, and orphaned children was a significant marker. The deaths frequently indicated a family that was repeatedly struck by consumption. Interrupted and periodically reconstructed career patterns provided other clues, particularly if they included a sea voyage or an overland journey west. Since invalids and health seekers congregated in specific regions or experimented with similar occupations, there was a strong likelihood that those whose careers evinced this pattern might have contracted the disease during adolescence.

In identifying women with the consumption or tuberculosis, the *Dictionary of Notable American Women* was especially helpful. Its editors self-consciously structured the entries to emphasize the links between women's public and private lives. Ever so conscious of the precariousness of female health, they included data on illness not only about the subject but her entire family. The new computer manuscript data bases, ARLIN and OCLC, made the tedious task of cross-checking less time-consuming.

Once I identified a manuscript collection and explained the project to archivists, they often recalled still other individuals and families. And so in an unanticipated and somewhat random manner, locating one manuscript collection often led to the identification of another. This occurred not only at major repositories, such as the American Antiquarian Society and the Huntington Library, which have meticulously catalogued all of their material, but at newer and smaller repositories such as the Whaling Museum of New Bedford, Massachusetts, or the Tutt Library at Colorado College. These archivists, often trained in social history and mandated to collect manuscripts from residents of their city, diligently catalogue material on ordinary citizens as well as eminent ones. The summaries of their collections generally pay special attention to health, career patterns, and family life.

Manuscript Collections

Below are the names of all the invalids, health seekers, and patients whose letters and diaries I read. Often their letters were buried among the correspondence of the more prominent members of the family. To guide future researchers I have identified the name of each person whose material I read. I have included the name of the collection (if it differed from the name of the subject) and the library where the collection is located.

Abiel Abbott, South Carolina Historical Society
David Abeel, New Brunswick Theological Seminary
Edwin A. Alderman, University of Virginia Library
William Appleton, Appleton Family Collection, Baker Library, Harvard
    Business School
Florence Merriam Bailey, The Bancroft Library, University of California at
    Berkeley
Zilpah Grant Banister, Mount Holyoke College Archives
Lucien Barbour Jr., Lucien Barbour Family Papers, Library of Congress
John Bell, Dinsmore Farm Collection, Arizona Historical Society;
Bell Family Papers, New Hampshire Historical Society
D. M. Berry, Huntington Library
Priscilla Bond, Louisiana and Lower Mississippi Valley Collections,
    Louisiana State University Library
Cyrus P. Bradley, New Hampshire Historical Society
Charles J. Braden, Illinois State Historical Society
David Brainerd, Manuscripts and Archives, Yale University Library; Con-
    necticut Historical Society
Francis Brown, Dartmouth College Archives
Maria Bryan, South Caroliniana Library

Francis Ann Brace Bunce, Connecticut Historical Society

William H. Burroughs, Rutgers College Library

John Calhoun Jr., John C. Calhoun Papers, South Caroliniana Library

Patrick Calhoun, John C. Calhoun Papers, South Caroliniana Library

Robert Campbell, Missouri Historical Society

George Champion, Edwards Family Papers, Manuscripts and Archives, Yale University Library

Henry G. Chapman, Chapman Family Collection, Boston Public Library

Nathaniel Cheever, Cheever-Wheeler Family Papers, American Antiquarian Society

Nathaniel Cheever II, Cheever-Wheeler Family Papers, American Antiquarian Society

Henry R. Cleveland, Cleveland-Perkins Family Papers, Rare Books and Manuscripts, New York Public Library

George Collier, Hitchcock Family Papers, Missouri Historical Society

Boyd Cornick, Southwest Collection, Texas Technical University

Charles Burnett Cory, Cory Family Papers, Whaling Museum of New Bedford

Isaac Cory, Cory Family Papers, Whaling Museum of New Bedford

Bronson Cutting, Library of Congress

Jeremiah Day, Day Family Papers, Manuscripts and Archives, Yale University Library

Emma Carter Dickinson, courtesy of Helen Dickinson Baldwin, Private Collection

Silas Dinsmore, Dinsmore Farm Collection, Arizona Historical Society

Arthur Earle, Hammond Family Papers, South Caroliniana Library

Ellen Peabody Eliot, Charles W. Eliot Papers, Harvard University Archives

Joseph Emerson, Mount Holyoke College Archives

Jeremiah Evarts, Evarts Family Papers, Manuscripts and Archives, Yale University Library

Robert M. Ferguson, University of Arizona

Anna Leonard Webb Ferris, Shaw-Webb Family Papers, American Antiquarian Society

Matthew C. Field, Missouri Historical Society

Irving Fisher, Manuscripts and Archives, Yale University Library

Deborah Vinal Fiske, Helen Hunt Jackson Papers, Tutt Library, Colorado College

Nathan Welby Fiske, Helen Hunt Jackson Papers, Tutt Library, Colorado College

Lawrence Flick, Catholic University Library

Harriet Fowler, Emily Ford Papers, Rare Books and Manuscripts, New York Public Library

Edwin Davis French, New York Historical Society

Mae Goodwin, Illinois State Historical Society

Donald Graham, Margaret Collier Graham Papers, Huntington Library

Sally Baxter Hampton, South Caroliniana Library

Catharine M. Haun, Huntington Library

Margaret Hereford, Sublette Family Papers, Missouri Historical Society

Thomas Hereford, Sublette Family Papers, Missouri Historical Society

Edwin Bliss Hill, Huntington Library

Frank Holm, Edwin Bliss Hill Collection, Huntington Library

Arthur Hunt, Hunt Family Papers, Peterborough Historical Society

Ernest Hunt, Hunt Family Papers, Peterborough Historical Society

Harriet Boardman Hunt, Myron Hunt Papers, Huntington Library

Bessie Huntting-Rudd, Huntting-Rudd Family Papers, Schlesinger Library

Helen Hunt Jackson, Library of Congress, Rare Books and Manuscripts, New York Public Library; Minnesota Historical Society; Trinity College; Tutt Library, Colorado College.

Maria Rutherford Jay, John Jay Collection, Columbia University Special Collections

Charles Henry Kilton, Kilton Family Papers, Whaling Museum of New Bedford

Francis Albert Kilton, Kilton Family Papers, Whaling Museum of New Bedford

Joseph Horace Kimball, New Hampshire Historical Society

Julia Ann Draper Lazelle, Draper-White Family Papers, American Antiquarian Society

Benjamin Lincoln, Harvard Medical Library

Maria White Lowell, James Russell Lowell Collection, Houghton Library

Mary Macrery, Louisiana State University

Elisa Ann Washburn Moen, Washburn Family Papers, American Antiquarian Society

Augustus Olcott Moore, Augustus Olcott Moore Family Papers, Minnesota Historical Society

Daniel Mulford, Manuscripts and Archives, Yale University Library

Josiah Obear, Obear Family Papers, South Caroliniana Library

Alexander Fisher Olmsted, Denison Olmsted Papers, Manuscripts and Archives, Yale University Library

Frederick Allyn Olmsted, Denison Olmsted Papers, Manuscripts and Archives, Yale University Library

John Howard Olmsted, Denison Olmsted Papers, Manuscripts and Archives, Yale University Library

Denison Olmsted II, Denison Olmsted Papers, Manuscripts and Archives, Yale University Library

John Hull Olmsted, Frederick Law Olmsted Papers, Library of Congress

Theodore Parker, Massachusetts Historical Society

Ephraim Peabody, Derby-Peabody Family Papers, Massachusetts Historical Society

Harriet Peck, Peck Family Papers, Guilford College Library

L. Garnet Pelton, Richard C. Cabot Collection, Harvard University Archives

Alfred Perkins, Manuscripts and Archives, Yale University Library

Amos Augustus Phelps, Boston Public Library

Emeline Draper Rice, Draper-White Family Papers, American Antiquarian Society

Rebecca Scott Salisbury, Salisbury Family Papers, American Antiquarian Society

Charles Schwalb, Boyd Cornick Papers, Southwest Collection, Texas Technical University

Sarah Louisa Sheppard, Sheppard Family Collection, New England Genealogical and Historical Society

Jonathan Smith Jr., Smith Family Papers, Peterborough Historical Society

Amy Fay Stone, Fay Family Papers, Schlesinger Library

Martha Snell, Snell Family Papers, Amherst College Library

Sarah Josephine Stoughton, American Antiquarian Society

John Ward Stimson, Stimson Family Papers, New York Historical Society

Andrew Sublette, Sublette Family Papers, Missouri Historical Society

William Sublette, Sublette Family Papers, Missouri Historical Society

Henry Sumner, Charles Sumner Papers, Houghton Library

Mary Sumner, Charles Sumner Papers, Houghton Library

John Todd, Manuscripts and Archives, Yale University Library

Edward Livingston Trudeau, Trudeau Institute

Joseph Tuckerman, Tuckerman Family Papers III, Massachusetts Historical Society; Salisbury Family Papers, American Antiquarian Society

Charles Turner Torrey, Boston Public Library

Eliza Wadsworth, Henry W. Longfellow Collection, Longfellow National Historic Site

Harriot Wadsworth, Daniel Wadsworth Papers, Connecticut Historical Society

Philip Washburn, Washburn Family Collection, Special Collections, Tutt Library, Colorado College

Jenny Webb, Gerald B. Webb Papers, Courtesy of Mrs. John W. Stewart, Webb Memorial Library, Penrose Hospital

Kate M. Webb, James Joshua Webb Papers, Missouri Historical Society

James T. Williams, Jr., James T. Williams Papers, South Caroliniana Library

Sophia Draper White, Draper-White Family Papers, American Antiquar-
    ian Society
Charles Dwight Willard, Huntington Library
William Channing Woodbridge, Manuscripts and Archives, Yale Univer-
    sity Library
Jeffries Wyman, Wyman Family Papers, Harvard Medical Library

NOTES

Introduction

1. See Arthur Kleinman, *The Illness Narratives: Suffering, Healing, and the Human Condition* (New York: Basic Books, 1988). On the case record, see Kathryn Montgomery Hunter, "Remaking the Case," *Literature and Medicine* 11 (Spring 1992): 164. For a fascinating discussion of the way the technical language of medicine shapes these documents and the physician-patient relationship, see Rita Charon, "To Build a Case: Medical Histories as Traditions in Conflict," *Literature and Medicine* 11 (Spring 1992): 115–32. For an analysis of the psychoanalytic case history, see Stephanie Kiceluk, "The Patient as Sign and Story: Disease Pictures, Life Histories, and the First Psychoanalytic Case History," *Journal of Clinical Psychoanalysis* 1 no. 3 (1992): 333–67.

2. Charles E. Rosenberg, "Framing Disease: Illness, Society, and History," in Charles E. Rosenberg and Janet Golden, eds., *Framing Disease: Studies in Cultural History* (New Brunswick, N.J.: Rutgers University Press, 1992), pp. xiii–xxvi; Megan Vaughan, *Curing Their Ills: Colonial Power and African Illness* (Stanford, Calif.: Stanford University Press, 1991). For another fascinating essay on the way a society frames disease, see Bert Hansen, "American Physicians: 'Discovery' of Homosexuals, 1880–1900: A New Diagnosis in a Changing Society," in Rosenberg and Golden, *Framing Disease*, pp. 104–25. For an effort to frame a contemporary disease, see Robert A. Aronowitz, "Lyme Disease: The Social Construction of a New Disease and Its Social Consequences," *Milbank Quarterly* 69 (1991): 79–110.

3. William Sweetser, *Treatise on Consumption* (Boston: T. H. Carter, 1836), pp. 65, 68, 73.

4. Mary Douglas, *Purity and Danger: An Analysis of Concepts of Pollution and Taboo* (New York: Praeger, 1966), has described the way societies inform members of what types of behavior are clean and acceptable and which are dirty and polluted.

5. For a fine historical analysis of how gender influenced the medical treatment of men and women with neurasthenia in the late nineteenth century, see F. G. Gosling, *Before Freud: Neurasthenia and the American Medical Community, 1870–1910* (Urbana, Ill.: University of Illinois Press, 1987).

6. There are several excellent recent historical studies documenting the fluid relationships between physicians and patients. See, for example, Dorothy Porter and Roy Porter, *Patient's Progress: Doctors and Doctoring in Eighteenth-Century England* (Stanford: Stanford University Press, 1989); and Judith Walzer Leavitt, *Brought to Bed: Childbearing in America, 1750–1950* (New York: Oxford University Press, 1986).

7. Talcott Parsons, "Definitions of Health and Illness in the Light of American Values and Social Structure," in *Patients, Physicians, and Illness,* ed. E. Gartly Jaco, (Glencoe, Ill.: Free Press, 1972) pp. 107–27.

8. Susan Sontag, *Illness as Metaphor* (New York: Farrar, Straus and Giroux, 1978); and Thomas Mann, *The Magic Mountain* (New York: Alfred A. Knopf, 1927). For an interesting study on the way culture shaped personal and public behavior toward cancer, see James T. Patterson, *The Dread Disease: Cancer and Modern American Culture* (Cambridge: Harvard University Press, 1987).

9. See David Rosner and Gerald Markowitz, *Deadly Dust: Silicosis and the Politics of Occupational Disease in Twentieth-Century America* (Princeton: Princeton University Press, 1991).

10. While mortality rates were declining for whites in the 1920s and 1930s, they were rising dramatically among blacks, but, in contrast to whites, few resources were allocated for their treatment. See Louis I. Dublin, "Decline of Tuberculosis: Present Death Rates and Outlook for the Future," *American Review of Tuberculosis* 43 (1941): 227–28. This disparity may have led Barbara Bates, *Bargaining for Life: A Social History of Tuberculosis, 1876–1938* (Philadelphia: University of Pennsylvania Press, 1992), pp. 289–310, to examine the plight of blacks with tuberculosis in Philadelphia during the first decades of the twentieth century separately from whites. Bates notes that despite the fact that large numbers had the disease, "hospitals and sanatoriums often excluded blacks, and neither money nor personal recommendations could assure them acceptable care" (p. 292). For another historical examination of the experience of blacks and disease in the pre–Civil War era, see Todd E. Savitt, *Medicine and Slavery: The Diseases and Health Care of Blacks in Antebellum Virginia* (Urbana, Ill.: University of Illinois Press, 1978). Native Americans also contracted tuberculosis, but until the 1940s few resources were allocated for their treatment either. Even when they gained admission to a sanatorium, their experience was also different. For a poignant narrative of illness of a Lakota woman, see *Madonna Swan: A Lakota Woman's Story*, as told to Mark St. Pierre (Norman, Okla.: University of Oklahoma Press, 1991).

Chapter 1: The Dreaded Disease

1. Physicians themselves often noted these facts. "Fully one-half the deaths from consumption," wrote Sir James Clark, "occur between the twentieth and fortieth years. . . . Mortality is about its maximum at thirty." Quoted in William Sweetser, *Treatise on Consumption* (Boston: T. H. Carter, 1836), p. 45. Sweetser noted that females were more prone to consumption than males (p. 43).

2. Larry Gara, *The Presidency of Franklin Pierce* (Lawrence, Kan.: University of Kansas Press, 1991), p. 31. See also Ivor D. Spencer, *The Victor and the Spoils: A Life of William L. Marcy* (Providence, R. I.: Brown University Press, 1959).

3. Lemuel Shattuck, *Report of the Sanitary Commission of Massachusetts* (Boston: Dutton

and Wentworth, 1850; Cambridge, Mass.: Harvard University Press, 1948), p. 94. Shattuck also notes that in Massachusetts between 1845 and 1858 the disease claimed 3,502 men and 5,458 women (p. 94).

4. See Katharine Park, *Doctors and Medicine in Early Renaissance Florence* (Princeton, N.J.: Princeton University Press, 1985).

5. On the prehistory and early history of tuberculosis, see William D. Johnston, "Tuberculosis," in *The Cambridge World History of Human Disease*, ed. Kenneth F. Kiple (New York: Cambridge University Press, 1993), pp. 1062–64; and John Bunyan, *The Life and Death of Mr. Badman* (London: J. A. for Nath Ponder, 1680), ed. James F. Forrest and Roger Sharrock (Oxford: Clarendon Press, 1988), p. 148.

6. During the last decades of the century, physicians began to comment on the increasing number of those who died from consumption. See Edward A. Holyoke, "A Bill of Mortality for the Town of Salem for the Years 1782 and 1783," in *Memorials of the American Academy of Arts and Sciences* (Boston: Adams and Nourse, 1785), p. 546. At the turn of the century the comments were more frequently accompanied by a sense of panic; see Joseph H. Gallup, *Sketches of Epidemic Diseases in the State of Vermont* (Boston: Bradford and Reed, 1816), p. 76. The large migration that occurred during the last quarter of the century may have also had a role. For a sense of the scope and impact of the migration generally, see Bernard Bailyn, *Voyages to the West: A Passage in the Peopling of America on the Eve of the Revolution* (New York: Alfred A. Knopf, 1986).

7. Orra Hitchcock to Deborah Fiske, July 18, 1843, Helen Hunt Jackson Papers, Special Collections, Tutt Library, Colorado College. On the dread of consumption, see David Donald, *Charles Sumner and the Coming of the Civil War* (New York: Alfred A. Knopf, 1960), pp. 94–97. Within a year Sumner's brother Henry, his sister Mary, and his friend Henry Cleveland all died of consumption.

8. Thomas Beddoes, *Essay on the Causes, Early Signs, and Prevention of Pulmonary Consumption* 2d ed. enlarged (London: Longman and Rees, 1799), p. 6.

9. On the response of European governments to epidemics, such as the plague, and contagious diseases, such as leprosy, see Ann G. Carmichael, "History of Public Health and Sanitation in the West before 1700," in Kiple, *Cambridge World History*, pp. 192–99.

10. John Weiss, *Life and Correspondence of Theodore Parker* (New York: Appleton and Company, 1864), pp. 513–15.

11. Sweetser, *Treatise on Consumption*, pp. 56–57.

12. Ibid., pp. 65, 68.

13. Ibid., pp. 36, 60.

14. The stethoscope was invented in 1816 and became available in this country in the 1830s. See Luther Vose Bell, *"A Practical Treatise in the Use of the Stethoscope in the Diagnosis of Consumptive Diseases"* (Manuscript, Harvard Medical Library, Boston, 1836). There is some evidence that medical students were taught how to use the stethoscope in the 1840s. See Henry I. Bowditch, *The Young Stethoscopist, or the Student's Aid to Auscultation* (New York: J. and H. G. Langley, 1846). But there is also widespread anecdotal evidence that even into the 1880s some physicians still preferred to rely on their eyes or more directly on their ears to judge when the person had entered stage two or stage three. Sweetser, *Treatise on Consumption*, pp. 72–73.

15. Sweetser, *Treatise on Consumption*, pp. 81–82.

16. On medical practices in this era, see Charles E. Rosenberg, "The Therapeutic Revolution: Medicine, Meaning and Social Change in Nineteenth-Century America,"

in *Sickness and Health in America*, ed. Judith Walzer Leavitt and Ronald Numbers (Madison, Wis.: University of Wisconsin Press, 1985), pp. 39–52.

17. John Harley Warner, *The Therapeutic Perspective: Medical Practice, Knowledge and Identity in America, 1820–1885* (Cambridge, Mass.: Harvard University Press, 1986), p. 58, provides an important analysis on the specificity of treatment.

18. The recommendation of constitutional treatment does not imply that physicians ceased to treat individual symptoms through bleeding, leeching, and so forth. Rather, constitutional treatment was at times given in conjunction with the heroic interventions and was expected to continue when the medical crisis abated. Charles J. B. Williams, *Lectures on the Physiology and Diseases of the Chest: Including the Principles of Physical and General Diagnosis* (Philadelphia: Haswell, Barrington and Haswell, 1839), pp. 246–47.

   Physicians endorsed these principles over many centuries. British and American physicians subscribed to them. Sir James Clark assured readers of *The Sanative Influence of Climate: With an Account of the Best Places of Resort for Invalids in England and the South of Europe* 3d London ed. (Philadelphia: A. Wadel, 1841), that "influence of climate over disease has been long established . . . and physicians have from a very early period considered change of climate and change of air as remedial agents of great efficacy" (p. 5). See also René Dubos and Jean Dubos, *The White Plague: Tuberculosis, Man, and Society* (Boston: Little, Brown, 1952), pp. 3–10.

19. On the tendency of physicians to link diseases to specific regions, see Warner, *The Therapeutic Perspective*. Treatment regimens were also linked to the gender and socioeconomic status of the sick; thus, it was appropriate for some to take long voyages and for others to take short trips. Some invalids were advised to go to the West Indies for the winter, while others with less money and more familial obligations were advised to go to the mountains or to the seacoast for a shorter time.

20. Although there was medical evidence to the contrary, until the late 1840s consumption was presumed to be primarily a disease of those who resided in cold climates. Sweetser, *Treatise on Consumption*, p. 82; John Eberle, *A Treatise on the Practice of Medicine*, 3d ed. (Philadelphia: Grigg and Elliot, 1835), 1:361.

21. Samuel George Morton, *Illustrations of Pulmonary Consumption, Its Anatomical Characters, Causes, Symptoms, and Treatment* (Philadelphia: Key and Biddle, 1834), p. 150; Clark, *The Sanative Influence of Climate*, pp. 39–40; Robert Thomas, *The Modern Practice of Physic*, (New York: S. B. Collins, Co., 1824), p. 522.

22. Quoted in Christopher Lloyd, ed., *The Health of Seamen* (London: Navy Records Society, 1965), p. 313; Sweetser, *Treatise on Consumption*, p. 172.

23. Sweetser, *Treatise on Consumption*, pp. 168–69; the quote of John Locke can be found in Dubos and Dubos, *The White Plague*, pp. 146–47.

24. Henry I. Bowditch, "Open Air Travel as a Curer and Preventer of Consumption," *Science* 14 (Oct. 1889): 230–32. As we shall see, rumors of the fabulous and often seemingly miraculous cures that occurred when consumptives went to the dry western deserts led to a revision of Sydenham's cure to fit with the conditions of Western travel.

25. Dr. James Thacher endorsed long overland journeys if they offered "a proper degree of exercise on horseback, or in an open carriage." Thacher, *American Modern Practice, or, A Simple Method of Prevention and Cure of Diseases*, new ed. (Boston: Cottons and Barnard, 1826), p. 365. Sweetser, *Treatise on Consumption*, p. 169.

26. Clark, *The Sanative Influence of Climate*, p. 40; Thomas, *The Modern Practice of Physic*, p. 512.

27. Clark, *The Sanative Influence of Climate*, pp. 14–15.

28. Williams, *Lectures on the Physiology and Diseases of the Chest*, p. 247.

29. D. J. T. Francis, *Change of Climate Considered as a Remedy in Dyspeptic, Pulmonary, and Other Chronic Affections* (London: John Churchill, 1853), p. 46.

30. Clark, *The Sanative Influence of Climate*, pp. 152, 154, 155; Sweetser, *Treatise on Consumption*, p. 252. Warner, *The Therapeutic Perspective*, demonstrates that climate was only one aspect of medical therapeutics (pp. 70–71).

31. Clark, *The Sanative Influence, of Climate*, pp. 154–55. The choice of destination was further complicated by testimonials that some climates were better in one season than another. Nice, for example, was recommended for its mild winters but to be avoided when the mistral arrived.

32. Dubos and Dubos argue that the theories of irritation and counterirritation were nothing more than "fads and counterfads" that led to unnecessary suffering and death. "All the tragedy of consumption," they contended, "the perverted attitude of the romantic era toward the disease, and the ignorance of nineteenth-century medicine . . . are exemplified in the story of John Keats, dead tuberculous in 1821 at the age of twenty-six." But to view nineteenth-century therapeutics from the perspective of twentieth-century advances is to violate the most basic principles of historical analysis. The question is not whether these physicians were right or wrong but how they arrived at their theories and translated them into practice, and, most important for us, how individuals with a life-threatening disease responded to them. See Dubos and Dubos, *The White Plague*, p. 11.

33. Robert Louis Stevenson, "Health and Mountains," in *Essays of Travel and in the Art of Writing* (New York: Charles Scribner's Sons, 1907), p. 230.

34. Men and women who lived in the second half of the nineteenth century and suffered from a constellation of symptoms called neurasthenia were also invalids. For an excellent study on the disease, see F. G. Gosling, *Before Freud: Neurasthenia and the American Medical Community, 1870–1910* (Urbana, Ill.: University of Illinois Press, 1987). See also Alice James to Alice Howe Gibbens James February 5, 1890, in *The Death and Letters of Alice James*, ed. Ruth B. Yeazell (Berkeley, Calif.: University of California Press, 1981), p. 181.

35. Sweetser, *Treatise on Consumption*, pp. 196–97.

36. Robert Means to Elizabeth Appleton, February 15, 1816, Jane A. Pierce and Family Papers, Library of Congress.

37. Henry S. Kelsey, "An Account of the Last Two Years of Martha Snell's Life," is an unpublished manuscript in the Snell Family Papers, Amherst College library. Martha, the daughter of an Amherst professor, was in the final stage of consumption when she became engaged to Henry Kelsey. Henry's detailed account of their engagement and Martha's death makes clear that the disease did not alter their plans. Stephen Longfellow, the father of Henry Longfellow, was engaged to marry Eliza Wadsworth when she contracted the disease. The engagement continued until her death. For the courtship of Ellen Tucker and Ralph Waldo Emerson, see Edith W. Gregg, *Our First Love: The Letters of Ellen Louisa Tucker to Ralph Waldo Emerson* (Cambridge, Mass.: Harvard University Press, 1962). *The Lowell Offering* contains several stories about brides who died of consumption. See, for example, E. W. J., "Ella Howard," *The Lowell Offering* 5 (June 1845).

38. The narratives confirm the presence of deep and emotive familial relationships that have been documented by other historians. See Mary P. Ryan, *Cradle of the Middle*

Class: The Family in Oneida County, New York, 1790–1865 (New York: Cambridge University Press, 1981), pp. 145–85; and Daniel Blake Smith, "Autonomy and Affection: Parents and Children in Chesapeake Families," in Michael Gordon, ed., *The American Family in Social-Historical Perspective* (New York: St. Martin's Press, 1978), pp. 209–28.

Chapter 2: Manhood and Invalidism

1. For the experiences of healthy men of the same status, see E. Anthony Rotundo, *American Manhood: Transformations in Masculinity from the Revolution to the Modern Era* (New York: Basic Books, 1993).
2. See David Allmendinger, Jr., *Paupers and Scholars: The Transformation of Student Life in Nineteenth-Century New England* (New York: St. Martin's Press, 1975); Lawrence A. Cremin, *American Education: The National Experience, 1783–1876* (New York: Harper and Row, 1980), pp. 404–9; Rotundo, *American Manhood*, pp. 63–69; Cyrus Bradley, Journal, August 1834, Cyrus Bradley Papers, New Hampshire Historical Society.
3. Nathaniel Cheever II, Private Journal, April 28, 1829; August 2, 1829; July 21, 1829, Cheever-Wheeler Family Papers, American Antiquarian Society.
4. Joseph Horace Kimball, Journal, September 11, 1836, Joseph Horace Kimball Papers, New Hampshire Historical Society.
5. John Gould, *Private Journal of a Voyage from New York to Rio de Janeiro*, ed. Edward S. Gould (New York: no publisher, 1839), pp. 3–4.
6. Samuel A. Eliot to Charles W. Eliot, September 1, 1849, Charles W. Eliot Papers, Harvard University Archives. Joseph Kett maintains that the type of parental concern Eliot articulated was an effort of fathers to assure their sons' continuing subordination. Given the prevalence of consumption and the propensity for men in college to evince its symptoms, this interpretation seems to ignore the real danger to health that college life presented. See Joseph Kett, *Rites of Passage: Adolescence in America, 1790 to the Present* (New York: Basic Books, 1977), p. 45.
7. John Howard Olmsted, Diary, October 1837, in Denison Olmsted, "Family Memoirs," Denison Olmsted Papers, Natural Sciences Manuscript Group Manuscripts and Archives, Yale University Library.
8. Ibid., Spring 1838.
9. Ibid., September 14, 1840.
10. *John Todd: The Story of His Life Told Mainly by Himself*, comp. and ed. by John E. Todd (New York: Harper and Brothers, 1876), p. 77. Bradley, Journal, August 31, 1833.
11. Cheever, Private Journal, April 13, 1843.
12. Although establishments offering the water cure were popular in this era, travel for health was the preferred treatment for those with primarily respiratory ailments.
13. Henry R. Cleveland to Horace Cleveland, October 20, 1842, Cleveland-Perkins Papers, Rare Books and Manuscripts, New York Public Library. George S. Hilliard, *A Selection from the Writings of Henry Russell Cleveland* (Boston: Freeman and Bolles, 1844).
14. For an extensive discussion of the reciprocal relationships between physicians and well-to-do patients, see Dorothy Porter and Roy Porter, *Patient's Progress: Doctors and Doctoring in Eighteenth-Century England* (Stanford, Calif.: Stanford University Press, 1989). The relationships between physicians and patients in their study have much in common with the men and their physicians here.

15. On gender obligations and privileges of men in this era, see E. Anthony Rotundo, "Learning about Manhood: Gender Ideals and the Middle-Class Family in Nineteenth-Century America," in J. A. Mangan and James Walvin, eds., *Manliness and Morality: Middle-Class Masculinity in Britain and America, 1800–1940* (New York: St. Martin's Press, 1987), pp. 35–51, and Joseph H. Pleck, "The Male Sex Role: Definitions, Problems and Sources of Change," *Journal of Social Issues* 32, no. 3 (1976): 155–64.

16. See Samuel Eliot Morison, *The Maritime History of Massachusetts, 1783–1860* (Boston: Houghton Mifflin, 1941); Robert G. Albion, *Square-Riggers on Schedule* (Princeton, N.J.: Princeton University Press, 1938); and Robert G. Albion, William A. Baker, and Benjamin W. Labaree, *New England and the Sea* (Middletown, Conn.: Wesleyan University Press, 1972).

17. On the economic prosperity of New England maritime commerce, see George Rogers Taylor, *The Transportation Revolution: 1815–1860* (New York: Rinehart, 1951), pp. 104–10; Albion, Baker and Labaree, *New England and the Sea;* Morison, *Maritime History*, pp. 3–16. On the effects of the sea on American culture, see Francis Otto Matthiessen, *American Renaissance: Art and Expression in the Age of Emerson and Whitman* (New York: Oxford University Press, 1941).

18. Joseph Tuckerman to Elisabeth Salisbury, October 28, 1836, Salisbury Family Papers, American Antiquarian Society; William Ellery Channing to Joseph Tuckerman, October 24, 1836, William Ellery Channing Papers, Massachusetts Historical Society. See also Joseph Tuckerman, "Observations on the Climate &c. of Santa Cruz," *Boston Medical and Surgical Journal* 16 (1837): 357–64, 373–79.

19. Mills Day to Thomas Day, August 17, 1801, Day Family Papers, Manuscripts and Archives, Yale University Library.

20. Sarah Caldwell Colt to Samuel Colt, October 1834, Samuel Colt Papers, Connecticut Historical Society.

21. On the romantic and adventurous aspects of life on the high seas, see Thomas Philbrick, *James Fenimore Cooper and the Development of American Sea Fiction* (Cambridge, Mass.: Harvard University Press, 1961).

22. For discussions of the meaning of the sea in men's imagination, see Philbrick, *James Fenimore Cooper;* and W. H. Auden, *The Enchafed Flood, or The Romantic Iconography of the Sea* (New York: Random House, 1950). See also James Fenimore Cooper, *The Red Rover* (Philadelphia: Carey, Lea and Blanchard, 1836), p. 348.

23. Jonathan Smith, Jr., Journal, October 1836–January 1837, Smith Family Papers, Peterborough Historical Society.

24. Nathaniel Cheever to Charlotte Cheever, October 30, 1818, Cheever-Wheeler Family Papers.

25. Jonathan Smith, Jr., Journal, November 27, 1836.

26. Ibid.

27. Ibid.

28. Henry Cleveland to Mrs. Guild, February 24, 1843, Cleveland-Perkins Papers.

29. Nathan Fiske, Diary, November 19 and 24, 1846. Helen Hunt Jackson Papers, Special Collections, Tutt Library, Colorado College.

30. James Fenimore Cooper, *The Pilot, A Tale of the Sea* (New York: D. Appleton and Company, 1873). On women at sea, see Suzanne J. Stark, "The Adventures of Two Women Whalers," *American Neptune* 44 (Winter 1984): 22–24; Julia C. Bonham, "Feminist and Victorian: The Paradox of the American Seafaring Woman in the Nineteenth Century," *American Neptune* 38, no. 3 (July 1977): 203–18.

31. Marcus Rediker, *Between the Devil and the Deep Blue Sea: Merchant Seamen, Pirates, and the Anglo-American Maritime World, 1700–1750* (Cambridge: Cambridge University Press, 1987), provides an exploration of life at sea from the vantage of the forecastle and integrates maritime history into working-class history. For a literary exploration of this same experience, see David S. Reynolds, *Beneath the American Renaissance: The Subversive Imagination in the Age of Emerson and Melville* (New York: Alfred A. Knopf, 1986).

32. Hugh H. Davis, "The American Seamen's Friend Society and the American Sailor, 1828–1838," *American Neptune* 39 (January 1979): 45. There are surviving records of many cases in the Southern District of New York that seamen brought against owners for both lack of compensation and cruel and unfair punishment.

33. Invalids also joined the U.S. Navy in an effort to cure their disease. For example, Denison Olmsted wrote to George Bancroft, the secretary of the navy, asking if Frank could have a position. See Olmsted, "Family Memoirs."

34. Morison, *Maritime History*, pp. 314–26, equates life on a whaler with "peonage." "Whaling skippers," Morison maintained, "had been proverbial for cruelty and whale-ship owners for extortion, since colonial days; but the generation of 1830–60 surpassed its forbears" (p. 319).

35. Olmsted, "Family Memoirs." Francis Allyn Olmsted, *Incidents of a Whaling Voyage* (New York: D. Appleton, 1841), pp. 5–6.

36. Olmsted, *Incidents of a Whaling Voyage*, pp. 148–49.

37. Ibid., pp. 153, 183.

38. Ibid., pp. 71–72. I am indebted to Eugene F. Rice, Jr., for alerting me to recent studies that focus on the homosocial aspects of life in the forecastle. See particularly Robert K. Martin, *Hero, Captain, and Stranger: Male Friendship, Social Critique and Literary Form in the Sea Novels of Herman Melville* (Chapel Hill, N.C.: University of North Carolina Press, 1986).

39. Olmsted, *Incidents of a Whaling Voyage*, p. 8.

40. Richard Henry Dana, Jr., *Two Years Before the Mast* (New York: Harper and Brothers, 1840; New York: Penguin edition, 1981), p. 40.

41. Thomas Philbrick, "Introduction," in Dana, *Two Years Before the Mast* (New York: Penguin, 1981), p. 19.

42. Gould, *Private Journal*, pp. 4, 5.

43. Gould, "My First and Last Flogging," *Knickerbocker Magazine*, December 1834, reprinted in Gould, *Private Journal*, pp. 117–32.

44. Gould, *Private Journal*, p. 5.

45. Frederick Law Olmsted to Frederick Kingsbury, August 5, 1851, Fredrick Law Olmsted Papers, Library of Congress.

Chapter 3: The Pursuit of Health

1. Two historical studies describe the way that the social and economic situations of students forced them to interrupt higher education. Joseph Kett maintains that the academy provided "a form of seasonal education to complement seasonal labor patterns in pre-industrial American society." See Joseph Kett, *Rites of Passage: Adolescence in America, 1790 to the Present* (New York: Basic Books, 1977), p. 19. David Allmendinger, Jr., connects sporadic attendance to economic circumstances and not health. See David Allmendinger, Jr., *Paupers and Scholars: The Transformation of Student Life in Nineteenth-Century New England* (New York: St. Martin's Press, 1975), pp. 38–41.

2. E. Anthony Rotundo, *American Manhood: Transformations in Masculinity from the Revolution to the Modern Era* (New York: Basic Books, 1993), observes that for middle-class men in the nineteenth century, "work was not just a personal matter. . . . It helped to connect a man's inner sense of identity with his identity in the eyes of others" (p. 171). The professions, Rotundo maintains, were callings that "rested on power, pride, and public eminence" (p. 173).

3. Ralph Emerson, *The Life of Reverend Joseph Emerson* (Boston: Crocker and Brewster, 1834). There is also a small amount of correspondence between Emerson and his first two wives in the archives of Mount Holyoke College.

4. Emerson, *Life of Reverend Joseph Emerson*, p. 300.

5. Ibid., p. 21.

6. Ibid., pp. 427, 429.

7. Quoted from Denison Olmsted, Diary, December 20, 1840, contained in Denison Olmsted, "Family Memoirs." Quoted from Howard Olmsted, Diary, March 11, 1843, in Olmsted, "Family Memoirs," Denison Olmsted Papers, Natural Sciences Manuscript Group, Manuscripts and Archives, Yale University Library.

8. See Howard Olmsted, Diary, September 24, 1843.

9. Although the final years of Wyman's life lie beyond the closing dates of this section, the cure he pursued was begun in this era and was one with that of other male invalids of his education and background.

10. Letter-statement of Morrill Wyman after learning of Jeffries's death in September 1874, Wyman Family Papers, Harvard Medical Library.

11. For a report on his research, see Jeffries Wyman, *Fresh Water Shell Mounds of the St. Johns River, Florida* (Salem, Mass.: Peabody Academy of Science, 1875).

12. Sidney Lanier, *Florida: Its Scenery, Climate and History* (Philadelphia: J. B. Lippincott and Company, 1875), p. 131.

13. Jeffries Wyman to Morrill Wyman, March 29, 1871, Wyman Family Papers.

14. Ibid., March 19, 1854.

15. Ibid., April 1, 1872.

16. Ibid., April 1, 1872.

17. There is extensive biographical material on Frederick Law Olmsted, and much of it describes portions of John's life. For a very thorough and detailed examination, see Charles E. Beveridge and Charles Capen McLaughlin, eds., *The Formative Years, 1822–1852: The Papers of Frederick Law Olmsted* vol. 1 (Baltimore: Johns Hopkins University Press, 1977); and idem, *Slavery and the South, 1852–1857: The Papers of Frederick Law Olmsted* vol. 2 (Baltimore: Johns Hopkins University Press, 1981).

   The final years of John Olmsted's life occur beyond the time frame of this section. I have included Olmsted because in terms of birth, education, and life-style he belonged to this cohort of educated and privileged New England invalids.

18. Frederick Law Olmsted to Charles Loring Brace, June 22, 1845, Frederick Law Olmsted Papers, Library of Congress.

19. Frederick Law Olmsted's biographers portray John Olmsted, Sr., as a distant and aloof man. Although he appears somewhat taciturn, he displayed a deep affection for his sons and continually sacrificed his own material welfare to ensure their comfort and enhance their careers. John Olmsted was exceedingly concerned about their health, and his letters are filled with admonitions. At the same time he also enjoyed the companionship of his sons.

20. John Hull Olmsted to Frederick Kingsbury, June 18, 1847, Frederick Law Olmsted Papers. In October 1847 John Hull Olmsted also tried a stint at a water-cure estab-

lishment in Northampton to cure his dyspepsia and reduce his nervousness. The treatment was not generally recommended for those with pulmonary ailments. See John Hull Olmsted to Frederick Kingsbury, October 7, 1847, Fredrick Law Olmsted Papers.

21. Quoted in Laura Wood Roper, *FLO: A Biography of Frederick Law Olmsted* (Baltimore: The Johns Hopkins University Press, 1973), p. 56.

22. John Hull Olmsted to Frederick Kingsbury, July 21, 1849, Frederick Law Olmsted Papers.

23. John Hull Olmsted to Frederick Kingsbury, August 18, 1851, Frederick Law Olmsted Papers.

24. Ibid.

25. Ibid.

26. John Hull Olmsted to Frederick Kingsbury, August 27, 1851, Frederick Law Olmsted Papers.

27. Frederick Law Olmsted, *A Journey through Texas; or, A Saddle-Trip on the Southwestern Frontier* (New York: Dix, Edwards and Company, 1857). The quotation from Frederick is in the preface, and from John in the note by the editor. When the book appeared, John was dying and Frederick was the author of record.

28. The pro-free-soil pages contrast the life-style of recent German immigrants, who espoused the free-soil cause, with "poor whites," who had migrated to Texas from the southern states. John found the German immigrants very appealing, and while he knew he could never live in a slave society, he thought he could settle in West Texas. See Olmsted, *A Journey through Texas*, pp. 66–67.

29. Frederick Law Olmsted, *A Journey through Texas*, p. 380.

30. Ibid. pp. 380–81.

31. Nathaniel Cheever to Elizabeth Cheever, March 8, 1843, quoted in Henry T. Cheever, *Memorials of the Life and Trials of a Youthful Christian in Pursuit of Health, as Developed in the Biography of Nathaniel Cheever, M.D.* (New York: C. Scribner, 1851), p. 287.

32. Nathaniel Cheever II, Diary, December 6, 1843, Cheever-Wheeler Family Papers.

33. Nathaniel Cheever II, Private Journal, March 15, 1844, Cheever-Wheeler Family Papers.

34. See Nathaniel Cheever, "Medical Examination and Licenses in Cuba," *Boston Medical and Surgical Journal* 31 (1844): 56–61.

35. Cheever, Diary, November 3, 1843.

36. Cheever, Private Journal, April 22, 1844.

Chapter 4: Body and Soul

1. The literature on the Second Great Awakening is voluminous. Especially useful for this study were Barbara Cross, *Horace Bushnell: Minister to a Changing America* (Chicago: University of Chicago Press, 1958); and William G. McLoughlin, *Revivals, Awakenings and Reform: An Essay on Religion and Social Change in America 1607–1977* (Chicago: University of Chicago Press, 1978), pp. 98–140.

2. There is a large literature on the importance of religious pilgrimages and the use of religious metaphors by Protestants in America. Perry Miller, *Errand into the Wilderness* (Cambridge: Harvard University Press, 1956), remains the most important study. See also Edmund S. Morgan, *Visible Saints: The History of a Puritan Idea* (New York: New York University Press, 1963). Also very useful is Charles Hambrick-

Stowe, *The Practice of Piety: Puritan Devotional Disciplines in Seventeenth-Century New England* (Chapel Hill, N.C.: University of North Carolina Press, 1982), pp. 54–90.

3. Ministers and educators encouraged keeping a diary that charted the spiritual journey. For example, Jacob Abbott, *The Young Christian* (New York: Harper and Brothers, 1849), encouraged young men to form this habit. Families often preserved both the public and the private diaries. During this era it was also popular to keep secular diaries. See Perry Miller, *Consciousness in Concord: The Text of Thoreau's Hitherto 'Lost Journal' 1840–41* (Boston: Houghton Mifflin, 1958).

4. John Bunyan, *The Pilgrim's Progress* (London: 1678; Baltimore: Penguin Books, 1965). For the Emerson quote, see Ralph Emerson, *The Life of Reverend Joseph Emerson* (Boston: Crocker and Brewster, 1834), p. 17.

5. George Barrell to Nathaniel Cheever, April 3, 1818, Cheever-Wheeler Family Papers, American Antiquarian Society.

6. Nathaniel Cheever, "Reflections on Immigration," *American Advocate and Kennebec Advertiser*, October 4, 1817.

7. Nathaniel Cheever to Charlotte Cheever, October 19, 1881, Cheever-Wheeler Family Papers.

8. Ibid., November 16, 1818.

9. Ibid. For the responses of other travelers, see Adam Hodgson, *Remarks during a Journey through North America in the Years 1819, 1820 and 1821* (New York: Samuel Whiting, 1823).

10. Nathaniel Cheever to Charlotte Cheever, November 16, 1818; December 18, 1818, Cheever-Wheeler Family Papers.

11. Ibid., November 16, 1818.

12. Ibid. Abiel Abbot, a Congregational minister from Beverly, Massachusetts, was in Charleston the same winter as Cheever. Unlike Cheever, Abbot delighted in visiting all the public institutions and the homes of the planters. See "The Abiel Abbot Journals: A Yankee Preacher in Charleston Society, 1818–1827," ed. John Hammond Moore, *South Carolina Historical Magazine* 68 (1967): 51–73, 232–54.

13. Nathaniel Cheever to Charlotte Cheever, November 23, 1818, Cheever-Wheeler Family Papers.

14. Nathaniel Cheever to Charlotte Cheever, November 16, 1818, Cheever-Wheeler Family Papers. Cheever's use of the term "impious" here points to some of the conflicts that he had with his medical prescription.

15. Nathaniel Cheever to Charlotte Cheever, December 6, 1818, Cheever-Wheeler Family Papers.

16. Ibid.; Nathaniel Cheever to Charlotte Cheever, January 2, 1819; December 18, 1818, Cheever-Wheeler Family Papers.

17. Nathaniel Cheever to Charlotte Cheever, January 7, 1819; January 30, 1819, Cheever-Wheeler Family Papers; For a description of Augusta in this era, see Charles C. Jones, *Memorial History of Augusta, Georgia* (Syracuse, N.Y.: D. Mason and Company, 1890).

18. James Bates and Samuel Weston to Charlotte Cheever, March 4, 1819, Cheever-Wheeler Family Papers.

19. Ebenezer C. Tracy, *Memoir of the Life of Jeremiah Evarts Esq.* (Boston: Crocker and Brewster, 1845), pp. 64–65, 41. On the linkage between religious goals and national unity, see McLoughlin, *Revivals, Awakenings and Reform*, esp. pp. 138–40. See also Martin E. Marty, *Righteous Empire: The Protestant Experience in America* (New York: Dial Press, 1970), pp. 68–99.

20. Nathaniel Cheever II and his brothers always distributed tracts on their voyages for health. Nathaniel Cheever II, Diary, August 23, 1835, Cheever-Wheeler Family Papers. See also David Abeel, *Journey of a Residence in China . . . from 1829 to 1833* (New York: Leavitt, Lord and Company, 1834).

Franklin Bowditch Dexter, Comp., *Biographical Notices of Graduates of Yale College* (New Haven: Yale University Press, 1913), includes many accounts of invalid men who became missionaries. When symptoms of consumption appeared, Issac Orr, class of 1818 and an ordained minister, became a missionary "among the colored people" for the American Colonization Society (pp. 38–39). Henry Gerrish French, class of 1834, was another minister who planned to become a missionary. He accepted a position with the American Board of Foreign Missions but died in 1842 en route to his assignment (p. 251). See also Franklin Bowditch Dexter, Comp., *Biographies and Annals of Yale College Graduates*, 3d–6th ser. (New Haven: Yale University Press, 1903–1912).

21. Emerson, *The Life of Reverend Joseph Emerson*, p. 4.

22. Joseph Conforti, "Jonathan Edwards's Most Popular Work: 'The Life of David Brainerd' and Nineteenth-Century Evangelical Culture," *Church History* 54 (1985): 192; idem, "David Brainerd and the Nineteenth-Century Missionary Movement," *Journal of the Early Republic* 5 (1985): 310. See also Ola Elizabeth Winslow, *Jonathan Edwards, 1703–1758* (New York: Macmillan Company, 1941).

23. See Jonathan Edwards, *The Life of David Brainerd*, ed. Norman Pettit (New Haven: Yale University Press, 1985), p. 146. The solution was so attractive to invalids that missionary societies frequently lamented about the poor health of their agents. Some tried to screen out feeble applicants.

24. Jeremiah Evarts to Roswell R. Swan, December 5, 1803, quoted in Tracy, *Memoir . . . Jeremiah Evarts*, pp. 42–43. Jeremiah Evarts to Eleazer Foster, October 24, 1804, Evarts Family Papers, Manuscripts and Archives, Yale University Library.

25. Tracy, *Memoir . . . Jeremiah Evarts*, p. 48.

26. Ibid., p. 99.

27. Jeremiah Evarts to Samuel Worcester, April 30, 1818, quoted in Tracy, *Memoir . . . Jeremiah Evarts*, p. 119. For an analysis of Evarts's work among the Cherokees, see William McLoughlin, *Cherokees and Missionaries, 1789–1839* (New Haven: Yale University Press, 1984).

28. Tracy, *Memoir . . . Jeremiah Evarts*, pp. 119, 126.

29. Evarts most forcefully articulates his views in the "William Penn Essays." See Jeremiah Evarts, *Cherokee Removal: The 'William Penn' Essays and Other Writings*, ed. and with an introduction by Francis Paul Prucha (Knoxville, Tenn.: University of Tennessee Press, 1981). McLoughlin, *Cherokees and Missionaries*, discusses Evarts's lobbying efforts with the War Department to gain funds and supplies and ensure schooling for the Cherokees. Evarts's efforts collided with sectional politics, and the American Board and other evangelical societies allied with the Indians against southern politicians, judges, and legislators.

30. Jeremiah Evarts to Mehitabel Evarts, March 12, 1831, Evarts Family Papers.

31. The dedication of these invalid-abolitionists approximates the zeal of John Brown. See Stephen B. Oates, *To Purge This Land with Blood: A Biography of John Brown* (New York: Harper and Row, 1970). See also Lawrence J. Friedman, *Gregarious Saints: Self and Community in American Abolitionism, 1830–1870* (New York: Cambridge University Press, 1982); and Bertram Wyatt-Brown, "Conscience and Career: Young Abolitionists and Missionaries," in *Anti-Slavery, Religion and Reform*, eds. Christine Bolt and Seymour Drescher (Folkestone, England: William Dawson and Sons, 1980), pp. 183–203.

32. Charlotte Phelps to Amos A. Phelps, August 29, 1835, Amos Augustus Phelps Papers, Boston Public Library.

33. Amos A. Phelps to Charlotte Phelps, August 31, 1835, Amos Augustus Phelps Papers.

34. Amos A. Phelps, Diary, September 9, 1838, quoted in Edward A. Phelps, Memoir of Amos A. Phelps, manuscript, Amos Augustus Phelps Papers.

35. Joseph Kimball, Diary, July 11, 1835, Joseph Horace Kimball Papers, New Hampshire Historical Society.

36. Kimball, Diary, November 2, 1836; James Thome to Mr. Horace Kimball, 1837, Joseph Horace Kimball Papers. See also James H. Thome and Joseph Horace Kimball, *Emancipation in the West Indies* (New York: American Anti-Slavery Society, 1838).

37. Joseph C. Lovejoy, *Memoir of Rev. Charles T. Torrey* (Boston: J. P. Jewett and Company, 1847), pp. 128, 149.

38. Abby Champion to Ruth Champion, December 4, 1841; Abby Champion to Jonathan Edwards, December 9, 1841; Abby Champion to Ruth Champion, December 12, 1841, Edwards Family Papers, Manuscripts and Archives, Yale University Library.

39. Eliza Smith Lentilhon, Journal, pp. 49–53, private collection of Anne H. Willard.

40. Henry Cleveland to Margaret Cushing, April 28, 1843, Cleveland-Perkins Family Papers, Rare Books and Manuscripts, New York Public Library.

41. Jeffries Wyman to Morrill Wyman, January 19, 1860, Wyman Family Papers, Harvard Medical Library.

42. Jonathan Smith, Jr., Journal, December 8 and 9, 1836, Smith Family Papers, Peterborough Historical Society.

43. Ibid., December 16, 1836. Joseph Tuckerman, the Unitarian minister who was also in St. Croix that winter, lived in the same boardinghouse as McCall and was assigned the task of informing McCall's family of the unexpected death. Sarah Tuckerman, who had accompanied her husband, was also distressed by McCall's seemingly unnecessary death.

44. Smith, Journal, December 21, 1836, and December 30, 1836.

45. Dexter, *Biographical Notices of Graduates of Yale College*, pp. 65–66, 345, 383.

46. Thomas Day to Jeremiah Day, October 17, 1801, Day Family Papers, Manuscripts and Archives, Yale University.

47. John Olmsted to Frederick Law Olmsted, November 28, 1857, Frederick Law Olmsted Papers, Library of Congress.

48. The letters Ralph Emerson sent to Sarah Cleveland are in George S. Hillard, *A Selection from the Writings of Henry Russell Cleveland* (Boston: Freeman and Bolles, 1844), pp. xxxiii–xxxiv. See also Ralph Emerson to Sarah Cleveland, June 8, 1843, Cleveland-Perkins Family Papers.

49. Sarah Perkins Cleveland to Mrs. Andrews Norton, June 19, 1843, Cleveland-Perkins Family Papers.

50. Henry T. Cheever, *Memorials of the Life and Trials of a Youthful Christian in Pursuit of Health, as Developed in the Biography of Nathaniel Cheever M.D.* (New York: C. Scribner, 1851), pp. v–vi, xii–xiii, xiv.

Chapter 5: Coming of Age

1. Marriage often provided an opportunity for invalid women to change climate. For example, Priscilla Munnikhuysen married Howard Bond to live in Louisiana. See Priscilla M. Bond, Diary, December 25, 1860, Louisiana State University Library.

This same motivation may have affected invalid women who married missionaries. See Clifford Merrill Drury, *First White Women over the Rockies*, 3 vols. (Glendale, Calif.: Arthur H. Clark, 1963–66); and Joan Jacobs Brumberg, *Mission for Life: The Story of the Family of Adoniram Judson* (New York: Free Press, 1980).

Some women combined antislavery sentiments with curative regimens. See Ray Allen Billington, ed., *The Journal of Charlotte Forten* (New York: Collier Books, 1961). I am grateful to Deborah Van Broecken for alerting me to the letters of Harriet Peck, a consumptive whose strong antislavery feelings led her to accept a teaching post in a remote southern town. See Harriet Peck Collection, Guilford College Archives.

2. Advice books and medical texts urged women to combine exercise with household tasks. See William A. Alcott, *The Young Wife* (Boston: George W. Light, 1837), pp. 250–53; and William Sweetser, *Treatise on Consumption* (Boston: T. H. Carter, 1836), pp. 196–97.

3. Historians of gender have analyzed these female networks. Two critical studies are Mary P. Ryan, *Cradle of the Middle Class: The Family in Oneida County, New York, 1790–1865* (New York: Cambridge University Press, 1981); and Nancy Cott, *The Bonds of Womanhood: "Woman's Sphere" in New England, 1780–1835* (New Haven: Yale University Press, 1977).

4. Office of the town clerk of Amherst, Massachusetts. For a comparison with other towns in western Massachusetts, see R. S. Meindl and A. C. Swedlund, "Secular Trends in Mortality in the Connecticut Valley, 1700–1850," *Human Biology* 49 (September 1977): 389–414. For comparative statistics on the deaths of women and men from consumption, see S. W. Abbott, "The Decrease of Consumption in New England," *Journal of the American Statistical Association*, new ser. 9, no. 65 (March 1904): 1–37.

5. Steven Ruggles, *Prolonged Connections: The Rise of the Extended Family in Nineteenth-Century England and America* (Madison, Wis.: University of Wisconsin Press, 1987), argues that extended kin relationships crossed socioeconomic classes.

6. Few women invalids fully recounted their experience in this era; perhaps their domestic duties or the constraints of the disease left them little time. Their lives were often recorded by sisters, husbands, or fiancés. The life of Elisa Ann Washburn Moen was chronicled for her children by her sister. The journey for health of Harriot Wadsworth was recorded by her brother and those of Rebecca Scott Salisbury and Ellen Peabody Eliot by their husbands.

7. For an illuminating essay on the way women chose to record their lives, see Patricia Meyer Spacks, "Selves in Hiding," in *Women's Autobiography: Essays in Criticism*, ed. Estelle C. Jelinek (Bloomington, Ind.: Indiana University Press, 1980), pp. 112–32. Spacks defined the "hidden" aspects of female autobiographical writing, and her essay is relevant to understanding the narratives of New England invalid women. Carolyn G. Heilbrun, *Writing a Woman's Life* (New York: W. W. Norton, 1988), also provides a useful construct. For Deborah Fiske's official biography, see Heman Humphrey, *The Woman That Feareth the Lord: A Discourse Delivered at the Funeral of Mrs. D. W. V. Fiske, February 21, 1844* (Amherst, Mass.: J. S. and C. Adams, 1844).

8. Nineteenth-century biographies are filled with tragic stories that begin with the death of a family member from consumption. See Louise H. Tharp, *The Appletons of Beacon Hill* (Boston: Little Brown, 1973); Joyce Antler, *Lucy Mitchell Sprague* (New Haven: Yale University Press, 1987); Gay W. Allen, *Waldo Emerson: A Biography* (New York: Viking Press, 1981).

9. The details of Deborah's childhood can be found in Ruth Odell, *Helen Hunt Jackson* (New York: D. Appleton-Century, 1939), pp. 8–9. Deborah talked with her friends about her mother's death from consumption and its implications for her future. See Harriet Webster Fowler to Eliza Jones, July 30, 1843, Emily Ford Papers. Rare Books and Manuscripts, New York Public Library.

10. Over the years, continuing material success and boardinghouse living made David Vinal treasure his independence. David Vinal to Martha Vinal, September 23, 1829. Deborah frequently chided her father for his unwillingness to profess his faith. For his response, see David Vinal to Deborah Fiske, August 12, 1829, Helen Hunt Jackson (HHJ) Papers, Special Collections, Tutt Library, Colorado College.

11. Deborah Vinal Fiske to Elisabeth Terry, August 20, 1841, HHJ Papers.

12. Deborah repeated these instructions to her daughters. See Deborah Fiske to Helen Maria Fiske, n.d., HHJ Papers.

13. Deborah Fiske to Martha Vinal, January 19, 1844, HHJ Papers.

14. Odell, *Helen Hunt Jackson*, p. 9.

15. Deborah Fiske to Nathan Fiske, November 4, 1841, HHJ Papers.

16. Information on the link between physiognomy and disease can be found in all the standard medical texts of the period. See, for example, Robert Thomas, *The Modern Practice of Physic* (New York: S. B. Collins and Company, 1824), pp. 509–10. John Collins Warren's correspondence at the Massachusetts Historical Society contains information on his practice. For the specific remedies he prescribed for Deborah, see Deborah Fiske to David Vinal, October 19, 1829, HHJ Papers.

17. On Deborah's relationship to Dr. Warren, see Deborah Vinal Fiske to David Vinal, October 19, 1829, HHJ Papers. See also John Collins Warren, *Physical Education and the Preservation of Health*, 2d ed. (Boston: William D. Ticknor and Company, 1846), pp. 89–90.

18. Odell, *Helen Hunt Jackson*, p. 9, suggests that Martha Vinal persuaded David Vinal to send Deborah to Saugus Academy.

19. Deborah was regularly homesick at both schools. Deborah Vinal to Ann Scholfield, May 14, 1823, and Deborah Vinal to Ann Scholfield, October 4, 1825, HHJ Papers.

20. In 1825, further debilitated by consumption, Emerson moved the school to Connecticut. See Ralph Emerson, *The Life of Reverend Joseph Emerson* (Boston: Crocker and Brewster, 1834), p. 298.

21. On the expectations of the students, see Edward Hitchcock, *The Power of Christian Benevolence Illustrated in the Life and Labors of Mary Lyon* (Northampton, Mass.: Hopkins, Bridgman, and Childs, 1852), pp. 33–34.

    Adams provided a very rigorous education and was the first seminary to offer young women a diploma. As Deborah wrote to her cousin Ellen, "I think this is the most pleasant as well as the most strict school I ever attended." Deborah Vinal to Ellen Scholfield, June 23, 1825, HHJ Papers.

22. For Emerson's style of teaching, see Joseph Emerson, *A Union Catechism Founded upon Scripture History* (Boston: S. T. Armstrong, 1821), p. 4; and idem, *Emerson's Lessons on the Old Testament* (Boston: S. T. Armstrong, 1842).

23. Joseph Emerson, *Female Education: A Discourse Delivered at the Dedication of the Seminary Hall in Saugus, January 15, 1822* (Boston: S. T. Armstrong, 1822), p. 13.

24. Ibid., p. 8.

25. Mary Lyon became the more noted educator, founding Mount Holyoke College. See Elizabeth Alden Green, *Mary Lyon and Mount Holyoke: Opening the Gates*

(Hanover, N. H.: University Press of New England, 1979). But among their contemporaries, Grant was the more admired. For a lengthy discussion about Zilpah
Grant's charisma and influence on Catharine Beecher and other women educators, see Kathryn K. Sklar, *Catharine Beecher: A Study in American Domesticity*
(New Haven: Yale University Press, 1973). See also Laura T. Guilford, *The Uses
of a Life: Memorials of Mrs. Z. P. Grant Banister* (New York: American Tract Society, 1885).

26. See Hitchcock, *The Power of Christian Benevolence*, p. 33; Guilford, *The Uses of a Life*,
pp. 36–37; and Mary Lyon to Zilpah Grant, July 25, 1826, Mary Lyon Papers. In
the Mount Holyoke College Library/Archives a catalog of the Adams Academy
notes that of the 116 students who attended in 1825 only 51 married. Seventeen
married ordained ministers.

27. For a detailed account of Grant's health and her relationship with Emerson, see
Guilford, *The Uses of a Life*, pp. 28–57; and Emerson, *The Life of Joseph Emerson*, pp.
426–27.

28. Zilpah Grant's strong religious sentiments eventually alienated the trustees at
Adams Academy. See Guilford, *The Uses of a Life*, pp. 86–87; for Grant's educational philosophy, see pp. 196–97. Grant was very concerned about the health of
students and teachers. See John P. Cowles, "Miss Z. P. Grant–Mrs. William B.
Banister," *American Journal of Education* 30 (1880): 617. Since ill health plagued
both Emerson and Grant, the lessons were not didactic.

29. For an example of the way Grant and Lyon responded to the illness and death of
students, see Mary Lyon to Zilpah Grant, April 12, 1839, Mary Lyon Papers; and
Green, *Mary Lyon*, p. 100. See also Deborah Fiske to Ann Scholfield, September
19, 1837, HHJ Papers. Illness and death stalked all New England seminaries. At
Miss Pierce's School in Litchfield, Connecticut, students read Mrs. Lydia Howard
(Huntly) Sigourney, ed., *The Writings of Nancy Maria Hyde* (Norwich, Conn.: Russell Hubbard, 1816), a tract that focused on the way religion aided the sick and
dying.

30. Deborah attended Adams for two terms. See Adams Female Academy, *Catalogue of
the Officers and Members*, 1824, 1825, 1826. (Concord, N. H.: n. p. 1827), p. 8. Just
why she left is unclear, but it was not unusual for female students to leave before
completing the course of study.

31. Park Street Church founded in 1808 espoused aggressive opposition to the liberal
Christian principles of Unitarianism. The ministers preached a literal interpretation of divine revelation and the veracity of the biblical word, and they actively
proselytized. Membership required evidence of faith and a profession of faith. See
Leonard Woods, *A History of Andover Theological Seminary* (Boston: James R. Osgood, 1885), pp. 147–49.

32. Membership at the Park Street Church gave Deborah a circle of friends and a rou-
tine. She attended prayer meetings and sewing circles and taught Sunday school.
The young women also witnessed examinations at Andover Theological Seminary
and met the students. Deborah Vinal to Martha Hooker, September 27, 1827, HHJ
Papers. On Deborah's friends, see Mrs. E. H. Washburn, "The Mother of 'H.H.,'"
Independent, September 17, 1885, p. 5.

33. Edward Hitchcock, *Reminiscences of Amherst College* (Northampton, Mass.: Hopkins,
Bridgman and Childs, 1863), pp. 30–31.

34. See Heman Humphrey, *Memoir of Reverend Nathan W. Fiske* (Amherst, Mass.: J. S.
and C. Adams, 1850), pp. 24–30, 88–89. See also Nathan Fiske, Diary, HHJ Papers;
and Heman Humphrey, *Revival: Sketches and Manual* (New York: American Tract
Society, 1859).

35. On the founding of the college, see William S. Tyler, *History of Amherst College during Its First Half Century, 1821–1871* (Springfield, Mass.: Clark W. Bryan and Company, 1873); and Edward W. Carpenter and Charles F. Morehouse, *The History of the Town of Amherst, Massachusetts* (Amherst, Mass.: Press of Carpenter and Morehouse, 1896), pp. 160–75.

    For some of the founders the college fulfilled a religious mission. Noah Webster believed that training a corps of missionaries to "raise the human race from ignorance and . . . establish the 'Empire of Truth'" was the grand goal of Christians. See Noah Webster, "A Plea for a Miserable World," a sermon delivered August 9, 1820, at the laying of the cornerstone of Amherst College, p. 8. See also Cynthia Griffin Wolff, *Emily Dickinson* (New York: Alfred A. Knopf, 1986), pp. 13–35.

36. Fiske's major piece of scholarship, a translation of J. J. Eschenburg, *Classical Antiquities, Being Part of the Manual of Classical Literature* (Philadelphia: Key and Biddle, 1836), demonstrates the links between his religious beliefs and scholarship. Philip Gura, *The Wisdom of Words* (Middletown, Conn.: Wesleyan University Press, 1981), eloquently describes the battle between the sects and the importance of language. Classroom lessons were reinforced in the daily prayers and periodic revivals. See Tyler, *History of Amherst College*, pp. 266–83.

37. Ellen K. Rothman, *Hearts and Hands: A History of Courtship in America* (New York: Basic Books, 1984), pp. 31–44. For Deborah and Nathan, shared religious goals were key.

38. Nathan Fiske to Deborah Vinal, December 5, no year, HHJ Papers.

39. See Tyler, *History of Amherst College*, pp. 34–35.

40. Lydia Maria Child, *Letters* (Boston: Houghton Mifflin and Company, 1883), p. 33.

41. Deborah's letters to her aunt during her first months in Amherst describe how much she missed her aunt's home and her friends in Boston. See Deborah Fiske to David Vinal, December 11, 1828, HHJ Papers.

42. Deborah Fiske to Martha Vinal, December 12, 1828, HHJ Papers.

43. Odell, *Helen Hunt Jackson*, pp. 11–12.

44. Deborah Fiske to David Vinal, June 14, 1829, and Deborah Fiske to David Vinal, June 19, 1829, HHJ Papers.

45. It appears that Deborah had a physician present at the delivery. Although many women used midwives, educated and prosperous New England women increasingly employed physicians. See Sylvia D. Hoffert, *Private Matters: American Attitudes towards Childbearing and Infant Nurture in the Urban North, 1800–1860* (Urbana, Ill.: University of Illinois Press, 1989), p. 65. Deborah Fiske to Martha Vinal, September 23, 1829, HHJ Papers.

46. Nathan Fiske to Martha Hooker, October 5, 1829, HHJ Papers. Naming the child and grieving for him conflicts with findings of other historians. See Lewis O. Saum, "Death in the Popular Mind of Pre–Civil War America," in *Death in America*, ed. David Stannard (Philadelphia: University of Pennsylvania Press, 1975), pp.38–39; and Wolff, *Emily Dickinson*, p. 47.

47. Nathan Fiske to Deborah Fiske, n.d., probably December 1829, and Nathan Fiske to Deborah Fiske, December 6, 1829, HHJ Papers. A lengthy bereavement for an infant was not uncommon. See Sylvia D. Hoffert, "'A Very Peculiar Sorrow': Attitudes toward Infant Death in the Urban Northeast, 1800–1860," *American Quarterly* 39 (1987): 601–16.

48. Nathan Fiske to Deborah Fiske, December 6, 1829, HHJ Papers.

49. Through prayer and fulfillment of his duties, Nathan hoped to reconcile his spirit, destroy his pride, and demonstrate his willingness to submit to the judgment of his

Maker. Nathan Fiske to Deborah Fiske, December 6, 1829, HHJ Papers.

50. Nathan also missed Deborah. "To tell the plain truth, I am tired of living without you; not for want of outward comfort . . . but I do wish to lean my head on your bosom, as my friend one with me." Nathan Fiske to Deborah Fiske, December 17, 1829, HHJ Papers.

51. Nathan Fiske to Deborah Fiske, December 17, 1829, HHJ Papers.

52. Deborah Fiske to Elisabeth Washburn, May 24, 1831, HHJ Papers.

53. During these years Nathan worried about Deborah's future. "I wish you to avoid company, *your health is a reason amply sufficient; keep to your bedroom*." Nathan Fiske to Deborah Fiske, August 17, 1832, HHJ Papers.

54. Deborah Fiske to David Vinal, September 9, 1833, HHJ Papers.

Chapter 6: Domestic Duties

1. Deborah Fiske to Elisabeth Washburn, May 24, 1831, Helen Hunt Jackson (HHJ) Papers, Special Collections, Tutt Library, Colorado College.

2. Ann Douglas, *The Feminization of American Culture* (New York: Alfred A. Knopf, 1977), defines the domestication of death in sociopolitical terms—strategies devised by ministers and female parishioners to gain the control over the dead that they lacked over the living. "Death, province of minister and mother, instead of marking the end of power, had become its source. . . . Death widened . . . the ministerial and maternal sphere of influence" (p. 207). Douglas notes that many ministers were consumptive but links their frailty to an intellectual and political impotency and ignores other implications (see pp. 88–109). Deborah Fiske to Nathan Fiske, n.d., probably 1836, HHJ Papers.

3. Deborah Fiske to Elisabeth Terry, August 20, 1841, HHJ Papers. The vision of a family reunion can also be found in Lewis O. Saum, "Death in the Popular Mind of Pre–Civil War America," in David E. Stannard, ed., *Death in America* (Philadelphia: University of Pennsylvania Press, 1975); and Maris A. Vinovskis, "Angels' Heads and Weeping Willows: Death in Early America," *Proceedings of the American Antiquarian Society* 86 (1977): 273–302.

4. Deborah Fiske to Hannah Terry, January 26, 1840, HHJ Papers.

5. Nathan Fiske to Ann and Helen Fiske, June 25, 1846, HHJ Papers. For Nathan's views on the course of consumption, see Nathan W. Fiske, *Obituary Address at the Funeral of the Reverend Royal Washburn* (Amherst, Mass.: J. S. and C. Adams, 1833).

6. On the hidden aspect of women's autobiography, see particularly Patricia Meyer Spacks, "Selves in Hiding," in *Women's Autobiography: Essays in Criticism*, ed. Estelle C. Jelinek (Bloomington: Indiana University Press, 1980), pp. 112–32; and Jean Strouse, "Semi-Private Lives," in *Studies in Biography*, ed. Daniel Aaron (Cambridge, Mass.: Harvard University Press, 1978).

7. Deborah Fiske to Helen Fiske, n.d., probably 1836, HHJ Papers.

8. Deborah Fiske to Nathan Fiske, November 1833, HHJ Papers.

9. Deborah Fiske to Martha Hooker, n.d., probably 1836, HHJ Papers.

10. Deborah Fiske to Helen Fiske, n.d., probably 1836, HHJ Papers.

11. Educated Bostonians interpreted the plight of these vagrants in moral terms, convinced that the poor habits of this intemperate lot had grave implications for the "future of the republic." To maintain social order, they constructed almshouses, workhouses, and orphan asylums, in which under the watchful eyes of Christian superintendents the inmates would acquire "habits of industry and

usefulness" and the future of the country would no longer be in jeopardy. See David J. Rothman, *The Discovery of the Asylum* (Boston: Little, Brown and Company, 1971).

12. Deborah Fiske to Helen Fiske, n.d., probably 1836, HHJ Papers.

13. Deborah Fiske to Martha Hooker, n.d., probably 1840, HHJ Papers.

14. Lydia Child, *The Mother's Book* (Boston: Carter and Hendee, 1831), p. 76.

   In the advice books graveyards are the transition between the temporal and eternal life and were to be elaborately adorned. In Douglas, *The Feminization of American Culture*, graveyards were a pawn in a power struggle. Women and ministers turned them into a "Disney World for the mortuary imagination of Victorian America" (p. 210).

15. Deborah wrote to Helen in 1836 about "little Mary Lothrop," as if she were a friend. See *Memoir of Mary Lothrop Who Died in Boston March 18, 1831* (Boston: Perkins and Marvin, 1832).

16. Deborah Fiske to Helen Fiske, n.d., probably 1835, HHJ Papers. Deborah also added short notes to Helen's letters in which she pretended she was a cat. These letters are more endearing and affectionate, and they were later published. See Helen Hunt Jackson, *Letters from a Cat* (Boston: Little Brown and Company, 1912).

17. Deborah Fiske to Ellen Scholfield, April 28, 1843, HHJ Papers.

18. Deborah Fiske to Adeline Scholfield, April 26, n.y., HHJ Papers.

19. Deborah Fiske to Hannah Terry, n.d., HHJ Papers. Deborah did not approve of either Mount Holyoke's mandate to educate the daughters of the working poor or the efforts of the faculty to expand women's sphere of influence. Deborah Fiske to Martha Hooker, April 21, 1837, HHJ Papers.

20. Deborah Fiske to Ellen Scholfield, n.d., probably 1839; Deborah Fiske to Martha Hooker, n.d., probably 1838, HHJ Papers.

21. The columns appeared in the *Youth's Companion* in 1839. Some of titles are "Ten Questions That I Wish Nobody Would Ever Ask Me Again," "Aunt Betsy's Answer," "A Little Letter of Very Bad Spelling from a Miss Who Did Nothing but Play." Deborah Fiske to Martha Hooker, April 14, 1839, HHJ Papers.

22. Deborah Fiske to Ann Scholfield, n.d., probably February 1835, HHJ Papers. For an account of how a consumptive woman with far fewer resources managed her domestic obligations, see the letters of Sarah Louisa Sheppard, Sheppard Family Papers, New England Genealogical and Historical Society, Boston.

23. Deborah Fiske to Martha Hooker, June 18 n.y.; Deborah Fiske to Martha Hooker, n.d., probably July 1836, HHJ Papers.

24. Deborah Fiske to Ann Scholfield, October 14, 1841, HHJ Papers.

25. Deborah Fiske to Martha Hooker, August 13, 1833; Deborah Fiske to Nathan Fiske, August 8, 1843, HHJ Papers.

26. Deborah Fiske to Nathan Fiske, August 8, 1843, HHJ Papers.

27. Deborah Fiske to Helen Fiske, September 1841, HHJ Papers. Deborah was eager to have Helen profess her faith, but Helen could not. Barbara Leslie Epstein, *The Politics of Domesticity: Women, Evangelism, and Temperance in Nineteenth-Century America* (Middletown, Conn.: Wesleyan University Press, 1981), found that many women of Helen's generation from pious families faced a similar predicament (pp. 45–65).

28. After reading an edition of Abigail Adams's letters, Deborah noted "those to her husband are good, only there is a little too much love and veneration in them . . . it never reads well in *print*. [I] do think letters between husbands and wives ought *never* to be *published*—if even so *proper*, they always seem ludicrous . . . to me."

Deborah Fiske to Ann Scholfield, May 26, 1841, HHJ Papers.

29. Deborah Fiske to Nathan Fiske, July 3, 1836. HHJ Papers.

30. Nathan Fiske to Deborah Fiske, n.d., probably 1836, HHJ Papers.

31. Ibid.

32. Deborah Fiske to Nathan Fiske, July 22, 1836, HHJ Papers.

33. Ibid., July 18, 1836; Ibid., July 27, 1836; Ibid., July 20, 1836, HHJ Papers.

34. Deborah Fiske to Nathan Fiske, n.d., probably 1836, HHJ Papers.

35. Ibid., n.d., probably August 1836, HHJ Papers.

36. Ibid., July 22, 1836, HHJ Papers.

37. Ibid., July 27, 1836, HHJ Papers.

38. Ibid., October 18, 1836, HHJ Papers.

39. Ibid., July 27, 1836; Ibid., July 18, 1836, HHJ Papers.

40. Nathan's solemn manner was apparent in daily conversations. Her father, Helen maintained, had a "gloomy view of little things. . . . Whenever we did wrong, he used to sigh so deeply, it sounded as if his breath would give out; and say—'My child! My child!' in a tone of what seemed to me then terrible grief." The sound of his voice at times so frightened her that she was convinced "that if I did not take care, I would . . . some day be the death of him by my misconduct." See "Saxe-Holme" "The First Time," *St. Nicholas*, May 1877, pp. 474–75. "Saxe-Holme" was one of the pen names used by Helen Hunt Jackson.

41. Nathan Fiske, Journal, HHJ Papers.

42. On February 14, 1839, Deborah noted in a letter to Ann Scholfield that Nathan has "a chronic difficulty in his throat which troubles him occasionally." And her letters to Nathan contained admonitions: "Look out well for your *health* . . . . Remember how *easy* it is to inflame your throat, and if you get sick the first of the winter, how difficult it will be to recruit again." Deborah Fiske to Nathan Fiske, December 1840. In 1843 Nathan told Deborah that he had "a real sore throat, the *old* attack in full." Nathan Fiske to Deborah Fiske, June 10, 1843, HHJ Papers.

Chapter 7: Deborah and Her Doctors

1. Judy Walzer Leavitt, *Brought to Bed: Childbearing in America, 1750–1950* (New York: Oxford University Press, 1986), provides an excellent discussion of the way women and physicians negotiated decisions related to birthing (pp. 200–207). For another excellent discussion of negotiated relationships between physicians and patients, see Dorothy Porter and Roy Porter, *Patient's Progress: Doctors and Doctoring in Eighteenth-Century England* (Stanford, Calif.: Stanford University Press, 1989), pp. 70–91. Although the Porters discuss relationships in an earlier era, the social class and values of their group have much in common with New England invalids like Deborah Fiske. For another fine study of the influence of women's values on medical practices, see Regina Markell Morantz Sanchez, *Sympathy and Science: Women Physicians and American Medicine* (New York: Oxford University Press, 1985).

2. The term "old complaints" was often used by invalids to refer to respiratory ailments that reappeared in a more ominous form. Deborah Fiske to David Vinal, October 29, 1829, Helen Hunt Jackson (HHJ) Papers, Special Collections, Tutt Library, Colorado College.

3. Ibid.
4. Dr. James Thacher, *American Modern Practice: or, a Simple Method of Prevention and Cure of Diseases* (Boston: Cottons and Barnard, 1826), pp. 361–62. See also William Sweetser, *Treatise on Consumption* (Boston: H. H. Carter, 1836), p. 83. Thacher also noted that not every woman with consumptive symptoms died after repeated pregnancies. There were isolated cases of women who did regain their health after several pregnancies. It is important to note that women also transmitted the disease to their infants through their coughs, their kisses, and breast feeding.
5. On the confluence of childbirth and maternal death from consumption, see *The Autobiography of Lyman Beecher*, ed. Barbara M. Cross (Cambridge: Belknap Press of Harvard University Press, 1961), pp. 102–103; and Kathryn Kish Sklar, *Catharine Beecher: A Study in American Domesticity* (New Haven: Yale University Press, 1973), pp. 20–21. Leavitt, *Brought to Bed*, pp. 68–69, provides additional examples.
6. Deborah Fiske to Martha Hooker, n.d., HHJ Papers.
7. Deborah Fiske to Nathan Fiske, n.d., probably 1833, HHJ Papers.
8. Ibid.
9. Deborah Fiske to Ann Scholfield, May 26, 1841, HHJ Papers.
10. Ibid., March 1841, HHJ Papers.
11. Deborah Fiske to Martha Hooker, March 12, 1837; Deborah Fiske to Martha Hooker, March 3, 1836, HHJ Papers.
12. Deborah Fiske to Ann Scholfield, September 19, 1837, HHJ Papers.
13. M. L. Bennett to Deborah Fiske, January 5, 1838, HHJ Papers.
14. Deborah Fiske to Ann Scholfield, October 14, 1841, HHJ Papers.
15. Deborah Fiske to Martha Hooker, July 19, n.y., HHJ Papers.
16. M. L. Bennett to Deborah Fiske, January 5, 1838, HHJ Papers.
17. Oliver Wendell Holmes, "The Young Practitioner," in *Medical Essays* (Boston: Houghton Mifflin, 1892), p. 388.
18. Deborah Fiske to Nathan Fiske, July 18, 1836, HHJ Papers.
19. Ibid., June 28, 1836, HHJ Papers.
20. Ibid., July 20, 1836, HHJ Papers.
21. Ibid., July 20, 1836; July 7, 1836, HHJ Papers.
22. Ibid., October 21, 1841, HHJ Papers.
23. Ibid. Drs. Steve Martin and Robert Michels used this passage to point out to me the complexities in interpreting a doctor-patient relationship. Since the historian is often one step removed from the exchange, it is not always possible to know if the patient's letters or account accurately report what the doctor said. They may be talking past each other, or there may be misinterpretations. On the whole, however, Deborah's reports are so consistent in themselves and with medical texts as to be entirely trustworthy.
24. Deborah Fiske to Ann Scholfield, October 14, 1841, HHJ Papers.
25. Deborah Fiske to Nathan Fiske, July 13, 1843, HHJ Papers.
26. While physicians such as Jay Katz, *The Silent World of Doctor and Patient* (New York: Free Press, 1984), have contended that doctors did not tell their patients the truth, historians have reported extensive communication between patients and physicians. See Leavitt, *Brought to Bed*, pp. 200–209.
27. John Collins Warren to Grace Webster, January 23, 1828, John Collins Warren Papers, Massachusetts Historical Society.

Chapter 8: Intensive Care

1. On the bonds between women in this era, see Carroll Smith-Rosenberg, "The Female World of Love and Ritual: Relations between Women in Nineteenth-Century America," in *Disorderly Conduct: Visions of Gender in Victorian America*, ed. Carroll Smith-Rosenberg (New York: Alfred A. Knopf, 1985).
2. Deborah Fiske to Martha Hooker, March 12, 1841, Helen Hunt Jackson (HHJ) Papers, Special Collections, Tutt Library, Colorado College.
3. Deborah Fiske to Elisabeth Terry, February 18, 1842, HHJ Papers.
4. Deborah Fiske to Martha Hooker, August 15, n.y., HHJ Papers.
5. Ibid., March 12, 1841, HHJ Papers.
6. Deborah Fiske to Ellen Scholfield, n.d., HHJ Papers.
7. Deborah Fiske to Martha Hooker, March 21, 1841, HHJ Papers.
8. Ibid.
9. Richard Rollins, *The Long Journey of Noah Webster* (Philadelphia: University of Pennsylvania Press, 1980); and Harry Warfel, *Noah Webster: Schoolmaster to America* (New York: MacMillan Press, 1936).
10. Harriet Fowler to Eliza Jones, February 1839, Emily Ford Papers, Rare Books and Manuscripts, New York Public Library.
11. The notes Deborah sent Harriet are identified only by the initials: D. W. V. F., Emily Ford Papers. They were probably written between November 1843 and February 1844.
12. Ibid.
13. Harriet Fowler to Deborah Fiske, n.d., but probably November 1843, HHJ Papers.
14. D. W. V. F., Emily Ford Papers.
15. Ibid.
16. Deborah Fiske to Elisabeth Terry, February 18, 1842, HHJ Papers.
17. Harriet Fowler to Deborah Fiske, n.d., probably November 1843, HHJ Papers.
18. D. W. V. F., Emily Ford Papers.
19. Harriet Fowler to Deborah Fiske, n.d., probably November 1843, HHJ Papers.
20. Deborah Fiske to Helen Fiske, November 1843, HHJ Papers.
21. On Deborah's fall, see Deborah Fiske to Martha Vinal, January 19, 1844, HHJ Papers.
22. Ibid.
23. Martha Vinal to Otis Vinal, February 1 and February 4, 1844, HHJ Papers.
24. Deborah Fiske to Elisabeth Terry, September 6, 1843, HHJ Papers.
25. Deborah Fiske to Martha Vinal, January 19, 1844, HHJ Papers.
26. Martha Vinal to Otis Vinal, February 1, 1844, HHJ Papers.
27. On Nathan's attentiveness, see Deborah Fiske to Martha Vinal, January 19, 1844, HHJ Papers. On his renewed faith, see Nathan Fiske, Journal, September 1844, HHJ Papers.
28. Deborah Fiske to Martha Vinal, January 19, 1844, HHJ Papers.
29. Deborah Fiske to Ann Scholfield, November 9, 1843, HHJ Papers.
30. D. W. V. F., Emily Ford Papers.
31. On the visit, see Henry Jones, ed., *Memorials of Mrs. Harriet W. Fowler Wife of Reverend William C. Fowler* (Bridgeport, Conn.: H. Jones, 1845), p. 40.
32. On Deborah's behavior, see Sabra Snell to Louisa Clark, February 28, 1844, Snell Family Papers, Amherst College Archives. Cynthia Griffin Wolff maintains that "watching" was a female occupation in Amherst; during Deborah's final days she called men and women to watch with her. See Cynthia Griffin Wolff, *Emily Dickin-*

son (New York: Alfred A. Knopf, 1986), pp. 49–50, 60. See also Nathan Fiske, Diary, HHJ Papers.

33. For an interesting analysis of the funeral orations of pious women and the power of female friendships, see Irene Quenzler Brown, "Death, Friendship, and Female Identity during New England's Second Great Awakening," *Journal of Family History* 12 (1987): 367–87.

Nathan Fiske noted that "Dr. Humphrey, who had often visited [Deborah] her in her sickness . . . had long been expecting her death, and without her knowledge or mine had prepared a funeral sermon." Nathan Fiske, Diary, HHJ Papers.

34. See Jones, *Memorials of Mrs. Harriet W. Fowler*, pp. 9–16; and Heman Humphrey, *The Woman That Feareth the Lord: A Discourse Delivered at the Funeral of Mrs. D. W. V. Fiske, February 21, 1844* (Amherst, Mass.: J. S. and C. Adams, 1844), pp. 45–46; and Nathan Fiske, Diary, HHJ Papers.

35. Emily Fowler to Eliza Fowler, March 31, 1844, Fowler Family Papers, Connecticut Historical Society.

36. Jones, *Memorials of Mrs. Harriet W. Fowler*, pp. 11, 12, 14.

37. Ibid., p. 15

38. Jones, *Memorials of Mrs. Harriet W. Fowler*, p. 16. Humphrey sanctioned the highly domesticized vision of life and praised the energy and the way it vitalized invalid Christian women. For a different view, see Ann Douglas, "Heaven Our Home: Consolation Literature in the Northern United States, 1830–1850" in *Death in America*, ed. David E. Stannard (Philadelphia: University of Pennsylvania Press, 1975), pp. 49–68.

Chapter 9: Come West and Live

1. Daniel M. Fox, "AIDS and the American Health Polity: The History and Prospects of a Crisis of Authority," in Elizabeth Fee and Daniel M. Fox, eds., *AIDS: The Burdens of History* (Berkeley: University of California Press, 1988), pp. 316–43, provides an excellent discussion of how the AIDS crisis shattered medical confidence and affected health policy.

2. See Frederick L. Hoffman, "The Decline of the Tuberculosis Death Rate, 1871–1912," *Transactions of the National Association for the Study and Prevention of Tuberculosis (TNA)* 9 (1913): 101–37. For the English experience, see F. B. Smith, *The Retreat of Tuberculosis, 1850–1950* (London: Croom Helm, 1988).

3. There is an extensive and inconclusive literature on this point. See René Dubos and Jean Dubos, *The White Plague: Tuberculosis, Man and Society* (Boston: Little, Brown, 1952); and Barbara Bates, *Bargaining for Life: A Social History of Tuberculosis, 1876–1938* (Philadelphia: University of Pennsylvania Press, 1992), pp. 317–27.

4. The developers pitched their promotional literature on the health-giving qualities of the West to Europeans and Americans. See National Jewish Hospital, *Annual Meeting*, 1915, p. 18.

5. U.S. Public Health Service, "Interstate Migration of Tuberculous Persons," *Public Health Reports* 30:745–54, 826–40, 1051–90, 1147–73, 1225–55, 1808–27. John Mack Faragher, *Women and Men on the Overland Trail* (New Haven: Yale University Press, 1979), pp. 16–18, sees health as one of the major reasons for migration but omits it from his analysis.

6. In the 1860s and 1870s dying consumptives could find a bed on the wards of public

and voluntary hospitals and in homes for incurables such as the Channing Home in Boston and the House of Rest in New York and in the home of the Protestant Episcopal Mission in Philadelphia.

7. For an example of how mortality from consumption affected Swedish migration, see Britt-Inger Puranen, "The White Death: Not only a Disease of the Poor," *Historielärannas Förenings Arsskrift [Sweden]* 19 (1984–85): 19–28.

8. For a new and interesting analysis of these myths, see Richard White, *"It's Your Misfortune and None of My Own": A History of the American West* (Norman, Okla.: University of Oklahoma Press, 1991), esp. pp. 182–211.

9. Using Frederick Jackson Turner's provocative study, *The Significance of Frontier in American History*, historians have debated the effect of the West on American institutions. Many have questioned the validity of so marked a dichotomy as "civilization" and "wilderness" and its relationship to a national character. See Ray Allen Billington, *The Far Western Frontier, 1830–1860* (New York: Harper and Row, 1956). Richard Slotkin, *Regeneration through Violence: The Mythology of the American Frontier, 1600–1860* (Middletown, Conn.: Wesleyan University Press, 1973), has explored a darker side, focusing on the blatant disregard of Native American rights and the "immersion in the elemental violence of the wilderness." Historians of gender have maintained that women's life-styles and sensibilities were shaped more by gender considerations than by the western environment or migration.

10. George Frederick Ruxton, *Ruxton of the Rockies*, ed. Le Roy R. Hafen (Norman, Okla.: University of Oklahoma Press, 1950), pp. 269–70. For the extent of the health seekers' migration, see Billy Mac Jones, *Health Seekers in the Southwest, 1817–1900* (Norman, Okla.: University of Oklahoma Press, 1967); and John E. Baur, *The Health Seekers of Southern California, 1870–1900* (San Marino, Calif.: Huntington Library, 1959). Esmond R. Long, "Weak Lungs on the Santa Fe Trail," *Bulletin of the History of Medicine* 8 (1940): 1041–54, contends that the medical promotion of the West demonstrated the lack of scientific knowledge of American physicians.

11. Josiah Gregg, *Commerce of the Prairies*, ed. Max L. Moorhead (Norman, Okla.: University of Oklahoma Press, 1954), pp. 3–4.

12. Josiah Gregg, *Diary and Letters*, ed. Maurice G. Fulton (Norman. Okla.: University of Oklahoma Press, 1941), p. 151.

13. Gregg, *Commerce of the Prairies*, p. 147.

14. Jones, *Health Seekers in the Southwest*, p. 52.

15. Baur, *The Health Seekers of Southern California*, p. 32.

16. Matthew C. Field, *Prairie and Mountain Sketches*, ed. Kate L. Gregg and John F. McDermott (Norman, Okla.: University of Oklahoma Press, 1957), p. xxxviii.

17. Jones, *Health Seekers in the Southwest*, p. 47.

18. Billy Mac Jones, "West Texas: A Haven for Health Seekers," *West Texas Historical Association Year Book* 42 (October 1966): 7; "Medical Topography of the Pike's Peak Region," *Kansas City Medical and Surgical Review* 1 (1860): 123.

19. George Catlin, *Illustrations of the Manners, Customs and Condition of the North American Indians*, 7th ed. (London: Henry G. Bohn, 1848) 2:228. Robert F. Berkhofer, Jr., *The White Man's Indian: Images of the American Indian from Columbus to the Present* (New York: Alfred A. Knopf, 1978), discusses changing American perception of Native Americans and its effects on domestic policies.

20. Jones, *Health Seekers in the Southwest*, pp. 50–51.

21. William Goetzmann, "The Mountain Man as Jacksonian Man," *American Quarterly* 15 (1963): 402–15, presents the mountain men as entrepreneurs. Henry

Lewis Carter and Marcia Carpenter Spencer, "Stereotypes of the Mountain Man," *Western Historical Quarterly* 6 (1975): 17–32, have tried to explain the diverse historical interpretations. By far the most fascinating effort to try to differentiate fact from myth remains Howard R. Lamar, *The Trader on the American Frontier: Myth's Victim* (College Station, Tex.: Texas A & M University Press, 1977).

22. Andrew guided a party of invalids into the mountains in 1843 and again in 1844. Andrew Sublette to William Sublette, April 6, 1845, and Margaret Hereford to Esther Hereford, October 13, 1859, Sublette Family Papers, Missouri Historical Society.

23. Catlin, *Illustrations*, 2:228–29. Glenda Riley, *Women and Indians on the Frontier, 1825–1915* (Albuquerque, N.M.: University of New Mexico Press, 1984), explores the pervasiveness of white women's sense of moral superiority (pp. 1–36). Gender historians have explored the experience of Native American women. See Patricia Albers and Beatrice Medicine, eds., *The Hidden Half: Studies of Plains Indian Women* (Washington, D.C.: University Press of America, 1983).

24. Stella M. Drumm, ed., *Down the Santa Fe Trail and into Mexico: The Diary of Susan Shelby Magoffin 1846–47* (New Haven: Yale University Press, 1926), p. 68.

25. Catherine Margaret Haun, "A Woman's Trip across the Plains," Manuscript, Huntington Library, San Marino, Calif., p. 1. For an exploration of how the journey confirmed and expanded the boundaries of nineteenth-century domesticity, see Julie Roy Jeffrey, *Frontier Women: The Trans-Mississippi West, 1840–1880* (New York: Hill and Wang, 1979); and Annette Kolodny, *The Land before Her: Fantasy and Experience of the American Frontiers, 1630–1860* (Chapel Hill, N.C.: University of North Carolina Press, 1984). For an analysis of the way religion and ethnicity shaped the experiences of western women, see Elizabeth Jameson, "Toward a Multicultural History of Women in the Western United States," *Signs* (Summer 1988): 762–91. A fine analysis of women's diaries can be found in Elizabeth Hampsten, *Read This Only to Yourself: The Private Writings of Midwestern Women, 1880–1910* (Bloomington, Ind.: Indiana University Press, 1982); and Lillian Schlissel, *Women's Diaries of the Westward Journey* (New York: Schocken Books, 1982), particularly pp. 165–85.

26. Margaret Hereford to Esther Hereford, October 13, 1850, Sublette Family Papers.

27. Mark Twain, *Roughing It* (New York: American Publishing Company, 1872; New York: Penguin Books, 1981), pp. 188–89.

28. Daniel Drake, *A Systematic Treatise, Historical, Etiological, and Practical, on the Principal Diseases of the Interior Valley of North America* (Cincinnati: Winthrop B. Smith and Company, 1850).

29. It was the advocacy of an entire section of the country that set Drake's treatise apart from climatological studies of local medical societies. For an excellent discussion of these tracts and their importance in this era, see John H. Warner, *The Therapeutic Perspective: Medical Practice, Knowledge, and Identity in America, 1820–1885* (Cambridge, Mass.: Harvard University Press, 1986), pp. 72–80.

30. Harriet Martineau, *Retrospect of Western Travel* (London: Saunders and Otley, 1838), p. 225.

31. The details of Drake's life and excerpts from his most important works can be found in Henry D. Shapiro and Zane L. Miller, *Physician to the West: Selected Writings of Daniel Drake on Science and Society* (Lexington, Ken.: University of Kentucky Press, 1970), quotations at pp. 242–43.

32. Quoted in Shapiro and Miller, *Physician to the West*, p. 239.

33. Drake, Preface, in *A Systematic Treatise*.

34. *Ibid.*, p. 175.

35. *Ibid.*, p. 175.

36. Quotes can be found in Jones, *Health Seekers in the Southwest,* pp. 36, 84.

37. Drake, *A Systematic Treatise,* p. 690.

38. Donald E. Everett, "San Antonio Welcomes the 'Sunset'—1877," *Southwestern Historical Quarterly* 65 (July 1961): 57. F. H. Taylor, "Through Texas," *Harper's New Monthly Magazine* 59 (1879): 714.

39. Marian McIntyre McDonough, "Quest for Health, Not Wealth, 1871," *Montana: The Magazine of Western History* 14 (1964): 26, 28.

40. The communities discussed here are not typical of most western towns, which tended to be more informal and even clannish. See White, *"It's Your Misfortune and None of My Own,"* esp. pp. 298–325; Everett, "San Antonio," p. 56.

41. John S. Fisher, *A Builder of the West: The Life of General William Jackson Palmer* (Caldwell, Idaho: Caxton Printers, 1939); and Fountain Colony of Colorado, *Prospectus* (Denver, Colo.: Denver Tribune Printers, 1871).

42. See James F. Willard and Colin B. Goodykoontz, eds., "Fountain Colony," in *Experiments in Colorado Colonization 1869–1872,* in University of Colorado, *Historical Collections* 3 (1926): 451–59. See also Fountain Colony, *Prospectus,* 1873.

43. Fisher, *A Builder of the West: Palmer,* p. 57.

44. Ibid., pp. 162–63.

45. Ibid., pp. 163–64.

46. Denver Board of Trade, *Report* (Denver, 1869), p. 94.

47. "Medical Topography of the Pike's Peak Gold Region," 123. Kansas Pacific Railroad, *Colorado Resorts and Attractions to the Pleasure Seeker, Tourist and Invalid* (n.p.: Kansas Pacific Railroad, 1873), p. 25.

48. Bayard Taylor, *Colorado: A Summer Trip* (New York: G.P. Putnam and Son, 1867) p. 166.

49. A. A. Hayes, Jr., *New Colorado and the Santa Fe Trail* (New York: Harper and Brothers, 1880), pp. 46–47.

50. Bell reported on his surveying expedition in William A. Bell, *New Tracks in North America: A Journal of Travel and Adventure whilst Engaged in a Survey for a Southern Railroad to the Pacific Ocean during 1867–68,* 2 vols. (London: Chapman and Hall, 1869).

51. Fountain Colony, *Prospectus,* 1873.

52. Rose Kingsley, *South by West or, Winter in the Rocky Mountains and Spring in Mexico* (London: W. Isbister, 1874), p. 143.

53. Fountain Colony, *Prospectus,* 1873.

54. Stewart H. Holbrook, *The Yankee Exodus: An Account of Migration from New England* (New York: MacMillan Company, 1950), pp. 220–21; Edward P. Tenney, *Colorado: New Homes in the New West* (Boston: Lea and Shepard, 1880), pp. 37, 40, 41.

55. Quoted in Baur, *The Health Seekers of Southern California,* p. 45.

56. Benjamin Cummings Truman, *Semi-tropical California: Its Climate, Healthfulness, Productiveness, and Scenery* (San Francisco: A. L. Bancroft, 1874), pp. 32, 34. Another popular guidebook was Charles Nordhoff, *California: For Health, Pleasure and Residence* (New York: Harper, 1873).

57. Baur, *The Health Seekers of Southern California,* p. 62.

58. Ibid., p. 58.

59. Ibid., p. 55.

60. Ibid., p. 32.

61. Ibid., pp. 118–25.

Chapter 10: The Physician as Living Proof

1. See, for example, Charles F. Gardiner, "Early Days in Colorado," *Journal of the Outdoor Life* 29 (June 1932): 355–57.
2. Ibid., and Charles Denison, "The Climatic Treatment of Pulmonary Consumption," *Denver Medical Times*, September 1883, pp. 1–7.
3. For biographical data on Solly, see "Discussion," in *Transactions of the American Climatological Association* (*TACA*) 6 (1889): 203; and see "In Memoriam: Samuel Edwin Solly, M.D., M.R.C.S.," *TACA* 24 (1907): xxv–xxviii.
4. S. Edwin Solly, *Manitou, Col. U.S.A.: Its Mineral Waters and Climate* (St. Louis: John McKittrick, 1875) pp. 31–32, 33, 34, 35, 36.
5. Ibid., p. 34.
6. Hermann Weber, "Manitou in Colorado (U.S.A.): A Health Resort in Consumption," *Lancet* 2 (August 4, 1877): 157.
7. Samuel Edwin Solly, *The Health Resorts of Colorado Springs and Manitou* (Colorado Springs: Gazette Publishing, 1883), p. 51.
8. Ibid., pp. 54–55.
9. For biographical information, see "Charles Denison: In Memoriam," *TACA* 25 (1908): xxiii; and "Discussion," *TACA* 6 (1889): 202. Charles Denison, "Colorado as a Health Resort," *Chicago Medical Examiner* (January 15, 1874): 37, 39, 40.
10. Charles Denison, *Rocky Mountain Health Resorts* (Boston: Houghton Osgood and Company, 1880), pp. 150, 154, 158.
11. Denison, "Discussion," pp. 202–3; idem, *Rocky Mountain Health Resorts*, pp. 161–72.
12. Gardiner, "Early Days in Colorado," p. 356.
13. Charles Denison, *Exercise for Pulmonary Invalids* (Denver, Colo.: Chain and Hardy, 1893), pp. 15, 17.
14. Charles Fox Gardiner, "The Sanatory Tent and Its Use in Pulmonary Consumption," *TACA* 9 (1902): 209.
15. Boyd Cornick to Louise Cornick, October 24, 1890, and Boyd Cornick to Louise Cornick, December 25, 1890, Boyd Cornick Papers, Southwest Collection, Texas Technical University.
16. Boyd Cornick to Louise Cornick, October 24, 1890, Boyd Cornick Papers.
17. Carl Schwalb to Boyd Cornick, January 17 and February 12, 1891, Boyd Cornick Papers.
18. Boyd Cornick, "The Influence of High Altitudes on the Arrest of Pulmonary Phthisis," *Journal of the American Medical Association* 20 (June 10, 1893): 634.
19. Mark A. Rodgers, "The Climate of Arizona," *TACA* 13 (1896): 97.
20. William A. Edwards, "The Climate of Southern California in Relation to Disease," *Climatologist* 1 (1891): 33.
21. Frederick I. Knight, "The Opening Address," *TACA* 1 (1884): 2–4.
22. Austin Flint, *A Treatise on the Principles and Practice of Medicine*, 5th ed. (Philadelphia: Henry C. Lea, 1881), p. 215.
23. Frederick L. Knight, "On the Selection of a Climate for Patients with Pulmonary Tuberculosis," *Boston Medical and Surgical Journal* 128 (April 5, 1888): 343–44.
24. Dio Lewis, *Gypsies; or Why We Went Gypsying in the Sierras* (Boston: Century Book Company, 1881), pp. 396, 397, 399.
25. Loomis, "Discussion," p. 202; Alfred Loomis, "The Adirondack Region as a Therapeutical Agent in the Treatment of Pulmonary Phthisis," *New York Medical Record* 15 (April 26, 1879): 387. In the 1860s the Adirondacks was promoted as a summer resort for invalids. See William Henry Harrison Murray, *Adventures in the Wilder-*

ness or Camp-life in the Adirondacks (Boston: Fields, Osgood and Company, 1869).

26. Loomis, "The Adirondack Region," pp. 386, 387. A detailed account of life in the Adirondacks during this era may be found in Alfred L. Donaldson, *A History of the Adirondacks* vol. 1 (New York: Century Company, 1921).

27. Edward Livingston Trudeau, *An Autobiography* (New York: Lea and Febiger, 1916), pp. 10, 11.

28. Ibid., pp. 71, 73, 77, 78, 79, 80.

29. Ibid., p. 87. Trudeau admired the strength and skills of the Adirondack guides but loathed their habits (drink and tobacco). For all his ambivalence, he considered them essential to his cure.

30. Trudeau, *Autobiography*, p. 97.

31. Ibid., pp. 252–53.

32. Ibid., p. 97.

33. Loomis, "The Adirondack Region," pp. 387–88. Loomis and Trudeau give different dates for Trudeau's trips to the Adirondacks. I have followed the dates given by Trudeau.

34. The quotations from Trudeau can be found in Loomis, "The Adirondack Region," pp. 386–87. Other physicians also promoted the region to consumptives. See Joseph W. Stickler, ed., *The Adirondacks as a Health Resort* (New York: G. P. Putnam's Sons, 1886).

35. Hugh M. Kinghorn, "Brehmer and Dettweiler: A Review of Their Methods of Treatment of Tuberculosis," *American Review of Tuberculosis* 5 (1921–22): 950–72.

Chapter 11: The Western Narrative

1. George Weeks, *California Copy* (Washington: Washington College Press, 1928), p. 333.

2. Ibid., p. 13.

3. Ibid., p. 46.

4. Ibid., pp. 52, 81.

5. Ibid., pp. 18–19.

6. D. M. Berry to Helen Elliott, November 24, 1873, D. M. Berry Papers, Huntington Library.

7. Ibid., September 23, 1873, D. M. Berry Papers.

8. Quoted in John E. Baur, *The Health Seekers of Southern California, 1870–1900* (San Marino, Calif.: Huntington Library, 1959), p. 122.

9. G. Wesley Johnson, "Dwight Heard in Phoenix: The Early Years," *Journal of Arizona History* 18 (1977): 259–78.

10. *Colorado Springs Gazette*, January 11, 1873.

11. Quoted in Baur, *Health Seekers of Southern California*, pp. 52.

12. Charles Nordhoff, *California: For Health, Pleasure, and Residence*, 1883 ed. (New York: Harper, 1873), pp. 77–78, acknowledges how primitive accommodations were in the 1870s.

13. Weeks, *California Copy*, p. 48.

14. Alfred Terry Bacon, "Ranch-Cure," *Lippincott's Magazine* 28 (July 1881): 91. But Bacon's tale was also one of cure.

15. Helen Raitt and Mary Collier Wayne, *We Three Came West* (San Diego, Calif.: Tofua Press, 1974), p. 133.

16. Ibid., 133; quoted in Baur, *Health Seekers of Southern California*, p. 119; Weeks, *California Copy*, p. 90.

17. D. M. Berry to Helen Elliott, November 24, 1873, D. M. Berry Papers; Weeks, *California Copy*, pp. 48–50.

18. Quoted in Baur, *Health Seekers of Southern California*, p. 34–35.

19. Raitt and Wayne, *We Three Came West*, pp. 131, 135.

20. Samuel A. Fisk, "Colorado for Invalids," *Popular Science Monthly* 25 (July 1884): 318.

21. Baur, *Health Seekers of Southern California*, p. 71.

22. Frank D. Y. Carpenter, "The Climate Cure," *Lippincott's Magazine*, new ser., 5 (1883): 394–402, is one of the few articles in this period that describes the interests of westerners in the perpetuation of the myth.

23. Charles Denison, *Rocky Mountain Health Resorts* (Boston: Houghton, Osgood and Company, 1880), pp. 161–62.

24. Baur, *Health Seekers of Southern California*, p. 56; Joyce Antler, *Lucy Sprague Mitchell* (New Haven: Yale University Press, 1987), pp. 34–41.

25. William A. Edwards and Beatrice Harraden, *Two Health-Seekers in Southern California* (Philadelphia: Lippincott Company, 1897), p. 91; idem, "Agriculture as an Occupation for Women in California," *Overland Monthly*, 2d ser., 9 (1887): 656.

26. S. Weir Mitchell, *Doctor and Patient* (Philadelphia: J. B. Lippincott, 1887) pp. 155–57.

27. Denison, *Rocky Mountain Health Resorts*, p. 117; Samuel A. Fisk, "President's Address," *Transactions of the Colorado State Medical Society* (1889), pp. 19, 20. Raitt and Wayne, *We Three Came West*, p. 132.

28. *Colorado Springs Gazette*, November 21, 1874; Edwards and Harraden, *Two Health Seekers in Southern California* pp. 31–32.

29. Helen Maria Fiske to Julius Palmer, March 8, 1850, HHJ Papers, Special Collections, Tutt Library, Colorado College.

30. Helen Maria Fiske to Julius Palmer, March 8, 1850, HHJ Papers.

31. For a description of the origins of the school and its faculty see, J. Smith, "Ipswich Female Seminary," *American Quarterly Register* 11 (1839): 368–75.

32. Helen Maria Fiske to Ann Scholfield, February 1, 1847, HHJ Papers.

33. Helen Maria Fiske to Julius Palmer, March 8, 1850, HHJ Papers. For details of Nathan Fiske's journey to Palestine see Heman Humphrey, *Memoir of Reverend Nathan Welby Fiske* (Amherst, Mass.: J. S. C. Adams, 1850), p. 35–75.

34. Helen Maria Fiske to Julius Palmer, December 16, 1849, HHJ Papers.

35. John Stevens Cabot Abbott was the brother of Jacob Abbott, a friend and colleague of Nathan's at Amherst. John S. C. Abbott, *The Mother at Home* (Boston: Crocker and Brewster, 1834), was one of Deborah's favorite child-rearing tracts. Helen Maria Fiske to Julius Palmer, December 16, 1849, HHJ Papers.

36. Helen did allow Dr. Green to take out her tonsils, which he had pronounced "diseased." Helen Maria Fiske to Julius Palmer, January 14, 1850, HHJ Papers.

37. Helen often signed her letters to Julius Palmer, "your affectionate ward."

38. Helen Maria Fiske to Julius Palmer, October 13, 1851, HHJ Papers.

39. For a detailed chronology of Helen's life, see Ruth Odell, *Helen Hunt Jackson* (New York: D. Appleton Century Company, 1939).

40. For an account of the life of Edward Bissell Hunt, see "Biographical Memoir of Edward B. Hunt," *National Academy of Sciences* 3 (1895): 29–41.

41. The James family also lived in Newport, in part for its healthful climate. See Jean Strouse, *Alice James: A Biography* (Boston: Houghton Mifflin, 1980), pp. 60–82.

42. Mary Thacher Higginson, ed., *Letters and Journals of Thomas Wentworth Higginson 1846–1906* (Boston: Houghton Mifflin, 1921), p. 244. On Higginson's admiration for Helen's writing, see Thomas Wentworth Higginson, *Contemporaries* (Boston:

Houghton Mifflin, 1899), pp. 142–67. See also Anna Mary Wells, *Dear Preceptor: The Life and Times of Thomas Wentworth Higginson* (Cambridge: Houghton Mifflin, 1963), pp. 198–214.

43. Helen Hunt to Mary (no last name), March 23, 1872, HHJ Papers, Huntington Library.

44. Helen Hunt to William Hayes Ward, May 11, 1873, HHJ Papers, Huntington Library. Helen published essays on the California summer; see Helen Hunt Jackson, "The Way to Ah-Wah-Ne," *Bits of Travel at Home* (Boston: Roberts Brothers, 1878), pp. 87–91.

45. Helen Hunt to Annie Adams Field, October 29, 1873, HHJ Papers, Boston Public Library; Odell, *Helen Hunt Jackson*, pp. 130–31.

46. Helen Hunt Jackson, "A Symphony in Yellow and Red," *Bits of Travel at Home*, p. 212. Helen Hunt Jackson, "Colorado Springs," *Bits of Travel at Home*, p. 224.

47. Helen Hunt to Ann Scholfield, June 16, 1874, HHJ Papers.

48. Helen Hunt to Moncure D. Conway, September 20, n.d., probably 1874, Columbia University Special Collections.

49. Helen Hunt Jackson, "Colorado Springs," p. 225.

50. Jackson, "A Symphony in Yellow and Red," pp. 212–13.

51. Jackson, "A Colorado Week," *Bits of Travel at Home*, pp. 234, 235–36; and idem, "Colorado Springs," p. 233.

52. Higginson, *Contemporaries*, p. 155.

53. Ibid. For a dark view of Helen's advocacy efforts, see Alan Nevins, "Helen Hunt Jackson: Sentimentalist vs. Realist," *American Scholar* 10 (1941): 269–85; Helen Hunt Jackson, *Century of Dishonor* (Boston: Roberts Brothers, 1885); idem, *Ramona* (Boston: Roberts Brothers, 1884).

Chapter 12: A Disease of the Masses

1. Robert Koch, "The Aetiology of Tuberculosis," *American Review of Tuberculosis* 25 (March 1932): 299, 306, 311. This is a translation of the paper that Koch read at the Berlin Physiological Society on March 24, 1882.

2. Ibid., pp. 319, 320, 322, 323.

3. James H. Cassedy, *Charles V. Chapin and the Public Health Movement* (Cambridge: Harvard University Press, 1963), p. 61.

4. In 1887 Charles Chapin, who promoted the new methodology, expressed his disdain for "old-fashioned" practitioners. "Until the majority of the medical profession learn how to study disease and its treatment in the impartial and accurate manner . . . the practice of medicine will be as it is chiefly . . . a trade." Cassedy, *Chapin*, p. 32. Even as Chapin wrote, a few medical schools were setting up laboratories.

5. Mark Caldwell has argued that the antituberculosis campaign was really a secular crusade. He shows how physicians joined those concerned with the problems of poverty to eradicate the disease. See Caldwell, *The Last Crusade: The War on Consumption, 1862–1954* (New York: Atheneum, 1988). Michael E. Teller, *The Tuberculosis Movement: A Public Health Campaign in the Progressive Era* (New York: Greenwood Press, 1988), focuses more on the complex interaction of medical and social factors. Lawrence Flick, *Consumption, A Curable and Preventable Disease* (Philadelphia: D. Mckay, 1903), p. 14; S. Adolphus Knopf, *Tuberculosis as a Disease of the Masses, and How to Combat It*, 4th ed. (New York: Fred P. Flori, 1907), p. 86.

6. Charles V. Chapin, "Dirt, Disease, and the Health Officer," in Frederic P.

Gorham, ed., *Papers of Charles V. Chapin, M.D.* (New York: The Commonwealth Fund, 1934), pp. 20–21.

7. See Theobald Smith, "Public Health Laboratories," *Boston Medical and Surgical Journal* 143 (November 15, 1900): 491–93.

8. Chapin, "Dirt, Disease, and the Health Officer," pp. 22–23.

9. "As a result of the collaboration of the laboratory and the epidemiologist," Chapin explained, "it has been fairly well determined that … contagious diseases are spread chiefly by means of the quite direct transfer of quite fresh infective material from person to person. … This is most commonly accomplished by the smearing of saliva and other body fluids on the fingers and … from hand to hand and from hand to mouth." Charles V. Chapin, "The Principles of Epidemiology," in Gorham, *Papers of Charles V. Chapin,* p. 184.

10. On the lag between Koch's discovery and changes in attitudes of American physicians, see Phyllis Allen Richmond, "American Attitudes towards the Germ Theory of Disease," *Journal of the History of Medicine and the Allied Sciences* 9 (October 1954): 428–54. For a fascinating study on how the popularization of germ theory affected women's lives, see Nancy Tomes, "The Private Side of Public Health: Sanitary Science, Domestic Hygiene, and the Germ Theory, 1870–1900," *Bulletin of the History of Medicine* 64 (Winter 1990): 509–39. On attitudes toward cleanliness in the prebacteriological era, see Richard L. Bushman and Claudia L. Bushman, "The Early History of Cleanliness in America," *Journal of American History* 74 (1988): 1213–38.

11. T. Mitchell Prudden, *The Story of the Bacteria and Their Relations to Health and Disease,* 1917 ed. (New York: G. P. Putnam's Sons, 1889), pp. 84–86, 90, 97–98.

12. Hermann Biggs, "To Rob Consumption of Its Terrors," *Forum* 16 (February 1894): 761.

13. C. E. A. Winslow, *The Life of Hermann Biggs* (Philadelphia: Lea and Febiger, 1929), pp. 149, 246.

14. Knopf, *Tuberculosis as a Disease of the Masses,* p. 43.

15. Godias J. Drolet and Anthony M. Lowell, *A Half Century's Progress against Tuberculosis in New York City, 1900–1950* (New York: New York Tuberculosis and Health Association, 1952), pp. iii, li–liv, quotes Billings. See also John S. Billings, *Vital Statistics of New York City and Brooklyn Covering a Period of Six Years Ending May 31, 1890* (Washington, D.C.: U.S. Census Office, 1894). Detailed statistics on the decline in the death rate from the disease can be found in Frederick L. Hoffman, "The Decline in the Tuberculosis Death Rate, 1871–1912," *Transactions of the National Association for the Study and Prevention of Tuberculosis (TNA)* 9 (1913): 130.

16. Historians, statisticians, charity organization workers, and physicians have maintained that Jews, even those who lived in the most crowded tenement districts, had lower mortality rates than other groups. Maurice Fishberg, "The Relative Infrequency of Tuberculosis among the Jews," *American Medicine* 2 (1901): 695–99. Two historians have interpreted this disparity. Deborah Dwork, "Health Conditions of Immigrant Jews on the Lower East Side of New York: 1880–1914," *Medical History* 25 (1981): 1–40; Jacob Jay Lindenthal, "Abi Gezunt: Health and the Eastern European Jewish Immigrant," *Jewish History* 60 (1981): 420–41.

17. Knopf, *Tuberculosis as a Disease of the Masses,* p. 16.

18. Ibid. Knopf sets down an elaborate strategy to attain this goal; see particularly, pp. 43–45, 83–86.

19. Ibid.

20. Edward von Adelung, "The Prevention of Tuberculosis," *California State Journal of Medicine* 1 (1903): p. 292.

21. Lawrence Veiller, "Tenement House Reform in New York City, 1834–1900," in Robert De Forest and Lawrence Veiller, eds., *The Tenement House Problem*, vol. 1 (New York: MacMillan, 1903), pp. 71–97.

22. De Forest and Veiller, *The Tenement House Problem*, p. 114. See also Charity Organization Society of New York, *A Handbook on the Prevention of Tuberculosis* (New York: Charity Organization Society, 1903).

23. Hermann M. Biggs, "Tuberculosis and the Tenement House Problem," in De Forest and Veiller, *The Tenement House Problem*, pp. 447, 453.

24. Arthur R. Guerard, "The Relation of Tuberculosis to the Tenement House Problem," in De Forest and Veiller, *The Tenement House Problem*, p. 470.

25. Knopf, "The Tenements and Tuberculosis," *Journal of the American Medical Association* 34 (May 12, 1900): 1154.

26. William H. Welch, "What May Be Expected from More Effective Application of Preventive Measures against Tuberculosis" (Address delivered in Albany, N.Y., January 27, 1908), reprinted in William H. Welch, *Papers and Addresses*, ed. Walter C. Burket (Baltimore: Johns Hopkins University Press, 1920), p. 632.

27. A copy of this circular can be in found in New York City Department of Health, *Annual Report* (1894): 95.

28. Charity Organization Society, *A Handbook*, p. 98.

29. John S. Billings, Jr., "The Registration and Sanitary Supervision of Pulmonary Tuberculosis in New York City," New York City Department of Health, *Monograph Series no. 1* (1912), p. 57.

30. On tactics the tubercular poor used to avoid detection see Hermann M. Biggs and John Henry Huddleston, "The Sanitary Supervision of Tuberculosis as Practiced by the New York City Board of Health," *American Journal of the Medical Sciences* 109 (1895): 25–26.

31. Over the next two decades most large cities and some states adopted many of the same measures. See James A. Tobey, *Public Health Law* (New York: Commonwealth Fund, 1947).

32. The New York City Department of Health was the most aggressive in enforcing these ordinances. For the efforts of other cities, see Lillian Brandt, "Summary of Existing Measures in the Principal Cities of the United States," in Brandt, Comp. *A Directory of Institutions and Societies Dealing with Tuberculosis in the United States and Canada* (New York: Charity Organization Society of the City of New York, 1904), pp. 220–21.

33. New York City Department of Health, *Annual Report* (1894): 96.

34. The law contained precise instructions for disinfection that became more stringent over time. At first landlords had ten days, later forty-eight hours. The costs were to be borne by the landlord, and the expense was the first lien upon the property. New York City Department of Health *Annual Report* (1894), p. 97. See also National Association for the Study and Prevention of Tuberculosis, Technical Series, *A Manual of Tuberculosis Legislation* 8 (1926): 37.

35. Biggs, "To Rob Consumption of Its Terrors," p. 767.

36. Winslow, *Life of Hermann Biggs*, p. 158; Charles V. Chapin, "Pleasures and Hopes of the Health Officer," in Gorham, *Papers of Charles V. Chapin*, p. 6.

37. For details, see Winslow, *Life of Hermann Biggs*, pp. 131–52. Public health officials defined tuberculosis as a communicable disease. "No reasonable sanitary officer," Biggs maintained, "would expect to put in force regulations requiring notification of tuberculosis, with the same conditions and in the same way that a similar one with regard to small pox would be enforced" (p. 151). For a fascinating analysis of the way Biggs's professional motivations shaped the battle, see Daniel M. Fox,

"Social Policy and City Politics: Tuberculosis Reporting in New York, 1889–1900," *Bulletin of the History of Medicine* 49 (Summer 1975): 169–95.

38. New York City Department of Health, *Annual Report (1894):* 98–99. In the 1930s the right of the insurance companies to have access to public health records was adjudicated in the courts, but earlier an official of a public or private institution could use the information to protect the public health. See Tobey, *Public Health Law*, pp. 136, 152–53. Some European companies, in Germany in particular, provided insurance against tuberculosis and the topic was debated here. See Lee K. Frankel, "Insurance against Tuberculosis," *TNA* 7 (1910): 35–61.

39. Winslow, *Life of Hermann Biggs*, pp. 144, 146. For an analysis of the composition of the city's medical profession in the city and its response to compulsory reporting, see Fox, "Social Policy and City Politics," pp. 169–95. For another view, see Paul Starr, *The Social Transformation of American Medicine* (New York: Basic Books, 1983), p. 187.

40. Winslow, *Life of Hermann Biggs*, p. 139; Edward Devine, "A Working Program," *TNA* 1 (1905): 53.

41. On the penalties contracting the disease imposed, see Teller, *The Tuberculosis Movement*, pp. 77–78, 109–10. For a discussion of particular exclusions, see J. S. Kerr and A. A. Moll, "Communicable Disease: An Analysis of the Laws and Regulations for the Control Thereof in Force in the United States," in United States Public Health Service, *Public Health Bulletin no. 62* (Washington, D.C.: U. S. G. P. O., 1914).

42. Winslow, *Life of Hermann Biggs*, p. 178.

43. De Lancey Rochester, "The Role of Local Sanatoria in Preventing the Spread of Tuberculosis," *Transactions of the American Climatological Association (TACA)* 1 (1903): 61; Charles Wilson Ingraham, "Control of Tuberculosis from a Strictly Medico-Legal Standpoint," *Journal of the American Medical Association* 27 (September 26, 1896): 693. Dr. J. F. A. Adams described tuberculosis as "the leprosy of our time; and, as leprosy is kept under control by the segregation of lepers, so may consumption be eradicated by the segregation of consumptives." See Dr. Adams, "The Segregation of Consumptives," *Medical Communications of the Massachusetts Medical Society* 20 (1907): 401.

44. The educational efforts became nationwide in the twentieth century. In 1910 the National Association for the Study and Prevention of Tuberculosis (NASPT) produced educational films with an unmistakable messages on hygiene and disease prevention. See Philip P. Jacobs, "Tuberculosis in Motion Pictures," *Journal of the Outdoor Life* 9 (1912): 302–5. The films educated the public about the danger of tuberculosis and led to a fear of associating with the tubercular. For an analysis of the films, see Martin S. Pernick, "Thomas Edison's Tuberculosis Films: Mass Media and Health Propaganda—The Ethics of Preventive Medicine," *Hastings Center Report* 8 (June 1978): 21–27.

45. The term appears to have originated in the 1890s; its spelling varied between phthisiophobia and phthisophobia. F. M. Pottenger, "Is Another Chapter in Public Phthisiophobia about to be Written?" *California State Journal of Medicine* 1 (1903): 81–84. According to some physicians, phthisiophobia grew more virulent in the early twentieth century. See S. Adolphus Knopf, "The Unjustified Prejudice of Tuberculous Patients against Sanatoria and Hospitals," *Medical Record* 82 (September 1912): 553–59. Knopf argues many of the tubercular were reluctant to enter a sanatorium because, as his fictional patient put it, "I will be ostracized. My former employers will not wish to take me back into their office or shop" (p. 553).

46. On the debate, see John E. Baur, *The Health Seekers of Southern California* (San Marino, Calif.: Huntington Library, 1959), pp. 150–73.

47. Ibid., p. 164.
48. In California the debate over quarantine was intense. Norman Bridge, "How Far Shall the State Restrict Individual Action of the Sick, Especially the Tuberculous," *California State Journal of Medicine* 1 (1903): 180.
49. Pottenger, "Another Chapter in Public Phthisiophobia," p. 82.
50. Edward von Adelung, "The Prevention of Tuberculosis," *op.cit.* p. 291. Tuberculosis Committee of the Medical Society of the State of California, "A Review of What Has Been Done for the Prevention of the Spread of Tuberculosis in the State of California, with Suggestions for Future Activity," *California State Journal of Medicine* 4 (1906): 164.
51. George H. Kress, "Tuberculosis," *Los Angeles Medical Journal* 1 (1904): 315.
52. Brandt, *Directory of Institutions and Societies,* p. viii.
53. National Tuberculosis Association, *A Manual of Tuberculosis Legislation,* p. 38, discusses the confinement laws. See also John Billings, "Discussion," *TNA* 3 (1907): 52. Some, but not all, public health nurses also advocated confinement. See Ellen N. La Motte, "The Unteachable Consumptive," *Journal of the Outdoor Life* 7 (1909): 105–7.
54. Tobey, *Public Health Law,* p. 152. Tobey has a very detailed discussion of these issues (pp. 153–59).
55. Ingraham, "Control of Tuberculosis," p. 694; William Welch, "Address," *TNA* 5 (1909): 36; John Billings, "Remarks," *TNA* 3 (1907): 52.
56. Biggs's categories were not unique to New York. See Rhode Island, *State Commission on Tuberculosis: Report on Hospitals for Advanced Cases* (Providence, R.I.: E. L. Freeman, 1911), pp. 35–36.
57. Walter H. Conley, "Detention of Consumptives in a City Hospital," *Journal of the Outdoor Life* 11 (1914): 104.
58. Some nurses and dispensary physicians were not willing to send a policeman to the home to remove a non-compliant patient. See Boston Health League, *Conference,* August 11, 1921 (Manuscript, Harvard Medical Library).
59. Billings, "Registration and Sanitary Supervision," p. 54.

Chapter 13: Confining for Cure

1. S. Adolphus Knopf, "The Centenary of Brehmer's Birth," *American Review of Tuberculosis* 14 (August 1926): 208.
2. Hugh M. Kinghorn, "Brehmer and Dettweiler: A Review of Their Methods of Treatment of Pulmonary Tuberculosis," *American Review of Tuberculosis* 5 (1921–22): 962.
3. S. Adolphus Knopf, *Geheimrath Dr. Dettweiler: Eulogy Pronounced on the Occasion of the First Anniversary of His Death* (New York: William Wood and Company, 1905), p. 3; Kinghorn, "Brehmer and Dettweiler," pp. 966–67, 968. Others have translated Dettweiler's regimen as "permanent open air treatment."
4. Paul H. Kretzschmar, "Public Health Resorts versus Institutions for the Treatment of Bacillary Phthisis," *Transactions of the American Climatological Association (TACA)* 5 (1888): 69–83; idem, "Dr. Dettweiler's Method of Treating Pulmonary Consumption," *New York Medical Journal* 47 (February 1888): 175–80; idem, "Institutions for the Treatment of Pulmonary Consumption in the United States," *TACA* 6 (1889): 165–79.
5. To make this combination of rest, rich diet, and intense medical oversight more

compelling to American physicians, Kretzschmar cited the similarities between Dettweiler's cure and that of S. Weir Mitchell and noted that Dettweiler "speaks very highly of the favorable results obtained through the latter." Kretzschmar, "Dr. Dettweiler's Method," p. 180.

6. Kretzschmar, "Public Health Resorts," p. 72.
7. Ibid., p. 75.
8. Kretzschmar, "Dr. Dettweiler's Method," p. 178.
9. Ibid., pp. 176, 178.
10. Samuel A. Fisk, "President's Address," *Transactions of the Colorado State Medical Society* (1889): 14–28; and idem, "The Cottage Plan of Treating Consumption in Colorado," *Medical News* 54 (May 4, 1889): 480–83. For Kretzschmar's rebuttal, see Kretzschmar, "Institutions for the Treatment of Pulmonary Consumption," 165–79. For Fisk's response, see Fisk, "Climatology," *Transactions of the Colorado State Medical Society* (1890): 58–64.
11. Fisk's defense of climate is contained in his "President's Address," pp. 14–28; idem, "Cottage Plan," p. 480.
12. Fisk, "Cottage Plan, p. 481.
13. Ibid.
14. Ibid., pp. 482, 483.
15. Godias J. Drolet, *Tuberculosis Hospitalization* (New York: New York Tuberculosis and Health Association, 1926), pp. 1–2.
16. Edward Livingston Trudeau, *An Autobiography* (Garden City, N.Y.: Lea and Febiger, 1916), pp. 77–78, 137.
17. Ibid., 154.
18. Ibid., pp. 175–76.
19. Ibid., pp. 175, 179, 180.
20. Edward Livingston Trudeau, "Environment in Its Relation to the Progress of Bacterial Invasion in Tuberculosis," *TACA* 4 (1887): 131–36.
21. Ibid., pp. 132–33.
22. Ibid., pp. 134–35, 136.
23. Kretzschmar, "Dr. Dettweiler's Method," p. 177; William Osler, *The Principles and Practice of Medicine*, 4th ed. (New York: D. Appleton and Company, 1901), p. 832; Alfred Loomis, "Remarks," *TACA* 4 (1887): 136. Loomis's ambivalence about bacteriology is evident in his textbook. See Loomis, *A Textbook of Practical Medicine* (New York: William Wood and Company, 1885), pp. 185–207.
24. Edward Livingston Trudeau, "The History of the Tuberculosis Work at Saranac Lake, New York" (Paper delivered at the Henry Phipps Institute for the Study, Treatment and Prevention of Tuberculosis," Philadelphia, October 22, 1903), p. 2. The paper was also published in *Medical News* 83 (October 24, 1903): 2.
25. Trudeau, *Autobiography*, p. 149.
26. Ibid., p. 157–58.
27. Ibid., pp. 157–58; Loomis, "Remarks," *TACA* 7 (1889): 181.
28. Trudeau, *Autobiography*, pp. 155, 157–58. Trudeau does not give a date when he sailed with Stokes, but it was probably the summer of 1882 or 1883.
29. Ibid., pp. 158, 160.
30. Ibid., pp. 167, 168.
31. Ibid., pp. 158–61, 163. Trudeau does not give dates for his year of "begging," but given the chronology it was probably 1883–84.
32. On the expansion of the sanatorium, see Trudeau, "The History of the Tuberculosis Work," pp. 3–4.

33. Edward Livingston Trudeau, "Sanitaria for the Treatment of Incipient Tuberculosis," *New York Medical Journal* 65 (1897): 278.
34. Trudeau, "Sanitaria," p. 277. Trudeau, "The History of the Tuberculosis Work," p. 4.
35. Adirondack Cottage Sanatorium, "Rules." This unpublished manuscript is in the papers of the Adirondack Cottage Sanatorium at the Trudeau Institute.
36. Trudeau, "The History of the Tuberculosis Work," pp. 4–5.
37. Adirondack Cottage Sanatorium, *Patients on Entering the Adirondack Cottages Subscribe to the Following Rules* (undated set of rules was probably pre-1900), Trudeau Institute.
38. Trudeau, "Sanitaria," p. 277.
39. Adirondacks Cottage Sanatorium, "Rules." Trudeau, "Sanitaria," p. 278; idem, "The History of the Tuberculosis Work," p. 5.
40. Trudeau, "The History of the Tuberculosis Work," p. 6.
41. Jacob H. Schiff, "Institutional Care for Early or for Advanced Consumptives," *Transactions of the Sixth International Congress on Tuberculosis (TRICT)* 3 (1908): 363.
42. Lillian Brandt, "Introduction," in Lillian Brandt, comp., *A Directory of Institutions and Societies Dealing with Tuberculosis in the United States and Canada* (New York: Charity Organization Society of the City of New York, 1904), p. ix.
43. See "The National Jewish Hospital for Consumptives," in Brandt, *Directory*, p. 34. For a detailed history of the sanatorium and its policies, see James R. Giese, *Tuberculosis and the Growth of Denver's Eastern European Jewish Community: The Accommodation of an Immigrant Group to a Medium-Sized Western City, 1900–1920* (Ph.D. thesis, University of Colorado, 1979), pp. 111–20.
44. *History of Stony Wold* (Manuscript, Stony Wold Sanatorium Archives, New York City), p. 6. Its founder, Mrs. James Newcomb, contracted tuberculosis "while working on the Board of the Working Girl's Vacation Bureau" (p. 3).
45. Barbara Bates, *Bargaining for Life: A Social History of Tuberculosis, 1876–1938* (Philadelphia: University of Pennsylvania Press, 1992), p. 123. Trudeau concurred: "It will be justly urged that in a great majority of cases among the poorer classes it is absolutely impossible to follow the advice given." See Trudeau, "Sanitaria," p. 279.
46. Irving Fisher, "Diet in Tuberculosis," *TRICT 3*, vol. 1, pt. 2 (1908): 694, 707. A second investigation by Richard Cole Newton, "The Diet and Regime in Vogue in Thirty-four Sanatoriums," *TRICT 3*, vol. 1, pt. 2 (1908): 709–15, elaborated on the attitudes and practices Fisher uncovered. See also Herbert Maxon King, "Diet in Tuberculosis," *Transactions of the National Association for the Study and Prevention of Tuberculosis (TNA)* 2 (1906): 394–411; King pleaded for metabolic studies to determine just what were the food requirements of consumptives and what was the most beneficial diet.
47. Marcus Paterson, the medical superintendent of Frimley Sanatorium, considered manual labor for patients to have therapeutic value. For British practices and the "pickaxe cure," see Linda Bryder, *Below the Magic Mountain: A Social History of Tuberculosis in Twentieth-Century Britain* (Oxford: Clarendon Press, 1988), pp. 54–61; "Rest and Exercise," *Journal of the Outdoor Life* 8 (1911): 160.
48. Remarks of Dr. Alexius M. Forster can be found in "Discussion," *TNA* 10 (1914): 129.
49. F. M. Pottenger, "The Application of Rest and Exercise in the Treatment of Tuberculosis," *TRICT 3* (1908): 920; Charles W. Mills and Herbert Maxon King, "Exercise as a Therapeutic Measure in Pulmonary Tuberculosis," *TNA* 10 (1914):

124–25. See Forster, "Discussion," p. 129; Pottenger, "The Application Rest," p. 921.

50. On the preference of not-for-profit facilities for the incipient case of tuberculosis, see Schiff, "Institutional Care," pp. 361–65. For a detailed examination of this dynamic in regard to other caretaker institutions in this era, see David J. Rothman, *Conscience and Convenience: The Asylum and Its Alternatives in Progressive America* (Boston: Little, Brown and Company, 1980).

51. Drolet, *Tuberculosis Hospitalization*, p. 12.

52. On facilities for the insane and prisoners and the compromises reached between discipline and treatment, see Brandt, *Directory*, pp. 171–205.

53. Joseph H. Pratt, "The Class Method of Treating Consumption in the Homes of the Poor," *TNA* 3 (1907): 59.

54. New York City Department of Health, *Report* (1893): 88–89.

55. Walter Sands Mills, *The Tuberculosis Infirmary*, (New York: M. B. Brown, 1908), pp. 22–28. New York was not the only city with a municipal hospital for advanced cases. See Edwin A. Locke and Simon F. Cox, "The Municipal Hospital for Advanced Consumptives in Boston," *TRICT* 3 (1908): 988–95.

56. Mills, *The Tuberculosis Infirmary*, p. 63. In 1926 Godias J. Drolet discovered that 17 percent of all the patients in the 221 sanatoriums remained less than a month. See Drolet, *Tuberculosis Hospitalization*, p. 14.

57. From 1906 to 1912 half of the patients were native-born (most of them Irish), the other half were immigrants (most of Eastern European origin). Two-thirds were male, the majority single, and almost all were between the ages of twenty and forty.

58. Hermann M. Biggs, "The Municipal Sanatorium at Otisville," in New York City Department of Health, *Reprint Series* 7 (New York: New York City Department of Health, 1914), pp. 4, 7.

59. Ibid., pp. 10, 18.

60. Riverside had both voluntary and involuntary admissions. It also had a very high death rate. See S. Adolphus Knopf, "Discussion," *TNA* 5 (1909): 151.

61. Robert J. Wilson, "Difficulties Encountered by Hospital Authorities in Detaining Homeless Consumptives," *Journal of the Outdoor Life* 11 (1914): 102.

62. *Ibid.*, p. 103. To improve discipline, Wilson advocated a form of medical parole.

63. Theodore Sachs, Charles Hatfield, Livingston Farrand, and Thomas Carrington, "Report on Hospitals for Advanced Cases of Tuberculosis," *TNA* 9 (1913): 54–66.

Chapter 14. In the Shadow of the Sanatorium

1. This change occurred gradually. By 1930 withholding the diagnosis had become a fit subject for a medical journal. L. R. Williams and Alice M. Hill, "The Patient's Reaction to a Diagnosis of Tuberculosis," *New England Journal of Medicine* 203 (December 4, 1930): 1129–31.

2. Sanatorium records indicate the delay between diagnosis and admission. See particularly the records of the National Jewish Hospital and the Jewish Consumptive Relief Society. There was, Lee K. Frankel maintained, "repugnance on the part of the working-men and women to accept treatment which puts them in the same category with the pauper and vagrant." Frankel, "Insurance against Tuberculosis," *Transactions of the National Association for the Study and Prevention of Tuberculosis* (*TNA*) 6 (1910): 37.

3. Irving Fisher to William Greenleaf Elliot, December 11, 1898, Irving Fisher Papers, Manuscripts and Archives, Yale University Library. In the nineteenth century, some invalids and health seekers perceived the physician's order to travel as banishment, but their primary emotion was remorse at having to leave family and career and face an abbreviated life. Because travel for health was considered a privilege, no one concealed the reason for the voyage. See Robert Louis Stevenson, "Ordered South," *Macmillan's Magazine*, May 30, 1874, pp. 68–73. Patients in the twentieth century, on the other hand, equated banishment with ostracism and isolation. The prescription reinforced their own sense of shame.

4. Edwin Davis French to Charles Dexter Allen, September 8, 1897, Edwin Davis French Papers, New York Historical Society.

5. James T. Williams, Jr., to James T. Williams, May 28, 1909, Williams Family Papers, South Caroliniana Library, University of South Carolina.

6. John Ward Stimson to Henry A. Stimson, September 4, 1894, Stimson Family Papers, New York Historical Society.

7. This information can be found in a file labeled "Queries," in the Edwin A. Alderman Papers at the University of Virginia. See also Bessie Alderman to Arthur W. Page, December 1, 1912, Edwin A. Alderman Papers.

8. Irving Fisher to William Greenleaf Elliot, December 11, 1898, Irving Fisher Papers.

9. Anne Ellis, *Sunshine Preferred: The Philosophy of an Ordinary Woman* (Boston: Houghton Mifflin Company, 1934; Lincoln: University of Nebraska Press, 1984), p. 58.

10. Patty Selmes to Julia Dinsmore, November 19, 1908, Robert Ferguson Papers, Arizona Historical Society.

11. Neil Cowan and Ruth Schwartz Cowan, *Our Parents' Lives: The Americanization of Eastern European Jews* (New York: Basic Books, 1989), p. 140.

12. For the difficulties the department encountered, see John S. Billings, Jr., "The Registration and Sanitary Supervision of Tuberculosis in New York City," New York City Department of Health *Monograph Series no. 1* (1912), pp. 14–17.

13. On gaining compliance in New York City, see Billings, "Registration and Sanitary Supervision," p. 86. For compliance in other cities, see Michael E. Teller, *The Tuberculosis Movement: A Public Health Campaign in the Progressive Era* (New York: Greenwood Press, 1988), p. 72–73.

14. For department's effort to track the tubercular, see Billings, "The Registration and Sanitary Supervision," pp. 56–57.

15. Although the New York City Department of Health registry of names increased annually, from 4,166 in 1893 to 29,736 in 1908, it was made up mainly of persons who went to outpatient dispensaries or applied for aid from charitable societies. Persons with tuberculosis who visited private physicians were far less likely to be registered. Of the 29,736 cases in 1908, only 6,053 were reported by private physicians. For strategies the poor employed, see Billings, "Registration and Sanitary Supervision," pp. 84–86; and Hermann M. Biggs and John Henry Huddleston, "The Sanitary Supervision of Tuberculosis as Practiced by the New York City Board of Health," *American Journal of the Medical Sciences* 109 (1895): 25–26.

16. Justine Cutting, *Biographical Material* pp. 2, 3, 4, 1910–1913, Bronson Cutting Papers, Library of Congress.

17. Philip Washburn to Mary Washburn, January 19, 1894, Washburn Family Papers, Tutt Library, Colorado College.

18. Philip Washburn to Mary Washburn, January 26, 1894, Washburn Family Papers.

19. A resident of Colorado, "Colorado as a Health Resort: Opportunities and Obliga-

tions of the Health Seeker on the Western Plateau," *Journal of the Outdoor Life* 8 (1911): 51, 52.

20. Ernest Sweet, "The Interstate Migration of Tuberculous Persons," *U.S. Public Health Reports* 30 (April 16, 1915): 1149.

21. Will Ross, *I Wanted to Live: An Autobiography* (Milwaukee, Wis.: Wisconsin Anti-Tuberculosis Association, 1953) p. 51.

22. Thomas C. Galbreath, *Chasing the Cure in Colorado* (Denver, Colo.: by the author, 1908), p. 29.

23. Ross, *I Wanted to Live*, pp. 54–56.

24. Ellis, *Sunshine Preferred*, p. 17.

25. Sydney C. Haley, "The True Experiences of a Consumptive, *The Independent* 64 (1908): 241. Caring for the utensils was so repugnant a task, Lucy Sprague Mitchell recalled several decades later, that "I often sent my breakfast down the toilet as a finish." See Mitchell, *Two Lives: The Story of Wesley Clair Mitchell and Myself* (New York: Simon and Schuster, 1953), p. 105. See also Gerald B. Webb and Desmond S. Powell, *Henry Sewall, Physiologist and Physician* (Baltimore: Johns Hopkins University Press, 1946), p. 276.

26. Mae Goodwin to Elizabeth Goodwin, December 7, 1905, and Mae Goodwin to Elizabeth Goodwin, March 14, 1906, Mae Goodwin Papers, Illinois Historical Society.

27. Mae Goodwin to Elizabeth Goodwin, January 22, 1906, Mae Goodwin Papers.

28. For a history of the policies of an interesting sanatorium (one of the few that readmitted patients on an as-needed basis), see Jeanne Lichtman Abrams, "Chasing the Cure: A History of the Jewish Consumptives' Relief Society of Denver" (Ph.D. thesis, University of Colorado, 1983).

29. Case #27, Dr. M. Ziselman to Dr. Charles Spivak, September 26, 1904, Beck Memorial Archives, Center for Judaic Studies, University of Denver, JRCS Collection.

30. Case #14, Beck Memorial Archives.

31. For a detailed description of life in these colonies, see Paul M. Carrington, "Economic Housing of Consumptives with Especial Reference to the Southwest," *Transactions of the Sixth International Congress on Tuberculosis* 3 (1908): 1042–50.

32. Dick Hall, "Ointment of Love: Oliver E. Comstock and Tucson's Tent City," *Journal of Arizona History* (Summer 1978): 112. See also Sharlot M. Hall, "The Burden of the Southwest," *Outwest* 28 (January 1908): 3–19.

33. Hester Shigley, "Without the Camp," *Journal of the Outdoor Life* 11 (July 1914): 207.

34. Ibid., p. 208.

35. Hall, "Ointment of Love," p. 112. There were advice books which warned persons with tuberculosis and limited means about the hostility they would encounter in the West, but they did not seem to deter many migrants. See George B. Price, *Gaining Health in the West* (New York: R. B. Huebsch, 1907). The *Journal of the Outdoor Life* frequently carried articles by people with tuberculosis who went west and were ostracized.

36. Frederick I. Knight, "What Shall We Do with Patients Having Pulmonary Tuberculosis?" *Boston Medical and Surgical Journal* 151 (September 8, 1904): 258.

37. Marshall McClintock, *We Take to Bed* (New York: Jonathan Cape and Harrison Smith, 1931), p. 23.

38. Elizabeth Mooney, *In the Shadow of the White Plague* (New York: Crowell, 1979), p. 35.

39. For an interesting discussion of the cottages, see Philip L. Gallos, *Cure Cottages of*

Saranac Lake: Architecture and History of a Pioneer Health Resort (Saranac Lake, N.Y.: Historic Saranac Lake, 1985).

40. McClintock, *We Take to Bed*, pp. 6–7.
41. John E. Lathrop, "Back to Life," *Collier's*, May 24, 1913, p. 69.
42. Gallos, *Cure Cottages*, p. 43. Edwin French describes similar parties. See Edwin Davis French to Charles Dexter Allen, February 28, 1898, Edwin Davis French Papers, New York Historical Society.
43. Patricia Meyer Spacks, *Gossip* (Chicago: University of Chicago Press, 1985), pp. 5, 257.
44. Charles M. Palmer to Robert M. Ferguson, March 1, 1914, and Charles M. Palmer to Robert M. Ferguson, March 20, 1912, Robert M. Ferguson Papers, Arizona Historical Society.
45. Edwin Davis French to Charles Dexter Allen, February 28, 1898, Edwin Davis French Papers.
46. For a description of carnival, see Mark Caldwell, *The Last Crusade: The War on Consumption, 1862–1954* (New York: Atheneum, 1988), pp. 127–29.
47. McClintock, *We Take to Bed*, pp. 24–25, 38.
48. Adirondack Cottage Sanatorium, *Annual Report (1901)*, p. 8.
49. See Gallos, *Cure Cottages*, pp. 18–21.
50. Ibid., p. 20.
51. Ibid., pp. 16–17.
52. Ibid., pp. 18–19, 58–61. See also John L. Ward, *Health Survey of Saranac Lake, New York* (Manuscript, October 1932, Trudeau Institute), pp. 14–15.
53. Louis R. Andrews, *The White Peril* (Danbury: White Peril Publishing Company, 1909), pp. 58–59.
54. Isabel Smith, *Wish I Might* (New York: Harper and Brothers, 1955), p. 36; Philo Lathyrus, "A Convalescent's Balcony Boxes," *Journal of the Outdoor Life* (1912): 274.
55. Philip Washburn to Mary Washburn, March 22, 1893, Washburn Family Papers.
56. Bayard Cutting, Jr., to Edward Livingston Trudeau, August 13, 1905, Trudeau Papers, Trudeau Institute.
57. Alexis Stein to Edward Livingston Trudeau, September 2, 1909, Trudeau Papers.
58. Edward Livingston Trudeau to Leila Wheeler, March 28, 1908, Trudeau Papers.
59. Edward Livingston Trudeau to Leila Wheeler, July 6, 1910, Trudeau Papers.
60. Philip Washburn to Mary Washburn, December 11, 1893, Philip Washburn Papers.
61. For a description of Rutland, see Vincent Y. Bowditch, "The Massachusetts State Hospital for Consumptives at Rutland," *Boston Medical and Surgical Journal* 142 (February 8, 1900): 127–30; and Herbert C. Clapp, "The Hygienic Treatment of Phthisis at the State Hospital at Rutland, Mass.," *New England Medical Gazette* 34 (September 1899): 397–410.
62. Although the town boosters called Rutland "the Saranac of Massachusetts," the two towns had little in common. Its partisans nevertheless drew comparisons, insisting that "what Trudeau did for Saranac, this sanatorium has done for Rutland." See "The Saranac of Massachusetts," in Gabriel Nadeau, "The Rutland State Sanatorium: Historical Notes" (Manuscript, Boston Medical Library, Harvard Medical School, n.d., probably 1940s), p. 201.
63. J. N. Taylor, "Good Air Is Bringing Great Fame to Rutland," *Boston Sunday Globe*, January 17, 1904.
64. Edward Otis, "Remarks," *Transactions of the American Climatological Association* 19 (1902): 24.

65. "Saranac of Massachusetts," p. 212.

66. Ibid., pp. 231–32.

Chapter 15. The Sanatorium Narrative

1. Mann did not capture the entirety of the German experience either. Beginning in the 1890s there were also "people's" sanatoriums, which treated the working classes with funds provided by Germany's system of social insurance. For a description of the organization of the German facilities, see S. Adolphus Knopf, *Tuberculosis as a Disease of the Masses and How to Combat It*, rev. ed. (New York: Fred P. Flori, 1907), pp. 71–72. On the American ambivalencei toward the appropriateness of sanatoriums for the wealthy, see Charles F. Gardiner, William H. Swan, and Herbert M. King, "Sanatoriums for the Well-to-do," *Transactions of the Sixth International Congress on Tuberculosis* 3 (1908): 1052–57.

2. Erving Goffman, *Asylums: Essays on the Social Situation of Mental Patients and Other Inmates* (Garden City, N.Y.: Anchor Books, 1961).

3. For an excellent exploration of life in British sanatoriums from the perspective of the patient, see Linda Bryder, *Below the Magic Mountain: A Social History of Tuberculosis in Twentieth-Century Britain* (Oxford: Clarendon Press, 1988), esp. pp. 199–226. Bryder also views these facilities at total institutions and discusses the stigma reported by former patients.

4. Barbara Bates, *Bargaining for Life: A Social History of Tuberculosis, 1876–1938* (Philadelphia: University of Pennsylvania Press, 1992), describes the changes that occurred in Pennsylvania's not-for-profit and public sanatoriums (pp. 269–87).

5. Neil M. Cowan and Ruth Schwartz Cowan, *Our Parents' Lives: The Americanization of Eastern European Jews* (New York: Basic Books, 1989), p. 139–40.

6. Anne Ellis, *Sunshine Preferred: The Philosophy of an Ordinary Woman* (Boston: Houghton Mifflin Company, 1934; Lincoln, Neb.: University of Nebraska Press, 1984), p. 4.

7. Betty McDonald, *The Plague and I* (Philadelphia: J. B. Lippincott Company, 1948), pp. 30–31. When MacDonald contracted tuberculosis and went to a sanatorium in 1938, she was not a published writer. By the time *The Plague and I* appeared, she had already acquired some fame, through her autobiographical account of her experiences as a chicken farmer in the 1920s, *The Egg and I*. It has been suggested to me that she published *The Plague and I* to further her fame, but the grimness of the story and its similarity to other narratives of illness make it seem more of an effort to explain how she contracted and coped with so stigmatized a disease than to further personal ambition.

8. Will Ross, *I Wanted to Live: An Autobiography* (Milwaukee, Wis.: Wisconsin Anti-Tuberculosis Society, 1953), pp. 1–2, 7.

9. MacDonald, *The Plague and I*, pp. 38, 40.

10. Ibid., p. 47.

11. Frank Burgess, "Portraits," *Ninety Eight Six* 40 (1929): 2.

12. Iva Marie Lowry, *Second Landing* (Philadelphia: Dorrance and Company, 1974), p. 53.

13. The biographical data on Leivick and the poem can be found in Irving Howe, Ruth R. Wisse, and Khone Shmeruk, eds., *The Penguin Book of Modern Yiddish Verse* (New York: Penguin Books, 1987), pp. 227, 232–34. The poem was translated from the Yiddish by Cynthia Ozick.

14. MacDonald, *The Plague and I*, pp. 49–50.

15. The only sanatoriums that seemed to be less rule-oriented were some run by religious organizations on the southwestern plateau. These facilities retained an allegiance to the climatic cure and had no physicians on staff. Since patients were expected to employ physicians who were to give them medical advice and treatment, rules and discipline were lax. See, for example, Anne Ellis's description of the Methodist Sanatorium in Albuquerque, in Ellis, *Sunshine Preferred*, pp. 37–62.

16. Marshall McClintock, *We Take to Bed* (New York: Jonathan Cape and Harrison Smith, 1931), p. 145.

17. Sadie Fuller Seagrave, *Saint's Rest* (St. Louis: C. V. Mosby Company, 1918), pp. 50–51.

18. MacDonald, *The Plague and I*, pp. 53–54. It was traumatic not only for persons with tuberculosis to be separated from their families, but for the families also. A number of memoirs and biographies recount these events. Elizabeth Mooney spent years reconstructing her mother's life at Saranac Lake; see Elizabeth Mooney, *In the Shadow of the White Plague* (New York: Crowell, 1979). Richard Feynman, the Nobel Prize winning physicist, married a woman knowing she had active tuberculosis. He periodically left Los Alamos to visit her at a nearby sanatorium. The way his wife's disease and death affected his career and private life are vividly recounted in James Gleick, *Genius: The Life and Science of Richard Feynman* (New York: Pantheon Press, 1992), pp. 132–35, 140–51, 200–202.

19. Everett Morris, "An Introductory Talk to Patients at the Cook County Tuberculosis Hospital," *Journal of the Outdoor Life* (October 1915): 319–20.

20. Ross, *I Wanted to Live*, p. 86.

21. MacDonald, *The Plague and I*, pp. 72–73, 43.

22. Seagrave, *Saints' Rest*, p. 56. The amount of rule breaking and rule enforcement varied with the type of institution. In the for-profit facilities, directors tended to be most lenient, unwilling to lose the fees. The not-for-profit facilities frequently screened patients for compliance, and so a skilled director would have a better chance of keeping control. In municipal and state facilities, there was often open warfare between patients and staff, with discharge for misconduct rivaling departures against medical advice.

23. From Pennsylvania Medical College, *Oral History Project*, unpublished interview with Katharine Sturgis, p. 47. See also MacDonald, *The Plague and I*, p. 231.

24. Malcolm Logan, "In a Besieged City," *Ninety Eight Six* 52 (July 1931): 2.

25. MacDonald, *The Plague and I*, pp. 164–65.

26. Ibid., p. 51.

27. Ernest Morris, "Sanatoria Magazines," *National Jewish Hospital Fluoroscope* 2 (November 1930): 6.

28. Frances Cross and Lucille Hardy, "What Every Pisko Girl Should Know," *Fluoroscope* 12 (December 1940): 7.

29. Ibid., p. 6; G. S. M. "Advice to the Lunglorn," *Ninety Eight Six* 40 (September 12, 1929): 8.

30. McClintock, *We Take to Bed*, p. 155. Even decades later cousining was still remembered as one of the most distinctive features of sanatorium life. Both Charlie Moses and Sol Meyerwitz commented at length to Ruth and Neil Cowan about it. For Charlie it was one more happy and secretive aspect of his life at the facility. His cousin was a young Polish woman (a relationship his parents would have forbidden), and they "broke up" before he left the facility. Sol Meyerwitz reported he was "raped" by a married woman who shared his cure porch. Although the relationship

continued for months, Sol still felt guilty. "I felt like the biggest shitheel that ever lived," and he believed that the intensity of their relationship impeded his progress. Cowan and Cowan, *Our Parents' Lives*, pp. 140, 142.

31. Arnold Lamden, "Love, Ethics and Tuberculosis," *Fluoroscope* 2 (July 1930): 5.

32. J. W. Taft, "Dave," *National Jewish Hospital Fluoroscope* 7 (February 1937): 5, 14.

33. Bill Haking, "Ah! Sweet Misery of Life," *National Jewish Hospital Fluoroscope* 6 (February 1935): 8. See also Joseph P. Walsh, "Love and Tuberculosis," *Rehabilitator* 3 (1934): 19.

34. Lamden, "Love, Ethics," p. 5; Haking, "Sweet Misery," p. 8.

35. For a discussion of just how common it was for physicians to urge women with tuberculosis to avoid bearing children, see Judith Walzer Leavitt, *Brought to Bed: Childbearing in America, 1750–1950* (New York: Oxford University Press, 1986), pp. 68–69. For an excellent discussion of how intertwined medical advice was with social norms, see Barron Lerner, *Confounding Medical and Social Prescriptions: The Sterilization of Women with Heart Disease and Tuberculosis 1915–1937* (unpublished manuscript).

36. MacDonald, *The Plague and I*, p. 164.

37. Lamden, "Love, Ethics," p. 5; Haking, "Sweet Misery," p. 8.

38. n.a., "My First Week," *Minnesota Moccasin*, (May 1928): 14.

39. The sanatorium gossip columns are filled with romances at the movies. See, for example, *National Jewish Hospital Fluoroscope* 1 (May 1929): 6.

40. "Private Lives," *Otisan Sunbeam*, April 1940, p. 8.

41. Ross, *I Wanted to Live*, p. 83.

42. MacDonald, *The Plague and I*, p. 67.

43. Robert McBlair, "Portraits," *Ninety Eight Six* 38 (July 18, 1929): 2.

44. John William Parker, "A Healthy Protest," *Ninety Eight Six* 42 (January 13, 1930): 2.

45. Ellis, *Sunshine Preferred*, pp. 58–59.

46. Ibid., p. 37.

47. Parker, "A Healthy Protest," p. 2.

48. *The Killgloom Gazette* was a mimeographed sheet published by patients at the state sanatorium in New Mexico. This undated, unpaged copy was found at the Huntington Library, San Marino, California.

49. McClintock, *We Take to Bed*, p. 214.

50. Seagrave, *Saint's Rest*, p. 47.

51. Eleanor R. Remy, "Doctor and Patient," *Journal of the Outdoor Life* (November 1913): 326.

52. n.a., "The Ward Rat," *Seaview Sun* 1, February 1922, p. 19.

53. Arnold Lamden, "The Sanatorium Magazine," *National Jewish Hospital Fluoroscope* 4 (January 1933): 5.

54. Arno Eldi, "Tuberculosis . . . A Fool's Paradise," *National Jewish Hospital Fluoroscope* 6 (December 1934): 2–3.

55. McClintock, *We Take To Bed*, pp. 119–20.

56. n.a., "Relapse," *Ninety Eight Six* 28 (July 18, 1929): 11.

57. MacDonald, *The Plague and I*, p. 60. Like the patients, the medical staff, who were often ex-patients, were expected to be grateful, cheerful and obedient. See Bates, *Bargaining for Life*, pp. 198–296. MacDonald also noted that "discipline was not limited to the patients." At the Pines the nurses also were expected to follow a set of rules which set the hours for rising and retiring, and included "no indulgence in SEX" (p. 125).

58. Ibid., p. 142.
59. The patient discontent of the 1920s and 1930s had an impact on policy. Following
    the lead of prisons and mental hospitals, sanatoriums also had "medical boards" (in
    prisons they were"parole boards") mandated to review all cases at set intervals
    (generally every six months) and provide the patients with information on their
    progress or lack of it. But some patients were still ignored: their cases did not come
    for review at the right time and their efforts to get it on the calendar were disre-
    garded.
        Some sanatoriums, like prisons and mental hospitals, instituted "formal classifi-
    cation systems," both to reduce patient complaints and to ensure maximum medical
    discretion. At admission the patients were given a rank that corresponded to the
    severity of their symptoms and the staff's judgment about just how long it would
    take for them to recover. At first the facilities instituted a seven-point system, which
    gave the staff great discretion; minute changes in behavior or disease could lead to a
    change in classification.
        Within the classification system were a series of privileges and restrictions, which
    formally cataloged the informal system so graphically described by Betty MacDon-
    ald. But in the sanatorium the staff always retained maximum discretion. Even with
    these new systems and review processes, some patients got privileges to which they
    were not formally entitled, and others complained that they did not get their due.
    "You never seem to get anywhere," one patient complained to Roth," because peo-
    ple here don't pay too much attention to the classifications. . . . *It's like an ungraded
    school room.*" See Julius A. Roth, *Timetables: Structuring the Passage of Time in Hospital
    Treatment and Other Careers* (Indianapolis: Bobbs-Merrill, 1963), p. 10.
60. Quoted in Bates, *Bargaining for Life*, p. 263.
61. Godias J. Drolet and Donald E. Porter, *Why Do Patients in Tuberculosis Hospitals
    Leave against Medical Advice* (New York: New York Tuberculosis and Health Asso-
    ciation, 1949). See also E. K. Johnson, "Voluntary Discharges from a Tuberculosis
    Sanatorium, *American Review of Tuberculosis* 44 (November 1941): 540–47.

Epilogue

1. The Trudeau Institute did participate in later research and in clinical trials. Selman
   A. Waksman, "Tenth Anniversary of the Discovery of Streptomycin, The First
   Chemotherapeutic Agent to Be Found Effective Against Tuberculosis in Humans,"
   American Review of Tuberculosis 70 (July 1954): 1–3. See also Selman Waksman, *The
   Conquest of Tuberculosis* (Berkeley: University of California Press, 1964), pp. 103–4,
   113.
2. W. H. Feldman and H. C. Hinshaw, "Effects of Streptomycin on Experimental
   Tuberculosis in Guinea Pigs: A Preliminary Report," in H. McLeod Riggins and
   H. Corwin Hinshaw, eds., *Streptomycin and Dihydrostreptomycin in Tuberculosis* (New
   York: National Tuberculosis Association, 1949), pp. 14–20.
3. Waksman, "Tenth Anniversary," p. 6. For a very detailed and fascinating account
   of the trials, see Waksman, *Conquest of Tuberculosis*, p. 119–38.
4. Waksman, *Conquest of Tuberculosis*, p. 190.
5. See Louis I. Dublin, "Decline of Tuberculosis: Present Death Rates and Outlook
   for the Future," *American Review of Tuberculosis* 43 (1941): 227–28. Edna E. Nicholson, *A Study of Tuberculosis Mortality among Young Women* (New York: National
   Tuberculosis Association, 1932), documents the disparity in mortality rates between white and black women in Detroit.

6. See Richard Shryock, *National Tuberculosis Association 1904–1954: A Study of the Voluntary Health Movement in the United States* (New York: National Tuberculosis Association, 1957), pp. 302–3.

7. See, for example, G. B. Mackaness and N. Smith, "The Bactericidal Action of Isoniazid, Streptomycin, and Terramycin on Extracellular and Intracellular Tubercle Bacilli," *American Review of Tuberculosis* 67 (March 1953): 322–40; and H. H. Fox, "The Chemical Approach to the Control of Tuberculosis,"*Science* 116 (August 8, 1952): 129–34. See also Shryock, *National Tuberculosis Association*, pp. 300–301. For discussion of the differential mortality rates, see Godias J. Drolet and Anthony M. Lowell, "Whereto Tuberculosis? The First Seven Years of the Antimicrobial Era, 1947–1953," *American Review of Tuberculosis* 72 (1955): 419–52. For a detailed discussion of the scientific discoveries, see Frank Ryan, *The Forgotten Plague* (Boston: Little, Brown, 1993).

8. Isabel Smith, *Wish I Might* (New York: Harper and Row, 1955), pp. 198–99.

9. Ibid., pp. 200–201.

10. "TB—and Hope," *Time*, March 3, 1952, p. 42.

11. "A Victim of Progress: Sanatorium Closes on Optimistic Note," *Life*, December 27, 1954, p. 77.

12. When the Trudeau Sanitorium closed in 1954, it had not only a dwindling number of patients but also insufficient funds. Given the fact that the hospital stays of the remaining patients were growing shorter with the new drugs, there appeared to be no other choice. See George M. Meade, executive director of the Trudeau Saranac Institute, to Dr. James Perkins, November 26, 1954, Trudeau Institute Collection, Trudeau Institute.

13. Thomas Mann's comments can be found in Esmond R. Long, "Tuberculosis in Modern Society," *Bulletin of the History of Medicine* 27 (July–August 1953): 315.

14. E. R. N. Grigg, "The Arcana of Tuberculosis," *American Review of Tuberculosis* 78 (1958): 595.

15. In 1964 Waksman and other researchers recognized the extent of tuberculosis in underdeveloped countries. In India in 1960 tuberculosis was the chief cause of death. Others believed that in many sub-Saharan African countries "more than a generation must pass before the infection becomes . . . rare." Quoted in Waksman, *Conquest of Tuberculosis*, p. 216.

16. Daniel M. Fox, "AIDS and the American Health Polity," in Elizabeth Fee and Daniel M. Fox, eds., *AIDS: The Burdens of History* (Berkeley: University of California Press, 1988), has an excellent discussion on just how unprepared physicians, policy makers, and hospitals were for the epidemic (pp. 317–19).

17. Ann G. Carmichael, *Plague and Poor in Renaissance Florence* (New York: Cambridge University Press, 1986); Allan M. Brandt, *No Magic Bullet: A Social History of Venereal Disease in the United States since 1880* (New York: Oxford University Press, 1985).

18. Historians have examined past epidemics to clarify some of the complex issues of the AIDS crisis. See Fee and Fox, *AIDS: The Burdens of History*.

19. There is an extensive literature on tuberculosis among medical students, physicians, and nurses in the 1930s and 1940s. See, for example, Leopold Brahdy, "Arrested Tuberculosis and Hospital Employment," *Journal of Industrial Hygiene and Toxicology* 24 (1942): 53–58; and John Steidl, "Tuberculosis among Medical Students," *American Review of Tuberculosis* 26 (1932): 98–103.

20. David J. Rothman and Eileen Tynan, "Advantages and Disadvantages of Special Hospitals for Patients with HIV Infections: A Report by the New York City Task Force on Single Disease Hospitals," *New England Journal of Medicine* 323 (September 1990): 764–68.

21. David J. Rothman and Harold Edgar, "AIDS, Activism and Ethics," *Hospital Practice* 26 (July 15, 1991): 135–42.
22. See New York State Assembly Committee on Health, *The Return of an Epidemic* (Albany: May 1991); and Karen Brudney and Jay Dobkin, "Resurgent Tuberculosis in New York City," *American Review of Respiratory Diseases* 144 (October 1991): 745–49.
23. For an understanding of the complex ethical issues in the new epidemic and the efforts to grapple with them, see David J. Rothman, "Recommendations on the Facilities Needed to Care for Patients with Tuberculosis," in United Hospital Fund, *The Tuberculosis Revival: Individual Rights and Societal Obligations in a Time of AIDS* (New York: United Hospital Fund, 1992), 43–49; and Nancy Dubler et al., "Tuberculosis in the 1990s: Ethical, Legal, and Public Policy Issues in Screening, Treatment, and the Protection of Those in Congregate Facilities," in United Hospital Fund, *The Tuberculosis Revival*, pp. 1–28.

INDEX

Martineau, Harriet, 138, 283*n*30
Marty, Martin E., 269*n*19
Massachusetts State Sanatorium (Rutland), 208; treatment community around, 223–25
Mather, Cotton, 14
Matthiessen, Francis Otto, 32, 265*n*17
Medicine, Beatrice, 283*n*23
Meindl, R. S., 272*n*4
Men, and consumption, 26–74; college education of, 26–30, 47–48, 54, 63–64; communities of invalids, 68–71; dying away from home, 71–74; invalid-abolitionists, 65–68; occupational choices, 45–56; overland voyages, 20, 47–50, 52–53; and pursuit of health, 45–56; religious beliefs, 57–65; sea voyages, 19–20, 31–44, 71; western migration, 132–56, 161–67. *See also* Tuberculosis
Meyerwitz, Sol, 300–301*n*30
Miller, Perry, 268–69*n*2, 269*n*3
Miller, Zane L., 283*n*31–32
Mills, Charles W., 294–95*n*49
Mills, Walter Sands, 295*n*55–56
Minnesota, 159
Minor, Dr. Charles, 232–33
Missionaries, and consumption, 14, 62–65
Mississippi Valley, as unhealthy place, 139, 145
Mitchell, Lucy Sprague, 167, 297*n*25
Mitchell, S. Weir, 167, 287*n*26, 292–93*n*5
Moll, A. A., 291*n*41
Mooney, Elizabeth, 218, 297*n*38, 300*n*18
Morehouse, Charles F., 275*n*35
Morgan, Edmund S., 268–69*n*2
Morison, Samuel Eliot, 265*n*16, 266*n*34
Morris, Ernest, 300*n*27
Morris, Everett, 232, 300*n*19
Morton, Dr. Samuel George, 19, 262*n*21
Moses, Charlie, 212, 227–28, 300–301*n*30
Mother at Home, The (Abbott), 91
Mother's Book, The (Child), 91
Murray, William Henry Harrison, 285–86*n*25

Nadeau, Gabriel, 298*n*62
Narratives of illness: case records versus, 1–2, 25; of Deborah Vinal Fiske, 79–127; of health seekers, 133–37, 139–40, 143–54, 157–75; of persons with consumption, 3–7, 24–25, 26–74, 79–127, 133–37, 139–40, 143–54, 157–75; of persons with tuberculosis, 6–7, 227–45; from sanatoriums, 227–45; as term, 1–2; variations in, reasons for, 3; on western frontier, 160–75
National Association for the Study and Prevention of Tuberculosis, 192, 209–10
National Jewish Hospital (Denver), 205, 235, 236, 242, 249
Native Americans: and consumption, 8, 9, 200–201; good health of, 135–36; and Helen Hunt Jackson, 174–75; women, health of, 136
Nevins, Alan, 288*n*53
Newcomb, Mrs. James, 294*n*44
New England: consumption as endemic to, 4; death from consumption, 8, 13, 25, 78, 125–27; female invalids from, 13, 14, 23, 24; male invalids from, 26–44, 146; maritime routes, 32; physician testimonials for, 156. *See also* Fiske, Deborah Vinal
New Mexico, migration to, 132, 134, 215, 240
Newton, Richard Cole, 294*n*46
New York City Department of Health: circulars for immigrants on contagion, 186–87; and compulsory confinement of tuberculosis patients, 191–93, 209; educational efforts, 183, 186–87; Otisville Municipal Sanatorium, 208–9; and private physicians, 188, 213; registration laws in, 188–91, 193, 213; regulations regarding disinfection of lodgings, 184–86, 189; Riverside Hospital tuberculosis wing, 192–93, 209; and tenement house reform, 185–86; and tuberculosis, 183–91, 208–10, 251–52
New York State Sanatorium (Raybrook), 208, 220–21, 227–28
New York Tuberculosis and Health Association, 207–8
Nicholson, Edna E., 302*n*5
Nordhoff, Charles, 162, 164, 284*n*56, 286*n*12
Norton, Catherine, 72
Nurses: and invalids, 159; as patients, 229, 251; relations to patients, 193, 220,